Resilience and Aging

Resilience and Aging

Research and Practice

HELEN LAVRETSKY, MD, MS

Johns Hopkins University Press

Baltimore

© 2014 Johns Hopkins University Press
All rights reserved. Published 2014
Printed in the United States of America on acid-free paper
9 8 7 6 5 4 3 2 1

Johns Hopkins University Press
2715 North Charles Street
Baltimore, Maryland 21218-4363
www.press.jhu.edu

Library of Congress Cataloging-in-Publication Data

Lavretsky, Helen, author.
 Resilience and aging : research and practice / Helen Lavretsky.
  p. ; cm.
 Includes bibliographical references and index.
 ISBN-13: 978-1-4214-1498-0 (hardcover : alk. paper)
 ISBN-13: 978-1-4214-1499-7 (electronic)
 ISBN-10: 1-4214-1498-8 (hardcover : alk. paper)
 ISBN-10: 1-4214-1499-6 (electronic)
 I. Title.
 [DNLM: 1. Aging—psychology. 2. Resilience, Psychological. 3. Aged. WT 145]
 RC451.4.A5
 618.97'689—dc23   2013050153

A catalog record for this book is available from the British Library.

Special discounts are available for bulk purchases of this book. For more information,
please contact Special Sales at 410-516-6936 or specialsales@press.jhu.edu.

Johns Hopkins University Press uses environmentally friendly book materials, including recycled text paper that is composed of at least 30 percent post-consumer waste, whenever possible.

To the power of human spirit

CONTENTS

PREFACE

This book targets a readership of clinicians, researchers, and members of the interested general public. It provides a concise update on recent advances in our conceptual understanding of resilience in the context of aging, as well as on the latest research on the neurobiological and psychosocial correlates of resilience in older adults. Also included is a detailed summary of the practical implications of evidence-based interventions, with descriptions of emerging interventions designed to enhance resilience.

Research on resilience has been struggling with differences in definitions and diverse approaches; yet now is exactly the right time to provide a summary of what is already known and to outline directions for future research. Consider the aging of our global population; over the next four decades the number of individuals aged 60 years and older *will nearly triple*; there will be two elderly persons for every child (www.un.org). In order to ensure healthy and successful aging and reduce the cost of care for this huge increase, building resilience among the aging becomes a top priority for individuals, families, and society at large.

This rapid change in the population created an urgent need for a book that addresses inquiries from geriatric mental health practitioners, researchers, and lay persons—one that broadly presents up-to-date information about the resilience construct, the newest data on neurobiology, and the latest approaches in preventive care for older adults. Some practical information is provided on resilience measurement, the role of spirituality on resilience, and resilience-enhancing interventions designed to be integrated into clinical practice or everyday life. This knowledge is especially timely because of the characteristics and needs of aging baby boomers, who are more inclined to be involved in preventive healthcare and more self-deterministic in directing their care compared to earlier generations.

Clinicians and researchers active in the care of older adults will have to understand the issues discussed here in order to help adults cope with the multiple adversities that aging brings—such as physical and mental illnesses, social isolation, cognitive decline, and end-of-life issues. More and more, clinicians and caregivers will need guidance in finding successful strategies to support resilience and effective coping with such adversities. More researchers will face the issue of inadequate treatment response in the presence of medical and neurological comorbid disorders and psychosocial issues like bereavement and caregiver stress, or in the presence of the social isolation and loneliness that often perpetuate a chronic course of depression and determine poor treatment outcomes.

This volume will increase clinicians' and researchers' literacy about recent research findings, broaden their diagnostic and therapeutic perspectives, and enhance their powers of observation—all of which will better prepare them to deal with the challenges of finding appropriate, effective treatments to boost resilience in older adults. It can help them select and integrate measures of resilience and spirituality, and redirect their traditionally illness-oriented practices and research toward emphasis on the positive aspects of aging and prevention. Those who are dedicated to preventing the stress-related diseases of aging might consider this volume an essential part of their libraries.

A key difference between this volume and other publications is that it brings together (1) a wide variety of clinical issues, (2) the latest neuroscientific discoveries, and (3) the issues most relevant for public policy makers to understand in pursuing resilience-building interventions for aging adults. Fourteen chapters bridge science and policy, identifying viable models of treatment and fruitful future directions for therapeutics and prevention-development—with direct relevance to reimbursement for quality and evidence-based interventions.

In sum, it is my hope that this book will disseminate important knowledge, point to exciting research possibilities, and increase both professional and public awareness of the complexity of resilience-based interventions—ultimately leading to improved treatment outcomes and quality of life for older adults and their families.

I thank Ann Reeves for her help in editing this manuscript.

Resilience and Aging

CHAPTER 1

What Is Resilience in the Context of Aging?

THE AGING OF OUR global population is testimony to one of the most remarkable success stories of medicine and of humankind, but it also introduces an array of challenges. By 2050, the number of individuals aged 60 years and older will nearly triple, increasing from 672 million in 2005 to almost 1.9 billion (Alzheimer's Research & Prevention Foundation [ARPF] 2011). By midcentury, projected life expectancy in developed countries will be 82 years, resulting in two elderly persons for every child (ARPF 2011).

Human life expectancy around the world has increased steadily for nearly 200 years. During the past century, the mean age of the population increased by about two years for every decade, driven in the first decades by improvements in sanitation, housing, and education—with a steady decline in early and midlife mortality mostly due to infections. The continuing increase in life expectancy in the latter half of the past century is almost entirely attributable to a decline in late-life mortality, in large part due to medical advances, such as the treatment of hypertension; however, improved socio-economic conditions also contribute to the increase.

Getting older can be stressful for many individuals because of multiple interpersonal and financial losses, losses of health and independence, and declining cognitive and functional abilities. What's more, many older adults are living longer with chronic illnesses, and they are trying to make the best of their later years. As George E. Vaillant pointed out in his now classic book *Aging Well*, that the major factors involved in negative personality change at midlife are the same factors that caused negative aging at 70: bad habits, bad marriage, maladaptive defenses, and disease (Vaillant 2002). An essential question facing clinicians and health advocates is, How do we reduce the deleterious effects of risk factors and enhance the individual's protective factors to encourage successful aging?

Defining Resilience

The pursuit of happiness and fulfillment in life are an individual's right and privilege regardless of age. An increasing number of aging baby boomers strive to remain youthful and to be self-sufficient until the very end of their lives. In responding to this phenomenon, it is important to develop an understanding of resilience as applied to stress and aging, as well as of the interventions that can promote optimal functioning and maintain individuals' independence. At the start we need to ask, What is resilience?

To begin to answer this question, we must recognize that resilience is a multifaceted and intricate concept. It demands attention to a virtually unlimited complex of interacting biological, psychosocial, and environmental variables, and these must be viewed within the context of life-span development. The multidimensionality of resilience includes a number of risk factors, protective factors, and adaptive processes (Bergeman & Wallace 1999). Irrespective of chronological age, resilience has typically been defined as a pattern of positive adaptation resulting from past or present adversity or risk that has posed a substantial threat to good adaptation (Kaplan 2006; Rutter 2007). In a broader sense, resilience refers to the ability to maintain biological and psychological homeostasis under stress. The adaptations required to achieve resilience may vary according to context, time, age, gender, and cultural origin.

The scientific study of resilience began in the 1970s when developmental researchers noticed positive adaptation among subgroups of children who were considered "at risk" for developing later psychopathology (Wright & Masten 2006). This early child-centered research explored the relationship between exposure to risk and adversity and both positive and negative outcomes (Vanderbilt-Adriance & Shaw 2008). Indeed, Lipsitt and Demick (2011) argue that a fuller understanding of resilience in later life can be achieved by exploring its antecedents in childhood and adolescence. To an extent, it could be argued that interest in resilience among adults and older persons has also likely been prompted by the positive psychology movement (Seligman & Csikszentmihalyi 2000) and is consistent with the notion of intra-individual *plasticity* (Baltes 1997; Bergeman & Wallace 1999). In older adults, resilience has been studied mostly in the context of aging (e.g., in centenarians) or in the context of recovery from injury or illness, which is frequently characterized by the absence of disability (Depp & Jeste 2006).

Specific examples of the application of resilience to later life are found in discussions of strength-based approaches to counseling and therapy (Areán & Huh 2006; Ronch & Goldfield 2003), grief and bereavement (Bonanno, Westphal, & Mancini 2011; Moore & Stratton 2002; Stroebe, Hansson, Schut, & Stroebe 2008), dying (Nakashima & Canda 2005), and the notion of cognitive reserve capacity (Staudinger, Marsiske, & Baltes 1995; Stine-Morrow & Basak 2011). Resilience to stress appears to be central to optimal health and function in aging.

Folk wisdom over the centuries has promoted the idea that positive emotions are good for one's health. Accumulating empirical evidence in the studies of resilience is providing support for this belief. A key question is, In what ways can we assist aging adults in achieving optimal resilience later in life?

Although it was asserted more than 60 years ago by the World Health Organization (1948) that human health must be seen as *more than the absence of illness*, most of what is studied or treated under the rubric of health remains overwhelmingly focused on illness. The fundamental advantage of having well-conceptualized, empirically tractable indicators of human flourishing is that these allow for mapping the physiological substrates of positive experience. Even considering the multiple aspects of well-being, indicators in a positive direction afford windows on human health as *health* rather than as illness or disease (Ryff & Singer 1998).

Resilience brings "challenge" or "adversity" into the equation, allowing emotional resilience to be studied as health protection and psychological well-being. In this perspective, resilience acts as a buffer that can lead to optimal health as an individual confronts adversity. The interest in resilience within gerontology is increasing rapidly, as evidenced by books on this subject (Fry & Debats 2010; Reich, Zautra, & Hall 2010) and scores of journal articles, along with an intense interest in successful aging (Rowe & Kahn 1999), spirituality (Atchley 2009), and wisdom (Brugman 2006).

This heightened interest in resilience research has produced a change from disease-orientated inquiry to inquiry turned toward wellness and prevention. The central focus has increasingly shifted to assisting individuals to develop their adaptive and coping strengths. The emphasis on resilience shifts health paradigms toward finding more positive links to health. Understanding and enhancing resilience in the later years of life is one strategy that has potential to assist individuals in achieving better coping abilities and discovering additional possibilities for attaining happiness.

Controversies in Definitions of Resilience

Despite extensive research, a consensus around the definition of resilience is lacking. Inquiry into resilience has evolved from descriptions of resilient qualities toward focus on the process of resilient adaptation. As noted above, in older adults research on resilience has been conducted mostly in the context of successful aging (e.g., in centenarians) or in the context of recovery from injury or illness, which is frequently characterized by the absence of disability (Depp & Jeste 2006). Only occasionally has resilience been studied in the context of trauma and post-traumatic stress disorder (Yehuda et al. 2007). However, several authors indicate that successful aging is associated with a positive psychological outlook in later years, general well-being, and happiness (Depp & Jeste 2006; Rowe & Kahn 1999; Vaillant 2002).

Controversies concerning definitions of resilience in relation to aging reflect a lack of clarity in the interpretation of resilience as a dynamic process, as well as of resiliency as an individual characteristic (Luthar, Cicchetti, & Becker 2000). Human resilience is most commonly defined as the ability to cope with stress and preserve functioning (Connor & Zhang 2006). Selye coined the term *stress* to define the alarm reaction, the stage of resistance, and the stage of exhaustion in animals and in humans (McEwen 2004). Selye also described the mechanisms of the general adaptation syndrome to characterize the stress response (McEwen 2004). In evolutionary terms, *stress response* is a dynamic resilience that sharpens our attention and mobilizes our bodies to cope with threatening situations. Once the stressor remits, the response returns to baseline, usually with no ill effects. Only when the organism is overwhelmed or derailed does the stress-response system possess the potential to cause disease (McEwen 2004).

Richardson broadens the definition of resilience to encompass developmental adaptation in the face of disruptive events encountered in everyday life (Richardson & Waite 2002). Two postulates underlie Richardson's resilience meta-theory: (1) the source for actuating resilience comes from one's ecosystem, and (2) resilience is a capacity every person possesses.

Richardson defines resilience as the motivational force within everyone that drives them to pursue wisdom, self-actualization, altruism, and harmony with a spiritual source of strength within a period of biopsychospiritual homeostasis. This process of adaptation affords positive physical, mental, and spiritual outcomes. As Richardson describes it, the process of reintegration in response to life disruptions can produce growth.

Considering the circumstances of aging, current authors have expanded the construct of resilience to include adaptation processes associated with normative developmental change. Not all aging adults adapt to the aging process easily and gracefully, especially in cultures that "worship youth" as the Western world does. Yet many people embrace regenerative opportunities and actively engage in the challenges of later life.

Resilience has been variably defined by positive psychologists as a self-righting force that drives individuals to pursue self-actualization, altruism, wisdom, happiness, and harmony with a spiritual source of strength (Connor & Zhang 2006). Ryff (1995) has defined dimensions of psychological well-being to include such factors as self-acceptance, positive relationships with others, autonomy, environmental mastery, purpose in life, and personal growth—and these overlap with resilience (Ryff 1989).

It remains to be seen whether psychological well-being requires enhanced resilience. Unlike seemingly similar concepts such as successful aging, productive aging, positive aging, and optimal aging, resilience is unique. Resilience focuses attention on (1) the development of multifaceted strategies to enable persons to overcome the realities and hardships of aging and (2) linking earlier developmental processes to physical and mental well-being in later life.

Domains of Resilience

The roots of resilience research trace back to two bodies of literature: the psychological aspects of coping and the physiological aspects of stress (Tusaie & Dyer 2004). Researchers argue that the concept of resilience may reside in a set of traits (Jacelon 1997), an outcome, or a process (Olsson, Bond, Burns, Vella-Brodrick, & Sawyer 2003). Resilience is most often considered a personality characteristic that moderates the negative effects of stress and promotes adaptation. Resilience is further defined as the ability to successfully cope with change or misfortune (Wagnild & Young 1993). Unfortunately, the literature is somewhat inconsistent in making the distinction between resilience as a state-like reaction to a specific event (e.g., recovering from a traumatic event) and a personality trait or style of coping.

Resilience is also a common physiological characteristic of organs and tissues that helps them tolerate and recover from an injury. Neuronal resilience of the structures and circuits involved in emotional processing underlies psychological resilience. Such neuronal resilience plays an important role in the pathophysiology of mood disorders linked to impairment of structural plasticity and of cellular resilience, which together result in regional reductions in central nervous system (CNS) volume, as well as in reductions in the numbers or sizes of glia and neurons in discrete brain areas

(Manji & Duman 2001). Therefore, treatment targets for mood and anxiety disorders include pharmacological and nonpharmacological interventions directed toward enhancing brain resilience (Manji & Duman 2001).

Within the context of aging, resilience shifts emphasis from negative circumstances—such as caregiver stress and/or losses in health, independence, and financial security—to positive factors such as strength, capabilities, mastery, wisdom, and successful coping. This shift becomes particularly important with the increasing number of aging baby boomers. For this particular population, prevention and emphasis on positive changes are critical because of the increasing cost of living longer, with associated concerns about health care, financial security, caregiving, and so on.

The focus on enhancing resilience in older adults becomes part of the effort to improve quality of life and preserve independence in later years. To address the need to strengthen adaptation, we must regard resilience as a dynamic process—something that can be improved—rather than consider it a static attribute or inherent personal characteristic. Our most salient questions focus on whether one can be trained to become more resilient and whether happiness is truly a choice.

Characteristics of Resilience

A coherent pattern of individual characteristics associated with resilience and successful adaptation has emerged. The predominant characteristics are *commitment, dynamism, humor in the face of adversity, patience, optimism, faith,* and *altruism,* but, most importantly, *perceiving adversity as an opportunity to learn and grow.* As such, resilience may represent an important opportunity for treatment and prevention of anxiety, depression, and abnormal stress reactions. Understanding the many possible biological determinants of resilience associated with neurobiological, genetic, temperamental, and environmental influences can lead to the development of new interventions that carry the potential to enhance resilience significantly. It is very likely that, with further research on resilience, these constructs will converge into a composite human quality that protects mental and physical health in the face of adversity.

Resiliency, then, can be understood as a process that fends off disruption of the physiological or psychological balance caused by change, adversity, stressors, or challenges and facilitates personal growth and coping via accessing personal characteristics and strengths (Connor & Zhang 2006; Richardson & Waite 2002). Resilient individuals and communities rely on

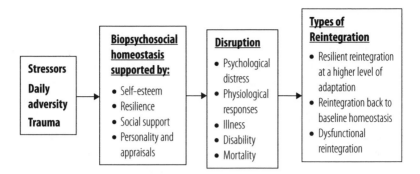

FIGURE 1.1 Theoretic model of resilience
Adapted from Richardson 2002

mutual support, are able to tolerate negative affect, are adaptive, identify meaningful goals, and implement same.

According to the model proposed by Richardson (figure 1.1), beginning at a state of biopsychospiritual balance or "homeostasis," an individual sets in motion a process to adapt mind, body, and spirit to her or his current life situation. The disruption of homeostasis presents an opportunity for growth and a higher-level adaptation. However, in the case of a dysfunctional psychological or physiological response, maladaptive behaviors could lead to decreased adaptation and the development of mental or physical illnesses (Connor & Zhang 2006).

Terminology and Constructs

The key elements of the resilience process are the interaction between *risk/adversity* or *protective factors* with *positive outcomes*. Resilient outcomes are the result of multiple risk and resilience factors that coalesce in a cumulative or additive manner, each contributing to or subtracting from the overall likelihood of a resilient outcome.

Risk factors are measurable characteristics of individuals or their environments that predict a negative outcome on specific criteria (Wright & Masten 2006). Common risk factors among older adults include negative events such as death of a spouse, caregiving, death of friends, being predisposed to an early death, declines in physical health and functioning, loss of social status and prestige, and financial insecurity (Staudinger, Marsiske, & Baltes 1995).

Vulnerability, by contrast, refers to the failure of resilience, which increases the probability of distress. Accordingly, Cohler, Stott, and Musick (1995) view vulnerability as a continuum in which inherited characteristics (e.g., innate affective or emotional styles) combine with subsequent life experiences (e.g., community relocation in later life) to determine the extent of resilience-related resources (be they dispositional or social/interpersonal) that individuals can master at any point in time in response to risk.

Although the requirement of *risk or adversity* is explicit in most definitions of resilience, the degree of adversity required for resilience to manifest is unclear. Furthermore, the types of adversities older adults face are often far different from those found in other age groups. These range from the likelihood of chronic illness experienced on a daily basis to the loss of important roles and relationships associated with retirement or widowhood, to more catastrophic experiences such as having dementia or being diagnosed with a terminal condition (Allen, Haley, Harris, Fowler, & Pruthi 2011).

Protective factors have been defined as characteristics of an individual or environment that predict or correlate with positive outcomes. They moderate the effects of individual vulnerabilities or environmental risks so that adaptation is more positive than would be the case if the protective factor were not available (Goldstein & Brooks 2005; Hess, Auman, Colcombe, & Rahhal 2003).

Another controversy in resilience literature involves the role of covariates or moderator variables in understanding the impact of resilience on a person's adaptive capacity. Luthar, Cicchetti, and Becker (2000) emphasize clarity in distinguishing the main effect of resilience on competence levels within specific risk conditions. Those who engage in resilience processes perform at greater levels of competence than those who do not engage in these processes, regardless of the level of risk associated with the protective or vulnerable characteristic. For example, in caregivers who deal with dementia, the influence of a protective-stabilizing attribute might be openness to learning new caregiving skills. Individuals in this at-risk group have been shown to use intervention strategies to maintain their well-being in the face of the deteriorating cognitive status of their care recipients (Pinquart & Sorensen 2004; Belle et al. 2006).

Resilience is demonstrated when caregivers using intervention strategies do not display decreased caregiving competence across time in comparison with caregivers in usual care or minimal support conditions, that is, without the benefit of skill-training interventions. In dementia caregivers, positive aspects of caregiving and the impact on response to intervention can also be protective (Duberstein et al. 2011).

Finally, resilience is not an all-or-nothing phenomenon (Rutter 2010; Vanderbilt-Adriance & Shaw 2008). As Cohler, Stott, and Musick (1995) state, "We all have a checkerboard of strengths and weaknesses leading to relative degrees of resilience across particular situations" (Hess et al. 2003). Resilience, as opposed to resiliency, is a dynamic process and not a static trait. It is important to examine the process by which a burdensome and adverse situation may lead to positive adaptations, emotions, and outcomes within particular domains.

Conclusion

This chapter has focused on trends and controversies in defining resilience in the context of aging. The interplay of personal predisposition and environmental conditioning leads to a dynamic process of resilience that tests individual strengths and weaknesses in everyday life, and it allows individuals to develop adaptive or resilient responses. When the burden of life circumstances becomes intolerable, even the most resilient older adults may benefit from some interventions boosting their resilience to stress that can shift maladaptive reactions to the health-promoting adaptation. Such a utilitarian view of resilience can empower individuals in taking control over their lives rather than feeling like the victims of circumstance. It can also help clinicians to broaden the range of the interventions to emphasize individuals' strengths and work in collaboration with them to enhance their quality of life.

Clinical Case

According to observations from our recent study of yogic meditation in family dementia caregivers (Lavretsky et al. 2012), the relief from distress after performing a daily 25- to 30-minute meditation can be strikingly beneficial for a person who provides around-the-clock unpaid intensive personal care to family members for many months or years. Many caregivers report relief in depression and insomnia and an improvement in coping ability. They shared similar stressors but differed in their personal vulnerability to stress (e.g., severity of perceived stress, social support, and personal characteristics). Fortunately, stress-reducing techniques can modify some of these characteristics.

For example, an African American woman, 65 years of age, who was caring for her mother with Alzheimer's disease and her sister with stroke-related dementia, came to participate in our meditation study. She scored 12—the moderate depression range—on the

Hamilton Depression Rating Scale (HDRS). She started daily meditation and demonstrated improvement in her distress within the first two weeks, with an HDRS score of only 1 at the second week. Her HDRS scores fluctuated between week two and week four, and then stabilized at a low improved score at the end of the study. She reported an increased ability to cope and to assess her stressful situation more objectively, without the level of anger and resentment she had prior to the meditation experience. She also learned to allocate time to her own pleasurable activities and did not feel "trapped" or like a "victim of circumstance."

With daily meditation and the recognition of her own psychological needs, this stressed caregiver increased her resilience and ability to cope with her life stressors. Also, she felt empowered by the idea of wellness, resilience, and self-reliance. Her strength was her openness to modifying her attitudes.

. . .

References

Allen, R. S., Haley, P. P., Harris, G. M., Fowler, S. N., & Pruthi, R. (2011). Resilience: Definitions, ambiguities, and applications. In B. Resnick, K. A. Roberto, & L. P. Gwyther (Eds.), *Resilience in aging: Concepts, research, and outcomes* (pp. 1–13). New York: Springer.

Alzheimer's Research & Prevention Foundation (2011). Kirtan Kriya: Practice the 12-Minute Yoga Meditation Exercise. Retrieved from www.alzheimers prevention.org/kirtan_kriya.htm.

Areán, P., & Huh, T. (2006). Problem-solving therapy with older adults. In S. H. Qualls & B. G. Knight (Eds.), *Psychotherapy for depression in older adults* (pp. 133–51). New York: Wiley.

Atchley, R. C. (2009). *Spirituality and aging.* Baltimore, MD: Johns Hopkins University Press.

Baltes, P. B. (1997). On the incomplete architecture of human ontogeny: Selection, optimization, and compensation as foundation of developmental theory. *Am Psychol, 52*(4), 366–80.

Belle, S. H., Burgio, L., Burns, R., Coon, D., Czaja, S. J., Gallagher-Thompson, D., . . . & I. I. Investigators Resources for Enhancing Alzheimer's Caregiver Health (2006). Enhancing the quality of life of dementia caregivers from different ethnic or racial groups: A randomized, controlled trial. *Ann Intern Med, 145*(10), 727–38.

Bergeman, C. S., & Wallace, K. A. (1999a). Resiliency in later life. In T. L. Whitman, T. V. Merluzzi, & R. D. White (Eds.), *Life-span perspectives on health and illness* (pp. 207–25). Hillsdale, NJ: Lawrence Erlbaum.

Bonanno, G. A., Westphal, M., & Mancini, A. D. (2011). Resilience to loss and potential trauma. *Annu Rev Clin Psychol, 7*(7), 511–35. doi: 10.1146/annurev-clinpsy-032210-104526.

Brugman, G. M. (2006). Wisdom and aging. In J. E. Birren & K. W. Schaie, *Handbook of the psychology of aging* (pp. 445–76). San Diego, CA: Academic.

Cohler, B. J., Stott, F. M., & Musick, J. S. (1995). Adversity, vulnerability, and resilience: Cultural and developmental perspectives. In D. Cicchetti & D. J. Cohen (Eds.), *Developmental psychopathology: Risk, disorder, and adaptation* (pp. 753–800). New York: Wiley.

Connor, K. M., & Zhang, W. (2006). Recent advances in the understanding and treatment of anxiety disorders. Resilience: determinants, measurement, and treatment responsiveness. *CNS Spectr, 11*(10 suppl 12), 5–12.

Depp, C. A., & Jeste, D. V. (2006). Definitions and predictors of successful aging: A comprehensive review of larger quantitative studies. *Am J Geriatr Psychiatry, 14*(1), 6–20.

Duberstein, P. R., Chapman, B. P., Tindle, H. A., Sink, K. M., Bamonti, P., Robbins, J., . . . & Franks, P. (2011). Personality and risk for Alzheimer's disease in adults 72 years of age and older: A 6-year follow-up. *Psychol Aging, 26*(2), 351–62.

Fry, P. S., & Debats, D. L. (2010). Sources of human life strength, resilience, and health. In P. S. Fry & C. L. M. Keyes (Eds.), *New frontiers in resilient aging* (pp. 15–59). New York: Cambridge University Press.

Goldstein, S., & Brooks, R. B. (Eds.). (2005). *Handbook of resilience in children.* New York: Kluwer Academic/Plenum Press.

Hess, T. M., Auman, C., Colcombe, S. J., & Rahhal, T. A. (2003). The impact of stereotype threat on age differences in memory performance. *J Gerontol B Psychol Sci Soc Sci, 58*(1), 3–11.

Jacelon, C. S. (1997). The trait and process of resilience. *J Adv Nurs, 25*(1), 123–29.

Kaplan, H. B. (2006). Understanding the concept of resilience. In Goldstein & Brooks (2006), 39–47.

Lavretsky, H., Siddarth, P., Nazarian, N., St. Cyr, N., Khalsa, D. S., Lin, J., . . . & Irwin, M. R. (2012). A pilot study of yogic meditation for family dementia caregivers with depressive symptoms: Effects on mental health, cognition, and telomerase activity. *Int J Geriatr Psychiatry, 28*(1), 57–65.

Lipsitt, L. P., & Demick, J. (2011). Resilience science comes of age: Old age that is. *PsycCRITIQUES, 36*(26).

Luthar, S. S., Cicchetti, D., & Becker, B. (2000). The construct of resilience: A critical evaluation and guidelines for future work. *Child Dev, 71*(3), 543–62.

Manji, H. K., & Duman, R. S. (2001). Impairments of neuroplasticity and cellular resilience in severe mood disorders: Implications for the development of novel therapeutics. *Psychopharmacol Bull, 35*(2), 5–49.

McEwen, B. S. (2004). Protection and damage from acute and chronic stress: Allostasis and allostatic overload and relevance to the pathophysiology of psychiatric disorders. *Ann N Y Acad Sci, 1032*, 1–7.

Moore, A. J., & Stratton, D. C. (2002). *Resilient widowers: Older men speak for themselves*. New York: Springer.

Nakashima, M., & Canda, E. R. (2005). Positive dying and resiliency in later life: A qualitative study. *J Aging Stud, 19* (1), 109–25.

Olsson, C. A., Bond, L., Burns, J. M., Vella-Brodrick, D. A., & Sawyer, S. M. (2003). Adolescent resilience: A concept analysis. *J Adolesc, 2626* (1), 1–11.

Pinquart, M., & Sorensen, S. (2004). Associations of caregiver stressors and uplifts with subjective well-being and depressive mood: A meta-analytic comparison. *Aging Ment Health, 8*(5), 438–49.

Reich, J. W., Zautra, A. J., & Hall, J. S. (2010). *Handbook of adult resilience*. New York: Guilford.

Richardson, G. E. (2002). The metatheory of resilience and resiliency. *J Clin Psychol, 58*(3), 307–21.

Richardson, G. E., & Waite, P. J. (2002). Mental health promotion through resilience and resiliency education. *Int J Emerg Ment Health, 4*(1), 65–75.

Ronch, J. L., & Goldfield, J. (2003). *Mental wellness in aging: Strength-based approaches*. Baltimore, MD: Health Professions Press.

Rowe, J. W., & Kahn, R. L. (1999). *Successful aging*. New York: Dell.

Rutter, M. (2007). Resilience, competence, and coping. *Child Abuse Negl, 31*(3), 205–9.

Rutter, M. (2010). From individual differences to resilience: From traits to processes. Presented at the 118th Convention of the American Psychological Association, San Diego, CA.

Ryff, C. D. (1989). Happiness is everything, or is it? Explorations on the meaning of psychological well-being. *J Pers Soc Psychol, 57* (6), 1069–81.

Ryff, C. D. (1995). Psychological well-being in adult life. *Curr Dir Psychol Sci, 4*(4), 99–104.

Ryff, C. D., & Singer, B. H. (1998). The contours of positive human health. *Psychol Inq, 9* (1), 1–28.

Ryff, C. D., Singer, B. H., & Dienberg Love, G. (2004). Positive health: Connecting well-being with biology. *Philos Trans R Soc Lond B Biol Sci, 359*(1449), 1383–94.

Seligman, M. E., & Csikszentmihalyi, M. (2000). Positive psychology: An introduction. *Am Psychol, 55*(1), 5–14.

Staudinger, U. M., Marsiske, M., & Baltes, P. B. (1995). Resilience and reserve capacity in later adulthood: Potentials and limits of development across the lifespan. In D. Cicchetti & D. J. Cohen (Eds.), *Developmental psychopathology, vol. 2: Risk, disorder, and adaptation* (pp. 801–47). New York: Wiley.

Stine-Morrow, E. A. L., & Basak, C. (2011). Cognitive interventions. In K. W. Schaie & S. L. Willis (Eds.), *Handbook of the psychology of aging* (pp. 153–70). New York: Elsevier.

Stroebe, M. S., Hansson, R. O., Schut, H., & Stroebe, W. (2008). Bereavement research: 21st-century prospects. In *Handbook of bereavement research and practice: Advances in theory and intervention* (pp. 577–605). Washington, DC: APA.

Tusaie, K., & Dyer, J. (2004). Resilience: A historical review of the construct. *Holist Nurs Pract, 18*(1), 3–8; quiz 9–10.

Vaillant, G. E. (2002). *Aging well: Surprising guideposts to a happier life from the landmark Harvard study of adult development.* Boston: Little, Brown.

Vanderbilt-Adriance, E., & Shaw, D. S. (2008). Conceptualizing and re-evaluating resilience across levels of risk, time, and domains of competence. *Clin Child Fam Psychol Rev, 11*(1–2), 30–58.

Wagnild, G. M., & Young, H. M. (1993). Development and psychometric evaluation of the Resilience Scale. *J Nurs Meas, 1*(2), 165–78.

World Health Organization (1948). *Constitution of the World Health Organization.* Geneva: WHO.

Wright, M. O., & Masten, A. S. (2006). Resilience processes in development: Fostering positive adaptation in the context of adversity. In S. Goldstein & R. B. Brooks (Eds.), *Handbook of resilience in children* (pp. 17–37). New York: Springer.

Yehuda, R., Golier, J. A., Tischler, L., Harvey, P. D., Newmark, R., Yang, R. K., & Buchsbaum, M. S. (2007). Hippocampal volume in aging combat veterans with and without post-traumatic stress disorder: Relation to risk and resilience factors. *J Psychiatr Res, 41*(5), 435–45.

CHAPTER 2

Psychological Emotional Resilience and Cognitive Resilience

THE CAPACITY TO MAINTAIN, or regain, psychological well-being in the face of challenges is known as *psychological emotional resilience*, whereas *cognitive resilience* is the innate and acquired reserve that buffers against cognitive decline (Ryff, Elliot, Friedman, Morozink, & Tsenkova 2012). This chapter provides examples from research on various challenges of later life, including chronic experiences (e.g., caregiving), acute events (e.g., relocation), and disadvantaged socioeconomic status. The need to emphasize individual human strengths in confronting adversity is discussed in outlining interventions to enhance emotional and cognitive resilience.

There are emotional and cognitive aspects of resilience that can be innate or learned. The innate affective or emotional styles that are likely to influence resilience refer to the individual style of affect regulation, which is usually a part of personality structure (e.g., optimism or pessimism) or "social intelligence." Temperament appears to be one of the determinants of resilience that is at least partially heritable. Protective temperamental factors include sociability, intelligence, social competence, internal locus of control, warmth and closeness of affectional ties, and active emotional support within the family network or religious group (Werner 1992).

Folk beliefs indicate that positive emotions can improve health. Empirical evidence increasingly supports this belief. The broaden-and-build theory of positive emotions (Fredrickson 2001; Fredrickson & Levenson 1998) provides a framework to demonstrate that positive emotions contribute to psychological and physical well-being through more effective coping. Individual differences in psychological resilience (the ability to bounce back from negative events by using positive emotions to cope) and positive emotional granularity (the tendency to represent experiences of positive emotion with precision and specificity), this theory suggests, play a crucial role in enhancing coping resources in the face of negative events (Tugade, Fredrickson, & Barrett 2004).

The definition of resilience is tightly linked to psychological and emotional well-being. Ryff (1989) has put forth six key dimensions of what constitutes well-being:

1. *autonomy* (capacity for self-determination),
2. *environmental mastery* (ability to manage one's surrounding world),
3. *personal growth* (realization of potential),
4. *positive relations with others* (high-quality relationships),
5. *purpose in life* (meaning and direction in life), and
6. *self-acceptance* (positive self-regard).

Other formulations of well-being deal with hedonic aspects, such as positive affect and life satisfaction (Ryan & Deci 2001).

Each of these components constitutes human strengths that are important in the encounter with life difficulties and that may be honed by adversity (Ryff & Singer 2003). Often a newly developed disability, such as poor balance, can discourage an individual from pursuing their previous hobbies. However, a resilient response to such challenge would be beating the odds (as disabled athletes do) or accepting the limitations and mastering a new activity that does not require having a skill such as perfect balance (e.g., swimming, painting, or writing). Purpose in life involves the capacity to find meaning and direction, especially when confronting life challenges. Meaning, as Frankl (1992) expresses it, comes from the struggle with trial and tribulation. Similarly, personal growth is about the continual realization of one's talent and potential. Not surprisingly, the development of new resources and strengths often occurs when individuals are faced with adversity. Therefore, adversity can be viewed positively as an opportunity to change and grow. Autonomy includes the capacity to march to one's own drum, even when personal convictions may go against conventional beliefs; so doing underscores having the courage of one's own convictions. Positive relations with others involve close connections, intimacy, and unconditional love. Aspects of well-being represent strengths that require active engagement with life.

Well-Being and Ill-Being in Aging

Similar to resilience, the individual sense of well-being is an important characteristic of successful aging. Ryff and colleagues described two key types of well-being: eudaimonic and hedonic (Ryff et al. 2006; Ryff, Singer, & Dienberg Love 2004). *Eudaimonic* involves self-development and self-acceptance, personal growth, positive relationships, and purposeful engagement, whereas *hedonic* is concerned with positive feelings such as happiness and contentment. Ill-being refers to all pathological states, such as negative affect, depression, anxiety, post-traumatic stress, and anger. Different biological systems relate to the states of well- or ill-being, including neuroendocrine (cortisol, epinephrine, norepinephrine); immune (IL-6, vaccine antibody response); cardiovascular (blood pressure, waist-hip ratio, cholesterol, glycosylated hemoglobin); sleep (duration and latency of REM); and neural circuitry (cerebral asymmetry) (Ryff et al. 2004, 2006).

Fredrickson and colleagues (2013) have found gene expression profile differences in 80 distinguishing hedonic and eudaimonic well-being, as well as potentially confounded negative psychological and behavioral factors. Hedonic and eudaimonic well-being showed similar affective correlates but highly divergent transcriptome (gene expression) profiles. Peripheral blood mononuclear cells from people with high levels of hedonic well-being showed up-regulated expression of a stress-related conserved transcriptional response to adversity (CTRA) involving increased expression of proinflammatory genes and decreased expression of genes involved in antibody synthesis and interferon type I response. In contrast, high levels of eudaimonic well-being were associated with CTRA down-regulation. Promoter-based bioinformatics implicated distinct patterns of transcription factor activity in structuring the observed differences in gene expression associated with eudaimonic well-being (reduced NF-κB and AP-1 signaling and increased IRF and STAT signaling). Transcript origin analysis identified monocytes, plasmacytoid dendritic cells, and B lymphocytes as primary cellular mediators of these dynamics. The finding that hedonic and eudaimonic well-being engage distinct gene regulatory programs despite their similar effects on total well-being and depressive symptoms implies that the human genome may be more sensitive to qualitative variations in well-being than are our conscious affective experiences. These findings are pioneering in elucidating the powerful epigenetic mechanisms of well-being.

Psychological ill-being has been extensively linked with biology. For example, depressive symptoms and negative affect have been correlated with elevated cortisol and norepinephrine (Brown, Varghese, & McEwen 2004; Hughes, Watkins, Blumenthal, Kuhn, & Sherwood 2004; Polk, Cohen, & Doyle 2005; Rubin, Poland, Lesser, Winston, & Blodgett 1987), as well as with increased cardiovascular risk (Ahlberg et al. 2002; Barefoot et al. 1998; Markovitz, Matthews, Wing, Kuller, & Meilahn 1991). Trait anxiety and anger have been associated with elevated glycosylated hemoglobin, elevated waist-hip ratio, increases of visceral adipose tissue, and lower levels of HDL cholesterol (Ahlberg et al. 2002; Landen et al. 2004; Raikkonen, Matthews, Kuller, Reiber, & Bunker 1999; Schuck 1998).

Preliminary findings on a sample of aging women showed that those with higher levels of eudaimonic well-being had lower levels of daily salivary cortisol, proinflammatory cytokines, cardiovascular risk, and longer-duration REM sleep compared with those showing lower levels of eudaimonic well-being. Hedonic well-being, however, showed minimal linkage to biomarker assessments (Ryff et al. 2006). These results add to the growing literature on how psychological well-being and mental maladjustment are exemplified in biology.

Cognitive Resilience

Cognitive development shows wide variation among aging adults, with some being more successful or resilient than others. The cascade of biological processes associated with senescence creates risk for cognitive decline in later adulthood. *Senescence* (the biological process of aging) certainly circumscribes limits on cognitive components requiring speedy information processing and executive control in later life, and it increases vulnerability to pathological processes that can compromise cognitive health. However, as a natural part of the life cycle, senescence itself is not so much a threat to successful development as it is a cultural context that does or does not accommodate the developmental period of later life. Attitudes about aging can be internalized in the form of negative aging stereotypes, which can compromise cognition by discouraging the recruitment of effort to maintain cognition (Hess et al. 2003). Another threat to successful development in aging is the lack of resources to prepare people to live long lives (Riley & Riley 2000) and to promote resilience.

Cognitive resilience is a multidimensional process in which resources and/or reserves buffer against late-life threats to cognitive health (Lachman & Agrigoroaei 2010). Cognitive resilience is usually expressed in a sense of personal agency, engendered by an array of individual factors (e.g., health; cognitive and motivational reserve), social factors (e.g., social support), and sociocultural factors (e.g., social equity, effective structures for life-span education) that nurture sustained intellectual engagement. Personal engagement, a sustained investment in mental stimulation, and personal agency, which enables one to construct a niche for successful life-span development, all contribute to cognitive resilience.

Block and Kremen (1996) conceptualized cognitive resilience as a subcategory of general intelligence that is responsible for individual competence, self-esteem, and "social IQ." A considerable body of evidence supports the persistence of general personality structure over time (Atchley 1999), but some growth can occur with aging, particularly in introspection and transcendence. The personality implications of "pure intelligence" and "pure ego-resilience," as measured by the Revised Wechsler Adult Intelligence Scale, revealed that persons relatively high on ego resilience (sometimes defined as emotional IQ) tend to be more competent and comfortable in the "fuzzier" interpersonal world. Persons with higher raw IQ scores may be more effective in the "clearer" world of structured work activities but are more likely to be uneasy in handling human affect and interactions expressed in emotional IQ (Wechsler 2008). In the latter group, therefore, cognitive decline associated with aging may disrupt individual cognitive resilience and increase vulnerability to stress due to a less-developed ability to navigate the "world of emotions and human interactions."

A range of factors at the individual level and within the broader sociocultural context contribute to life-span cognitive resilience, which can in turn affect factors promoting engagement and agency (e.g., health management, disposition affecting how experience is regulated) to support cognitive growth. Theoretical perspectives on successful aging and cognitive resilience have shifted their focus to principles that define individual differences in trajectories of development. It is important that researchers continue to explore the factors that buffer against internal and external threats to successful development in aging and find ways to translate those factors into effective intervention.

A booming area of exploration is the way buffering factors interact and reinforce one another in promoting cognitive reserve. For example, how do health promotion, healthy diet, and fitness enable individuals to maintain supportive social networks and to take advantage of opportunities for cognitive enrichment? How can social structures be arranged to promote the capacity for agency and offer opportunities for intellectual stimulation? What are effective translational models for intervention?

Assuming that resilience is an ongoing process in which different factors reciprocally reinforce one another (e.g., healthy sleep patterns and exercise habits promote effective coping with challenges to enable cognitive growth, which in turn enables self-regulatory efficacy in lifestyle management), what are the best options for intervening in this cycle when things go awry?

Effective translation will require research into dose-response functions for the resiliency factors. It is easy enough to feel inspired to make the relatively simple choices in lifestyle that have promise for cognitive resilience—to exercise, eat right, engage in activities that enrich the mind, or enjoy the comfort of friends and family. To the extent that agency is central to *sustained* engagement, practitioners find themselves having to strike a delicate balance between creating social and institutional structures and therapeutic interventions that embody principles of life-span resilience and affording sufficient personal choice.

Cognitive Reserve

An important factor contributing to lifelong cognitive resilience is an extended period of engagement in formal education early in the life span, an effect that has been attributed to "cognitive reserve" (Stern 2009). The explanation is that early educational experiences build neural networks and behavioral strategies that buffer against subsequent insults so that brain plasticity is enhanced and age-related degenerative processes are delayed.

Collectively, educational experiences early in life impact cognitive resilience via several routes. Education builds a cognitive and neural reserve that buffers late-life pathology. Knowledge continues to develop with continued investment in occupational activities and hobbies, which builds an arsenal of declarative knowledge, as well as skills in domain-related learning (Soederberg Miller 2009). Verbal ability, including vocabulary and reading skills, can show improvement with continued practice.

Approximately a quarter of community-dwelling individuals who show no obvious performance impairments before death will show evidence of brain pathology at autopsy. This proportion is greater for individuals with higher educational levels than it is for those with lower levels of education, reinforcing the suggestion that education builds a reserve, in terms of efficiency of neural networks, capacity, and/or flexibility in the use of networks or of strategies that enable individuals with incipient pathology to recruit this reserve to preserve function. Studies have shown that more highly educated individuals tend to be diagnosed with Alzheimer's disease at later ages than less-educated adults. One particular sort of early educational experience that shows evidence of wide-ranging effects on cognition is learning a second language (Bialystok, Craik, Green, & Gollan 2009).

Personality Style and Emotional and Cognitive Resilience

Historically, *neuroticism* (a tendency to worry and to feel anxious and threatened in ordinary situations) has been identified as a risk factor for cognitive impairment, whether by itself or in the presence of a mood disorder; this is likely due to higher levels of production of cortisol, a stress hormone known to damage the hippocampus. Neuroticism has been shown to be a risk factor for Alzheimer's (Duberstein et al. 2011). However, evidence for a negative relationship between neuroticism and cognitive function in a healthy sample has been mixed (Salthouse 2011; Soubelet & Salthouse 2011b), and the effect of neuroticism on cognition may depend on its context in the larger structure of personality (Crowe, Andel, Pedersen, Fratiglioni, & Gatz 2006).

A rich literature has been emerging that examines interrelationships between cognition and personality traits (Duberstein et al. 2011). For example, openness to experience—a trait marked by enjoyment of novelty, fantasy, and emotional experience; attunement to the environment; and mental flexibility—has been shown to be related to measures of cognitive performance (Parisi, Stine-Morrow, Noh, & Morrow 2009; Soubelet & Salthouse 2010, 2011a), as well as to reduced risk of Alzheimer's (Duberstein et al. 2011). In fact, there is evidence that those who are high in the facet of openness recruit more neural resources during a working memory task (DeYoung, Shamosh, Green, Braver, & Gray 2009).

Other dispositional factors related to motivation also have been related to cognition. Beliefs that one can influence the events in one's life and confidence that the investment of effort will pay off in performance gains, conceptualized as self-efficacy and perceived control (Lachman 2006; Valentijn et al. 2006), have often been shown to predict performance and have been targeted for intervention (West, Bagwell, & Dark-Freudeman 2008). Such beliefs are an important source of cognitive resilience via effective allocation of effort to activities that support and sustain cognition. For example, Payne and colleagues (2011) showed that self-efficacy at pretesting predicted perseverance in a 16-week program of reasoning training, as well as actual improvement in reasoning ability as a consequence of the training. Even as a resource for cognitive resilience, such beliefs are likely to be constructed over the life span (Forstmeier & Maercker 2008; Infurna, Gerstorf, Ram, Schupp, & Wagner 2011). For instance, Lachman and Leff (1989) have found fluid ability to predict perceived control five years later. Based on data from the German Socio-Economic Panel, a large-scale longitudinal study with a nationally representative sample, Infurna and colleagues (2011) showed that level of social participation contributed to control beliefs measured eight to ten years later.

Forstmeier and Maercker (2008) have coined the term *motivational reserve*, arguing that, analogous to cognitive reserve, motivational resources that underpin cognition and health constitute a set of abilities that buffer age-related neuropathological insults. They used the Occupational Information Network (O*NET) system to characterize work-related activities in midlife and relate the motivational reserve developed by these activities to current cognitive status. Although cognitive demands were correlated with a measure of premorbid intelligence, motivational demands were not, which is the basis for the claim that motivational reserve is a construct that is separable from cognitive reserve in contributing to cognitive resilience. They found that motivational reserve was predictive of cognitive status, as measured by a composite of processing speed, working memory, fluency, and inhibitory control.

Resilience and Successful Aging

In aging, the presence of comorbid medical and cognitive disorders may affect emotional resilience. In successful aging, people generally experience greater resolve and sense of agency. Emotional resilience helps older adults to maintain happiness and avoid hopelessness, and to deal with such feelings as irritability, sadness, anger, or fear. Because resilience depends, in part, on the inner continuity of ideas about self and personal goals, perceptions of inner continuity depend on memory and consciousness and therefore are susceptible to disintegration in dementia. However, with the presence of medical illnesses and functional disability, there may be a decline in the sense of agency, self-confidence, and self-reliance. When individuals reach very old age, accumulating negative conditions represent a serious challenge to their capacity to adapt and are likely to reduce the quality of life.

Depp and Jeste (2006) reviewed 28 studies with 29 definitions of successful aging and noted that the mean reported proportion of "successful agers" was 35.8% but varied widely. The most frequent significant correlates of the various definitions of successful aging were age (young-old), nonsmoking, and absence of disability, arthritis, and diabetes. Successful aging was moderately associated with greater physical activity, more social contacts, better self-rated health, absence of depression and cognitive impairment, and fewer medical conditions. Gender, income, education, and marital status did not generally relate to successful aging.

Data from the population-based Heidelberg Centenarian Study indicated high levels of happiness in the very old (Jopp & Rott 2006). Basic resources (i.e., job training, cognition, health, social network, extroversion) explained a substantial proportion of variance in happiness, but some resource effects were mediated through self-referent beliefs (e.g., self-efficacy) and attitudes toward life (e.g., optimistic outlook). Even in very advanced age, psychological resilience and the self-regulatory adaptation system maintains its efficiency (Jopp & Rott 2006).

The Umea 85+ study described the levels of resilience, sense of coherence, purpose in life, and self-transcendence in relation to perceived physical and mental health in 125 participants 85 years of age or older (Nygren et al. 2005). The findings showed significant correlations between perceived health and scores on the resilience scale, the sense-of-coherence scale, the purpose-in-life test, and the self-transcendence scale. The mean values of the different scales showed that the oldest old have scores the same as or higher than those for younger age groups (Nygren et al. 2005). The authors concluded that the patterns of resilience do not differ by age.

As has been shown in the Ohio Longitudinal Study of Aging and Adaptation (OLSAA), which involved a more than 20-year follow-up of a cohort of adults 50 years of age and older, continuity of resilience into retirement years is unaffected by gender and education (Atchley 1999). Likewise, in a study of 205 community-dwelling elderly, 92% of the participants rated themselves as aging successfully (Montross et al. 2006). A majority of them also met other research criteria for successful aging, such as independent living, mastery or growth, and positive adaptation—even in the presence of chronic medical illness or physical disability. It appears from the existing data that individual characteristics, rather than external events (e.g., co-morbid illness, income) determine happiness and successful aging. The search for biological determinants of positive versus negative predispositions is ongoing.

It is clear from these examples that several broad factors contribute to processes of lifespan emotional and cognitive resilience:

- health,
- education and cognitive reserve,
- knowledge,
- lifelong intellectual engagement,
- dispositions, temperament, and motivational reserve,
- social support, and
- sociocultural context.

Interventions directed at increasing these factors would likely boost emotional and cognitive resilience and ensure more successful aging, as the clinical case below demonstrates.

Conclusion

In this chapter, I have discussed the features of emotional and cognitive resilience and the importance of balancing both to ensure higher quality of life and successful aging. Our society has emphasized the need to be cognitively intact in order to maintain independence. The "A-word" (Alzheimer's) or the "D-word" (dementia) imply a frightening "sentence" of prolonged suffering in a nursing home that terrifies patients and their families. The diagnosis also can mean huge financial losses over many years of taking care of persons with dementia. Families wait for a miracle drug that would cure Alzheimer's, which is not coming anytime soon. As the number of those with cognitive decline and their caregivers grows, it is more productive and wise to emphasize the overall well-being and resilience in living with Alzheimer's, dementia, or any other chronic illnesses and disabilities.

Recent research has shown that the modifiable factors, such as lifestyle interventions, healthy diet, and fitness, play a critical role in promoting cognitive reserve. Lately, however, efforts have been directed to understanding the role of loneliness and supportive social networks, mind-body interventions, and stress-reduction to increase emotional resilience and resistance to stress. On the societal level, modification of social structures can and should be developed to promote the individual capacity for independent living and opportunities for intellectual stimulation in aging adults. We must educate the general public about the need to be responsible for own health since early adulthood in order to prevent chronic diseases of aging, but also remove the fear and stigma from aging-related diseases through active participation in self-management. At this point, it is unclear whether any pending changes with the Affordable Care Act (or "Obamacare"), or any new initiative concerning Medicare or Social Security can promote this orientation toward wellbeing and prevention for generation of aging baby boomers.

Clinical Case

Mrs. M., a 76-year-old Caucasian woman living alone with a full-time caregiver, came to see me about three years prior to this writing for depression and Parkinson's disease. She was confined to a wheelchair at that time. During the first appointment she also appeared demented, due to dilapidated mentation and psychomotor retardation. Her neck was bent down; she could not straighten it because of poor control of her parkinsonism symptoms. She was confined to home without any ability to enjoy life or pursue her hobbies.

We proceeded with a more aggressive treatment of her parkinsonism symptoms. Her motor control improved to the point that she could hold her head straight up and participate in physical therapy. However, she remained depressed, with a rapid loss of 20 pounds and with no will to live or do anything to improve her condition.

She was subsequently admitted to the hospital and received six treatments of electroconvulsive therapy (ECT), resulting in a rapid improvement in her mood and appetite and a return of her will to live. Physical therapy was also intensified, which improved her gait. ECT was then stopped because she started developing significant memory problems, a common adverse event in patients with coexisting neurodegenerative diseases (in her case, parkinsonism). At that time she also received treatment with antidepressants, as well as supplements like fish oil, B-vitamin complex, multivitamins, and donepezil to correct her ECT-related memory loss. She was discharged to her home and gradually became less depressed; her weight stabilized, and she was routinely engaged in physical exercise.

Over the course of the study—the next year—she demonstrated a remarkable improvement. Her parkinsonism and cognitive impairment were stabilized; her mood was euthymic. She started attending painting classes twice a week, which brought her great satisfaction. Later she started attending dance classes for older adults with parkinsonism and was quite proud of that accomplishment. She also took drumming classes that improved her coordination.

She proceeded to experience a good quality of life for the next several years and was always independent in her choice of activities. Although she moved to an assisted-living facility in March of 2013 (six month prior to this writing), she has been able to cope with this transition well and to enjoy new friends and activities, despite the existing daily challenges of coping with parkinsonism. She is still doing quite well.

Mrs. M. is an example of a highly resilient woman who overcame all odds of succumbing to either depression or parkinsonism with dementia. With some help, she has been able to maintain both her joy of living and a victorious attitude in her private battle with disease and disability. In her case, an integrative approach to wellness in the face of chronic disease brought success to managing emotional, cognitive, and physical problems. The patient's autonomy and choice were always respected and taken into account when selecting the components of intervention.

I could relate many other stories of my patients who have demonstrated amazing abilities to cope with their severe physical, mental, or cognitive adversities and disabilities. The quality they all share is the belief that anything is possible, that unfortunate circumstances represent a challenge and a life lesson, and that they can use the situation to strengthen their humanity—to feel themselves victors, not victims. They master their illnesses or disabilities, find solutions, and arrive at a higher level of adaptation with much personal satisfaction and reaffirmation of their human spirit.

. . .

References

Ahlberg, A. C., Ljung, T., Rosmond, R., McEwen, B., Holm, G., Akesson, H. O., & Bjorntorp, P. (2002). Depression and anxiety symptoms in relation to anthropometry and metabolism in men. *Psychiatry Res, 112*(2), 101–10.

Atchley, R. C. (1999). Incorporating spirituality into professional work in aging. *Aging Today, 20*(4), 17.

Barefoot, J. C., Heitmann, B. L., Helms, M. J., Williams, R. B., Surwit, R. S., & Siegler, I. C. (1998). Symptoms of depression and changes in body weight from adolescence to mid-life. *Int J Obes Relat Metab Disord, 22*(7), 688–94.

Bialystok, E., Craik, F. I. M., Green, D. W., & Gollan, T. H. (2009). Bilingual minds. *Psychol Sci Public Interest, 10*(3), 89–129.

Block, J., & Kremen, A. M. (1996). IQ and ego-resiliency: Conceptual and empirical connections and separateness. *J Pers Soc Psychol, 70*(2), 349–61.

Brown, E. S., Varghese, F. P., & McEwen, B. S. (2004). Association of depression with medical illness: Does cortisol play a role? *Biol Psychiatry, 55*(1), 1–9.

Crowe, M., Andel, R., Pedersen, N. L., Fratiglioni, L., & Gatz, M. (2006). Personality and risk of cognitive impairment 25 years later. *Psychol Aging, 21*(3), 573–80.

Depp, C. A., & Jeste, D. V. (2006). Definitions and predictors of successful aging: A comprehensive review of larger quantitative studies. *Am J Geriatr Psychiatry, 14*(1), 6–20.

DeYoung, C. G., Shamosh, N. A., Green, A. E., Braver, T. S., & Gray, J. R. (2009). Intellect as distinct from openness: Differences revealed by fMRI of working memory. *J Pers Soc Psychol, 97*(5), 883–92.

Duberstein, P. R., Chapman, B. P., Tindle, H. A., Sink, K. M., Bamonti, P., Robbins, J., . . . & Franks, P. (2011). Personality and risk for Alzheimer's disease in adults 72 years of age and older: A 6-year follow-up. *Psychol Aging, 26*(2), 351–62.

Forstmeier, S., & Maercker, A. (2008). Motivational reserve: Lifetime motivational abilities contribute to cognitive and emotional health in old age. *Psychol Aging, 23*(4), 886–99.

Frankl, V. (1992). *Man's search for meaning.* 4th ed. Boston: Beacon.

Fredrickson, B. L. (2001). The role of positive emotions in positive psychology: The broaden-and-build theory of positive emotions. *Am Psychol, 56*(3), 218–26.

Fredrickson B. L., Grewen, K. M., Coffey, K. A., Algoe, S. B., Firestine, A. M., Arevalo, J. M., . . . & Cole, S. W. (2013). A functional genomic perspective on human well-being. *Proc Natl Acad Sci U S A, 110*(33), 13684–89.

Fredrickson, B. L., & Levenson, R. W. (1998). Positive emotions speed recovery from the cardiovascular sequelae of negative emotions. *Cogn Emot, 12*(2), 191–220. doi: 10.1080/026999398379718.

Hess, T. M., Auman, C., Colcombe, S. J., & Rahhal, T. A. (2003). The impact of stereotype threat on age differences in memory performance. *J Gerontol B Psychol Sci Soc Sci, 58*(1), 3–11.

Hughes, J. W., Watkins, L., Blumenthal, J. A., Kuhn, C., & Sherwood, A. (2004). Depression and anxiety symptoms are related to increased 24-hour urinary norepinephrine excretion among healthy middle-aged women. *J Psychosom Res, 57*(4), 353–58.

Infurna, F. J., Gerstorf, D., Ram, N., Schupp, J., & Wagner, G. G. (2011). Long-term antecedents and outcomes of perceived control. *Psychol Aging, 26*(3), 559–75.

Jopp, D., & Rott, C. (2006). Adaptation in very old age: Exploring the role of resources, beliefs, and attitudes for centenarians' happiness. *Psychol Aging, 21*(2), 266–80.

Lachman, M. E. (2006). Perceived control over aging-related declines: Adaptive beliefs and behaviors. *Curr Dir Psychol Sci, 15*(6), 282–86.

Lachman, M. E., & Agrigoroaei, S. (2010). Promoting functional health in midlife and old age: Long-term protective effects of control beliefs, social support, and physical exercise. *PLoS One, 5*(10), e13297.

Lachman, M. E., & Leff, R. (1989). Perceived control and intellectual functioning in the elderly: A 5-year longitudinal study. *Dev Psychol, 25*(5), 722–28.

Landen, M., Baghaei, F., Rosmond, R., Holm, G., Bjorntorp, P., & Eriksson, E. (2004). Dyslipidemia and high waist-hip ratio in women with self-reported social anxiety. *Psychoneuroendocrinology, 29*(8), 1037–46.

Markovitz, J. H., Matthews, K. A., Wing, R. R., Kuller, L. H., & Meilahn, E. N. (1991). Psychological, biological, and health behavior predictors of blood pressure changes in middle-aged women. *J Hypertens, 9*(5), 399–406.

Montross, L. P., Depp, C., Daly, J., Reichstadt, J., Golshan, S., Moore, D., . . . & Jeste, D. V. (2006). Correlates of self-rated successful aging among community-dwelling older adults. *Am J Geriatr Psychiatry, 14*(1), 43–51.

Nygren, B., Alex, L., Jonsen, E., Gustafson, Y., Norberg, A., & Lundman, B. (2005). Resilience, sense of coherence, purpose in life and self-transcendence in relation to perceived physical and mental health among the oldest old. *Aging Ment Health, 9*(4), 354–62.

Parisi, J. M., Stine-Morrow, E. A., Noh, S. R., & Morrow, D. G. (2009). Predispositional engagement, activity engagement, and cognition among older adults. *Neuropsychol Dev Cogn B Aging Neuropsychol Cogn, 16*(4), 485–504.

Payne, B. R., Jackson, J. J., Hill, P. L., Gao, X., Roberts, B. W., & Stine-Morrow, E. A. (2011). Memory self-efficacy predicts responsiveness to inductive reasoning training in older adults. *J Gerontol B Psychol Sci Soc Sci, 67*(1), 27–35.

Polk, D. E., Cohen, S., & Doyle, W. J. (2005). State and trait affect as predictors of salivary cortisol in healthy adults. *Psychoneuroendocrinology, 30*(3), 261–72.

Raikkonen, K., Matthews, K. A., Kuller, L. H., Reiber, C., & Bunker, C. H. (1999). Anger, hostility, and visceral adipose tissue in healthy postmenopausal women. *Metabolism, 48*(9), 1146–51.

Riley, M. W., & Riley Jr., J. W. (2000). Age integration: Conceptual and historical background. *Gerontologist, 40*(3), 266–70.

Rubin, R. T., Poland, R. E., Lesser, I. M., Winston, R. A., & Blodgett, A. L. (1987). Neuroendocrine aspects of primary endogenous depression: I. Cortisol secretory dynamics in patients and matched controls. *Arch Gen Psychiatry, 44*(4), 328–36.

Ryan, R. M., & Deci, E. L. (2001). On happiness and human potentials: A review of research on hedonic and eudaimonic well-being. *Annu Rev Psychol, 52*, 141–66.

Ryff, C. D. (1989). Happiness is everything, or is it? Explorations on the meaning of psychological well-being. *J Pers Soc Psychol, 57*(6), 1069–81.

Ryff, C. D., Dienberg Love, G., Urry, H. L., Muller, D., Rosenkranz, M. A., Friedman, E. M., . . . & Singer, B. (2006). Psychological well-being and ill-being: Do they have distinct or mirrored biological correlates? *Psychother Psychosom, 75*(2), 85–95.

Ryff, C. D., Elliot, E. M., Friedman, M., Morozink, J. A., & Tsenkova, V. (2012). Psychological resilience in adulthood and later life: Implications for health. In B. Hayslip Jr. & G. C. Smith (Eds.), *Annual review of gerontology and geriatrics: Emerging perspectives on resilience in adulthood and later life.* New York: Springer.

Ryff, C. D., & Singer, B. H. (2003). Flourishing under fire: Resilience as a prototype of challenged thriving. In C. L. M. Keyes & J. Haidt (Eds.), *Flourishing: Positive psychology and the life well-lived* (pp. 15–36). Washington, DC: American Psychological Association.

Ryff, C. D., Singer, B. H., & Dienberg Love, G. (2004). Positive health: Connecting well-being with biology. *Philos Trans R Soc Lond B Biol Sci, 359*(1449), 1383–94.

Salthouse, T. A. (2011). Neuroanatomical substrates of age-related cognitive decline. *Psychol Bull, 137*(5), 753–84. doi: 10.1037/a0023262.

Schuck, P. (1998). Glycated hemoglobin as a physiological measure of stress and its relations to some psychological stress indicators. *Behav Med, 24*(2), 89–94.

Soederberg Miller, L. M. (2009). Age differences in the effects of domain knowledge on reading efficiency. *Psychol Aging, 24*(1), 63–74.

Soubelet, A., & Salthouse, T. A. (2010). The role of activity engagement in the relations between openness/intellect and cognition. *Pers Individ Dif, 49*(8), 896–901.

Soubelet, A., & Salthouse, T. A. (2011a). Correlates of level and change in the mini-mental state examination. *Psychol Assess, 23*(4), 811–18. doi: 10.1037/a0023401.

Soubelet, A., & Salthouse, T. A. (2011b). Personality-cognition relations across adulthood. *Dev Psychol, 47*(2), 303–10. doi: 10.1037/a0021816.

Stern, Y. (2009). Cognitive reserve. *Neuropsychologia, 47*(10), 2015–28.

Tugade, M. M., Fredrickson, B. L., & Barrett, L. F. (2004). Psychological resilience and positive emotional granularity: Examining the benefits of positive emotions on coping and health. *J Pers, 72*(6), 1161–90.

Valentijn, S. A., Hill, R. D., Van Hooren, S. A., Bosma, H., Van Boxtel, M. P., Jolles, J., & Ponds, R. W. (2006). Memory self-efficacy predicts memory performance: results from a 6-year follow-up study. *Psychol Aging, 21*(1), 165–72.

Wechsler, D. (2008). *Wechsler adult intelligence scale*, 4th ed. San Antonio, TX: Pearson.

Werner, E. E. (1992). The children of Kauai: Resiliency and recovery in adolescence and adulthood. *J Adolesc Health, 13*(4), 262–68.

West, R. L., Bagwell, D. K., & Dark-Freudeman, A. (2008). Self-efficacy and memory aging: The impact of a memory intervention based on self-efficacy. *Neuropsychol Dev Cogn B Aging Neuropsychol Cogn, 15*(3), 302–29.

CHAPTER 3

Resilience and Longevity

ADVANCED INTELLIGENCE, supplemented by social and industrial revolutions that have enhanced the capacity for DNA repair and stress resistance, has contributed to the extraordinary length of the human life span. As previously noted, human life expectancy has increased steadily over the past two centuries (Lavretsky, Siddarth, & Irwin 2010). In many developed countries today, 85% of newborn human babies can expect to attain their 65th birthday. The continuing increase in life expectancy since after World War II has been almost entirely due to people surviving until late life, aided by medical advances and improved living conditions. Aging has become more or less a universal experience.

Resilience, at least in part, is responsible for survival into old age, for it is associated with substantial physiological homeostasis and is strengthened by genes related to stress resistance that accommodate adaptation to stress (P. A. Parsons 1996). According to the stress theory of aging, selection of genes for stress resistance is the primary factor for longevity; genetic predisposition to a longer life span is secondary (P. A. Parsons 1996). In developed countries of the modern world, selection of genes for stress resistance has diminished in importance because of improved nutrition and decreased exposure to environmental stresses.

Human longevity is also strongly influenced by lifestyle and socioeconomic considerations. Thus, researchers into resilience and longevity have emphasized uncovering gene–environment interactions. Some genetic polymorphisms reflect the fact that studies of life span change over human history have been subject to statistical variations (e.g., temporal variations in causes of mortality such as epidemics, variations in food supply, and socioeconomic heterogeneity).

Research on resilience in centenarians has provided a source of information on protective mechanisms that lead to longevity. Although being a centenarian does not necessarily equate to the aged individual enjoying life, especially if he or she is bedridden in a nursing home, important lessons can be learned from community-dwelling centenarians. Extant literature has highlighted the particular relevance of healthy centenarians to longevity research, given that they have outlived most of their peers by several decades and thus represent a highly selected group.

The number of centenarians in most industrialized countries is about one in 10,000 and trending toward one in 5,000 (Poon & Perls 2007). Centenarians have met the two major requirements of being resilient. The first is surviving despite the presence of risks or threats. They have experienced a century of traumatic life events, including surviving the deaths of birth cohorts and family members, economic depressions, wars, and epidemics. The second requirement is that they have successfully adapted and survived in spite of a daunting number of daily positive and negative stressors. In this respect, longevity and resilience are immediately related. American centenarians born in 1900 lived to 2000 and beyond, while their birth cohort survived to an average of 46.3 years for men and 48.3 for women (National Center for Health Statistics 2007).

According to the U.S. Census Bureau, centenarians numbered 38,306 in 1990, rising to 50,454 in 2000 (Hetzel & Smith 2001). Current projections indicate that this number could increase to 324,000 in 2030 and 834,000 in 2050 (Krach & Velkoff 1999). Focusing on extreme cases is often a good way to gain research leverage at reasonable expense; thus, investigating centenarians (some of whom are healthy and demonstrate successful aging) and comparing them with younger age groups is an efficient way to identify factors that may contribute to healthy longevity.

An individual's vitality declines with chronological age. In a broad sense, vitality can also be viewed as resilience, as both grow out of an individual's ability to recover from "insults" such as accidents, infection, or psychological trauma (Selim et al. 2005). People who carry stress-resistant genes have an advantage in this regard. Furthermore, evidence shows that resistance to disease is inherited more directly than a long life span itself (Ju & Jones 1989), and high genetic control of frailty can be associated with a low heritability for longevity. Therefore, homeostatic mechanisms that reduce stress can slow the pace of the aging process.

Previous studies have demonstrated that resilience is generally positively correlated with cognitive function, physical health, and self-reported health among the elderly (Jeune 1995; Lamb 1999; Strehler & Mildvan 1960). In developed countries resilience is associated with self-rated successful aging (Hayflick 1994). Poon et al. (1992) discovered that common characteristics of a sample of centenarians in the country of Georgia are optimism and flexibility, which are documented to be associated with resilience (C. G. Parsons, Gruner, & Rozental 1994). Based on a Swedish sample, Nygren et al. (2005) found that mean resilience scores were higher in their oldest-old sample (over age 85) compared to the scores of the younger adults. Selim et al. (2005) discovered that centenarian veterans in the United States are psychologically resilient despite their poor physical health. Jopp and Rott (2006) also demonstrated that psychological resilience is sustained at the very end of the life span, based on the Heidelberg Centenarian Study.

However, research on centenarians and resilience has had several major limitations. Ethnic and cultural differences in mortality have only rarely been addressed in a single study. Most studies are based on small samples with limited numbers of centenarians and nonagenarians, which has re-stricted estimation efficiency (Lestienne 1988; Strehler 1977). Shen and Zeng (2010) reported on the positive association between resilience and survival among Chinese elderly aged 65 and older, but they did not investi-gate whether the association still held at extremely advanced ages (e.g., 95 and older). As Ju and Jones (1989) noted, in high-mortality populations the oldest elderly are those highly selected individuals who have survived dan-gers when being born, risks in infancy and childhood, and hunger, sickness, and accidents during youth and middle age. Stunning evidence of the im-portance of high-mortality selection is seen in the case of China, which had about five centenarians per million in the 1990s, compared with Western Europe, which had fifty per million (Jeune 1995).

Another factor that influences longevity is the availability of facilities to assist the oldest elderly in their daily lives. These are less prevalent in devel-oping countries than in industrialized nations. In the former, the oldest old are forced to perform daily activities by themselves or live with their families. The frequent physical activity may enable them to maintain their physical capacities for a longer time than their counterparts in developed countries. These factors may help explain why the elderly in Indonesia, Malaysia, the Philippines, Singapore, and Thailand have, in some comparative studies, been found to be more active than the elderly in developed countries (Ju & Jones 1989; Lamb 1999).

Similarly, the functional capacity of centenarians in Beijing, Hangzhou, and Chengdu has also been reported to be significantly higher than that of Danish centenarians (Wang, Zeng, & Jeune 1997). Thus, research on cente-narians from developing countries, including China, where the oldest old are highly selected from poor early-life conditions and severe adversities, may be useful for identifying factors that may affect exceptional longevity.

Aspects of resilience linked to longevity, quality of life, optimal functioning, and well-being in centenarians are "robust personality" with low levels of neuroticism and high conscientiousness, extraversion, cognitive reserve, and social and perceived economic resources. As Masten (2001) has noted, resilience occurs in the context of ordinary lives. Some of the resilience constructs have been tested in centenarians who successfully survived into a very old age despite many adversities (e.g., they outlived their families, have low incomes, and survived multiple chronic illnesses).

We don't know how resilient people become long-lived individuals, whether long-lived individuals inherently exhibit resilience or acquire these characteristics along the way. Further, we do not know what heritable and environmental influences combine to promote resilience among the oldest old. The general consensus to explain longevity covers multiple factors that range across distinct individual differences among centenarians (Gondo & Poon 2007; L. R. Martin, Friedman, & Schwartz 2007; Poon & Perls 2007). Their differences spread along the dimensions of physical, mental, cognitive, and functional health, as well as variations in family longevity, support systems, coping, personality, and lifestyles. This lack of a cohesive clustering of factors leaves us with no one "secret" to longevity (Poon &

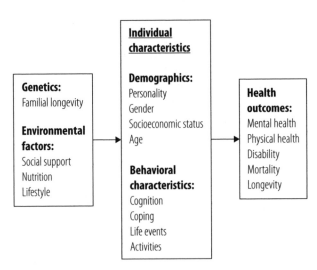

FIGURE 3.1 Modifiable components of resilience contributing to longevity
Adapted from P. Martin, MacDonald, Margrett, & Poon 2010

Perls 2007). Similarly, many factors contribute to resilience (Luthar, Cicchetti, & Becker 2000; Masten 2001) (figure 3.1). Interestingly, women compared to men are the champion survivors at all ages. Women account for 85% of centenarians, and the ten oldest people in the world are women. Is this because of superior resilience?

Successful adaptation is one aspect of resilience (Masten 2001). Poon and colleagues (1992) summarized the factors contributing to resilience in the Georgia Centenarian Study of cognitively intact and community-dwelling centenarians, octogenarians, and sexagenarians. The predictors in this model measure the direct and indirect impact of family longevity, environmental support, individual characteristics, coping abilities and styles, and nutrition on physical health, mental health, and life satisfaction.

Cognition

Aging can affect some aspects of cognition usually described as *fluid intelligence* or *fluid reasoning*, defined as the capacity to think logically and solve problems in novel situations, independent of acquired knowledge. These skills tend to peak during one's twenties and gradually decline afterward. Markedly different individual factors are found in "everyday problem solving" that depends on the constituent intellectual abilities. Abilities to solve everyday challenges are closely related to resilience in later life. However, "crystallized" abilities rely on accumulated knowledge and skills and are typically well maintained past age 70. *Crystallized intelligence* is the ability to use skills, knowledge, and experience. It should not be equated with memory or general knowledge, but it does rely on accessing information from long-term memory. Crystallized intelligence is one's lifetime or intellectual achievement, as demonstrated largely through one's vocabulary and general knowledge. This improves somewhat with age, as experiences tend to expand one's knowledge. Therefore, providing training that preserves crystallized cognition can provide the basis for building cognitive reserve and resilience.

Cognitive decline and dementia occur with disintegration of the protective resilient mechanisms of cognition, such as cognitive reserve. Dementia prevalence increases with age, from one in eight persons at age 65 to one in two among those 85 years and older. However, not all centenarians have dementia. Functional and cognitive reserves are responsible for the absence of dementia in the oldest old (P. Martin, MacDonald, Margrett, & Poon 2010; Perls 2004). In the Georgia Centenarian Study (Poon et al. 2000), cognition was one of four predictors of the number of days of survival after age 100 years. (The other predictors were female gender, father's age of death, and nutritional adequacy.) Therefore, intact cognition is a protective factor for longevity. Other factors—such as genetic (APOE-4 allele) makeup, physical and mental health, and the absence of depression—also can beneficially influence longevity (P. Martin et al. 2010).

Personality and Coping

Centenarians tend to have robust or resilient personalities (L. R. Martin, Friedman, & Schwartz 2007) and effective ways of coping with their limitations (P. Martin, Kliegel, Rott, Poon, & Johnson 2008). They tend to employ unique coping behaviors that help them adjust to aging-related challenges. In the Georgia Centenarian Study, centenarians had higher scores in dominance, suspiciousness, and shrewdness, whereas they were lower in imagination and tension compared with two younger groups (P. Martin, Long, & Poon 2002). "Openness to change" scores improved in the survivors of the same study (P. Martin et al. 2002). A relaxed but upfront personality, with low levels of neuroticism and high levels of extraversion, competence, and trust (described as "robust" among centenarians), is one factor that helps with adaptation in late life (P. Martin et al. 2002).

Similarly, Caspi (1998) suggested that three personality patterns are associated with longevity: (1) the "well-adapted" or resilient personality (i.e., persons who score moderately high on extraversion, openness, conscientiousness, and agreeableness and low on neuroticism); (2) the "overcontrolled" personality (i.e., persons low on extraversion and emotional stability); and (3) the "undercontrolled" personality (high on extraversion but low on agreeableness and conscientiousness) (Caspi 1998). Study results like these have suggested a common pattern of resilience: Low scores in neuroticism and relatively high scores in conscientiousness and extraversion aid effective coping and resilience in late life. Other features of successful adaptation include cognitive coping (e.g., analyzing the stressful situation first), acceptance, and religious coping (P. Martin et al. 2010). Pinquart and Sorensen (2000) suggested that the oldest people maintain their well-being through "downward age comparisons" and thus feel fortunate simply because they have survived. Therefore, promoting an "attitude of gratitude" and of counting one's blessings could be useful to encourage resilient coping (Pinquart & Sorensen 2000).

Social Resilience

The older-age individual faces an abundance of potential disadvantages and stressors related to social and economic resources. Physical disability and dependency often compound these difficulties. Pinquart and Sorenson (2000) in their meta-analysis of 286 empirical studies of subjective well-being reported the lack of age-associated decline and the important positive influence of social support related to subjective well-being. In their Berlin aging study, Smith and colleagues (1999) found that social activities had the strongest effect on overall well-being, along with subjective health.

Results of the Georgia Centenarian Study emphasize the influence of both social support and economic resources on mental health in community-dwelling elders (Shen & Zeng 2010). For example, centenarians had lower incomes compared to sexagenarians or octogenarians, and centenarians were more likely to get help in the form of in-kind assistance (e.g., meals, food, Medicaid) or income assistance (Goetting, Martin, Poon, & Johnson 1996). However, centenarians did not differ from younger-aged cohorts on their perceived economic status adequacy (e.g., they had "enough for emergencies"). In the same study, centenarians had fewer potential visitors and were less likely to talk on the phone compared to younger participants (P. Martin, Poon, Kim, & Johnson 1996). These measures of social resources were directly related to ratings of the activities of daily living and to mental health. At the same time, adverse life events were negatively related to economic resources and mental health (P. Martin et al. 2002). Perceived economic status mediated the negative influence of decreased functional ability on mental health and negative affect.

Conclusion

This chapter has focused on three aspects of resilience contributing to longevity that are modifiable, at least to some extent: cognition, personality, and social factors. Ideally, prevention should start in young adulthood with the understanding that good health practices, advanced education, and cognitive exercises, as well as maintenance of social network and economic resources, can lead to a more enjoyable later life. Building resources should be encouraged by government and policymakers, employers, and families. When asked, "Which would you prefer to have in later life: good health, wealth, or good cognition?," the overwhelming majority of younger individuals say they would prefer to end up with good cognition (P. Martin et al. 2010). The majority of older adults overwhelmingly agree with this choice.

Clinical Case

Although I have known a few centenarians living in long-term care facilities who were experiencing advanced dementia and numerous medical problems, including parenteral feeding devices, their longevity was mostly maintained by medical advances and frequent admissions to the hospital. I often wondered about the purpose of their long survival beyond being a medical miracle. However, the most striking individuals were those who maintained their cognitive and physical abilities, enjoyed all the benefits of accumulated wisdom, and even retained their ability to fall in love in their nineties.

An example is one such gentleman I met on his 99th birthday. He was recently married for the third time and came to the celebration with his 75-year-old wife, who had developed dementia. They lived independently, enjoyed their lives, and maintained an active lifestyle with a sufficient household income. His interpersonal manner was that of a curious, engaged, energetic 70-year-old rather than that of a 99-year-old. He had hobbies, was fairly healthy, and took only supplements and vitamins for osteoporosis and arthritis. (Admittedly, he had lost some inches in height.) He maintained a busy social schedule with his children and grandchildren, and occasionally accepted an engagement as an "extra" actor on a television show. He was certainly devastated by his wife's diagnosis, but he was determined to deal with it to the best of his ability.

However, caregiver stress became difficult for him to handle over time. He eventually moved his wife to a nursing home and himself to an assisted-living facility. He was able to deal with life stresses by keeping an open and flexible attitude of gratitude for each day that he lived pain free. Daily Bible reading and attendance at church became permanent tools in dealing with life. He always felt "close to God" and was not afraid of death or dying.

The last time I saw him, at the age of 101, he was looking forward to outings and exercise classes in his assisted-living facility. He visited his wife twice a week in the nursing home. Clearly, his optimism and personal resources, including his spirituality, determined his substantial resilience and survival into a very advanced age. I find this model of resilience to be inspiring. It illustrates a late-life experience full of the joy of life and adaptability to life challenges that many of us can aspire to in our advanced years.

. . .

References

Caspi, A. (1998). Personality development across the life course. In W. Damon & N. Eisenberg (Eds.), *Handbook of child development, vol. 3: Social, emotional, and personality psychology* (5th ed., pp. 331–88). New York: Wiley.

Goetting, M., Martin, P., Poon, L. W., & Johnson, M. (1996). The economic well-being of community-dwelling centenarians. *J Aging Stud, 10*(1), 43–55.

Gondo, Y., & Poon, L. W. (2007). Cognitive function of centenarians and its influence on longevity. *Annu Rev Gerontol Geriatr, 27*, 129–50.

Hayflick, L. (1994). *How and why we age.* New York: Ballantine.

Hetzel, L., & Smith, A. (2001). The 65 years and over population: 2000. Census brief, U.S. Census Bureau, Washington, DC.

Jeune, B. (1995). In search of the first centenarians. In B. Jeune & J. Vaupel (Eds.), *Exceptional longevity: From prehistory to the present* (pp. 11–24). Odense, Denmark: Odense University Press.

Jopp, D., & Rott, C. (2006). Adaptation in very old age: Exploring the role of resources, beliefs, and attitudes for centenarians' happiness. *Psychol Aging, 21*(2), 266–80.

Ju, C. A., & Jones, G. (1989). Aging in ASEAN: Its socio-economic consequences. Paper presented at the Institute of Southeast Asian Studies, Singapore.

Krach, C. A., & Velkoff, V. A. (1999). *Centenarians in the United States* (U.S. Census Bureau, Current Population Reports, P23-199RV). Washington, DC: U.S. Government Printing Office.

Lamb, V. L. (1999). *Active life expectancy of the elderly in selected Asian countries* (NUPRI Research Paper Series no. 69, Population Research Institute, Nihon University, Tokyo).

Lavretsky, H., Siddarth, P., & Irwin, M. R. (2010). Improving depression and enhancing resilience in family dementia caregivers: A pilot randomized placebo-controlled trial of escitalopram. *Am J Geriatr Psychiatry, 18*(2), 154–62.

Lestienne, R. (1988). On the thermodynamical and biological interpretation of the Gompertzian mortality rate distribution. *Mech Ageing Dev, 42*(3), 197–214.

Luthar, S. S., Cicchetti, D., & Becker, B. (2000). The construct of resilience: A critical evaluation and guidelines for future work. *Child Dev, 71*(3), 543–62.

Martin, L. R., Friedman, H. S., & Schwartz, J. E. (2007). Personality and mortality risk across the life span: The importance of conscientiousness as a biopsychosocial attribute. *Health Psychol, 26*(4), 428–36. doi:10.1037/0278-6133.26.4.428.

Martin, P., Kliegel, M., Rott, C., Poon, L. W., & Johnson, M. A. (2008). Age differences and changes of coping behavior in three age groups: Findings from the Georgia Centenarian Study. *Int J Aging Hum Dev, 66*(2), 97–114.

Martin, P., Long, M. V., & Poon, L. W. (2002). Age changes and differences in personality traits and states of the old and very old. *J Gerontol B Psychol Sci Soc Sci, 57B*, 144–52.

Martin, P., MacDonald, M., Margrett, J., & Poon, L. (2010). Resilience and longevity: Expert survivorship of centenarians. In P. S. Fry & C. L. M. Keyes (Eds.), *New frontiers in resilient aging: Life strengths and well-being in late life* (pp. 213–38). New York: Cambridge University Press.

Martin, P., Poon, L. W., Kim, E., & Johnson, M. A. (1996). Social and psychological resources in the oldest old. *Exp Aging Res, 22*(2), 121–39.

Masten, A. S. (2001). Ordinary magic: Resilience processes in development. *Am Psychol, 56*(3), 227–38.

National Center for Health Statistics (2007). *Health, United States, 2007, with chartbook on trend in the health of Americans*. Washington, DC: U.S. Government Printing Office.

Nygren, B., Alex, L., Jonsen, E., Gustafson, Y., Norberg, A., & Lundman, B. (2005). Resilience, sense of coherence, purpose in life and self-transcendence in relation to perceived physical and mental health among the oldest old. *Aging Ment Health, 9*(4), 354–62.

Parsons, C. G., Gruner, R., & Rozental, J. (1994). Comparative patch clamp studies on the kinetics and selectivity of glutamate receptor antagonism by 2, 3-dihydroxy-6-nitro-7-sulfamoyl-benzo(F)quinoxaline (NBQX) and 1-(4-amino-phenyl)-4-methyl-7,8-methyl-endioxyl-5H-2,3-benzodiaze pine (GYKI 52466). *Neuropharmacology, 33*(5), 589–604.

Parsons, P. A. (1996). The limit to human longevity: An approach through a stress theory of ageing. *Mech Ageing Dev, 87*(3), 211–18.

Perls, T. (2004). Dementia-free centenarians. *Exp Gerontol, 39*(11–12), 1587–93.

Pinquart, M., & Sorensen, S. (2000). Influences of socioeconomic status, social network, and competence on subjective well-being in later life: A meta-analysis. *Psychol Aging, 15*(2), 187–224.

Poon, L. W., Clayton, G. M., Martin, P., Johnson, M. A., Courtenay, B. C., Sweaney, A. L., . . . & Thielman, S. B. (1992). The Georgia Centenarian Study. *Int J Aging Hum Dev, 34*(1), 1–17.

Poon, L. W., Johnson, M. A., Davey, A., Dawson, D. V., Siegler, I. C., & Martin, P. (2000). Psycho-social predictors of survival among centenarians. In P. Martin, C. Rott, B. Hagberg & K. Morgan (Eds.), *Centenarians: Autonomy versus dependence in oldest old* (pp. 77–89). New York: Springer.

Poon, L. W., & Perls, T. (2007). The trials and tribulations of studying the oldest old. *Annu Rev Gerontol Geriatr, 27*, 1–10.

Selim, A. J., Fincke, G., Berlowitz, D. R., Miller, D. R., Qian, S. X., Lee, A., . . . & Kazis, L. E. (2005). *Comprehensive health status assessment of centenarians: Results from the 1999 large health survey of veteran enrollees*. Center for Health Quality, Outcomes & Economic Research, Veterans Affairs Medical Center, Bedford, MA. *J Gerontol A Biol Sci Med Sci, 60*(4), 515–19.

Shen, K., & Zeng, Y. (2010). *The association between resilience and survival among Chinese elderly*. 4th ed. New York: Springer.

Smith, J., Fleeson, W., Geiselmann, B., Settersten Jr., R., & Kunzmann, U. (1999). Sources of well-being in very old age. In P. B. Baltes and K. U. Mayer (Eds.), *The Berlin aging study: Aging from 70 to 100* (pp. 450–71). New York: Cambridge University Press.

Strehler, B. L. (1977). *Time, Cells, and Aging*. 2d ed. New York: Academic.

Strehler, B. L., & Mildvan, A. S. (1960). General theory of mortality and aging. *Science, 132*(3418), 14–21.

Wang, Z. L., Zeng, Y., Jeune, B., & Vaupel, J. W. (1997). A demographic and health profile of centenarians in China. In J. M. Robine, J. W. Vaupel, B. Jeune, & M. Allard (Eds.), *Longevity: To the limits and beyond* (pp. 92–104). New York: Springer.

CHAPTER 4

Biomarkers and the Neurobiology
of Resilience

R ESILIENCE ENCOMPASSES a virtually unlimited array of interacting biological, psychosocial, and environmental variables that are best examined within the context of different interdisciplinary and life span developmental perspectives. Biomarkers of resilience may shed light on underlying biological processes and coping abilities, and these may lead to developing tools for early detection of mental diseases in vulnerable populations, as well as treatments and preventive approaches. Several areas of biomarker development have a longstanding tradition (e.g., stress biology), while others are just emerging (e.g., neuroimaging, genetics).

A growing number of resilience scholars have shifted from person-focused and variable-focused research, both of which examine correlates of positive outcomes, to a more meaningful emphasis on the processes and mechanisms that actually produce resilient outcomes in animal models and in human children and adults (Goldstein & Brooks 2005; Ong, Bergeman, & Boker 2009; Rutter 2007, 2010; Wright & Masten 2006). The state of the art has progressed quickly in this research. Factors that influence resilience are briefly summarized in figure 4.1.

Stress, Endocrine Function, and Resilience

Stressors are defined as stimuli that are arousing, aversive, and unpredictable (Kim & Diamond 2002) or chronic (Koolhaas et al. 2011). They can induce multiple hormonal and behavioral responses. Additionally, exposure to stressors is considered a precipitating factor for many illnesses (Juster, McEwen, & Lupien 2010), including mood disorders. Indeed, in animal models of mood disorders, particularly depression, stress paradigms are

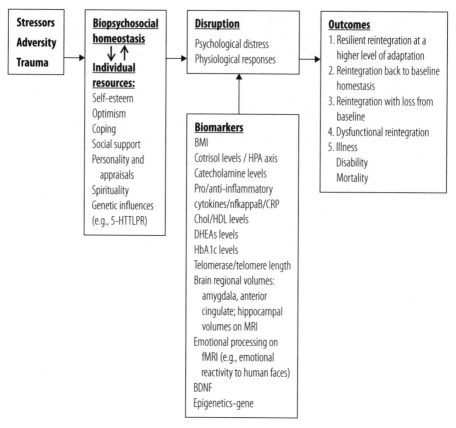

| Stressors Adversity Trauma | Biopsychosocial homeostasis ↓ ↑ Individual resources: Self-esteem Optimism Coping Social support Personality and appraisals Spirituality Genetic influences (e.g., 5-HTTLPR) | Disruption Psychological distress Physiological responses | Outcomes 1. Resilient reintegration at a higher level of adaptation 2. Reintegration back to baseline homestasis 3. Reintegration with loss from baseline 4. Dysfunctional reintegration 5. Illness Disability Mortality |

Biomarkers
BMI
Cotrisol levels / HPA axis
Catecholamine levels
Pro/anti-inflammatory
cytokines/nfkappaB/CRP
Chol/HDL levels
DHEAs levels
HbA1c levels
Telomerase/telomere length
Brain regional volumes:
amygdala, anterior
cingulate; hippocampal
volumes on MRI
Emotional processing on
fMRI (e.g., emotional
reactivity to human faces)
BDNF
Epigenetics-gene

FIGURE 4.1 Theoretic model of resilience. Key: Chol/HDL: Ratio of total cholesterol to high density lipoprotein' BMI: body mass index; DHEAs: Dehydroepiandrosterone sulfate; HBA1c: Glycosylated hemoglobin. Adapted from Lavretsky & Irwin 2007

often the principal manipulation (Nestler & Hyman 2010). Appropriately, these stress paradigms lead to adaptations in endocrine and immune systems, as well as behavior.

Exposure to stress can be characterized in several ways: by *duration* (acute, chronic); *responsiveness* (adaptive, hyperadaptive, nonresponsive); and *severity* (mild, moderate, extreme) (M. M. Miller & McEwen 2006).

Human responsiveness to stress may be attenuated by learned or adaptive skills, retraining, or indifference to future stress. A single stressful episode can cause a temporary upregulation of the hypothalamic-pituitary-adrenal (HPA) axis. Increased amounts of circulating glucocorticoids, catecholamines, serotonin, and cytokines modulate activity in areas of the brain that express high receptor density for these neurochemicals, such as the hippocampus, amygdala, and prefrontal cortex (M. M. Miller & McEwen 2006). Relatively less resilience research has focused on neurobiological processes related to psychological stress that may afford a protective buffer to developing neuropsychiatric disorders.

The neuroendocrine system, autonomic nervous system, and immune system are mediators in adapting to the challenges of daily life, referred to as *allostasis* (Sterling & Eyer 1988), meaning "maintaining stability through change." The adaptive physiological response to acute stress involves a process in which the internal milieu varies to meet perceived and anticipated demand (Sterling & Eyer 1988). McEwen (2002) extended the concept to include a set-point that changes because of the process of maintaining homeostasis. Physiological mediators—such as adrenalin from the adrenal medulla, glucocorticoids from the adrenal cortex, and cytokines from cells of the immune system—act upon receptors in various tissues and organs to produce effects that are adaptive in the short run but that can be damaging if the mediators are not shut off when no longer needed (table 4.1). When release of the mediators is not efficiently terminated, their effects on target cells are prolonged, leading to other consequences that may include receptor desensitization and tissue damage. This process of "allostatic load" is the price the tissue or organ pays for an overactive or inefficiently managed allostatic response. Therefore, allostatic load refers to the "cost" of adaptation.

TABLE 4.1   Measures of allostatic load

Allostatic load measurement
12-hour overnight urinary cortisol excretion
12-hour overnight urinary excretion of norepinephrine
12-hour overnight urinary excretion of epinephrine
Serum DHEAs level
Mean systolic blood pressure
Mean diastolic blood pressure
Ratio of waist-hip circumference
Serum HDL cholesterol
Ratio of total cholesterol to HDL cholesterol
Blood-glycosylated hemoglobin

SOURCE: Adapted from Seeman et al. 2001
    Note: DHEAs: dehydroepiandrosterone sulfate; HDL: high-density lipoprotein

The integrative model of resilience and vulnerability incorporates neuro-chemical response patterns to acute stress along with neural mechanisms that mediate reward, fear conditioning, social behavior, and important functional interactions among these systems (Bremner et al. 1997; Charney 2004; Connor & Zhang 2006). Some neurotransmitters, neuropeptides, and hormones work to promote resilience—for example, dehydroepiandrosterone (DHEA), neuropeptide Y, galanin, serotonin (5HT), brain-derived neurotrophic factor (BDNF), and benzodiazepine receptors—while others, including corticotropin-releasing hormone (CRH) and the locus coeruleus-norepinephrine system, undermine it.

Some neurotransmitters serve both functions (e.g., cortisol, dopamine) depending on circumstances. CRH is released from the hypothalamus with stress, activating the release of cortisol and DHEA via the hypothalamic-pituitary-adrenal axis. High levels of CRH have been persistently found in association with major post-traumatic stress disorder (PTSD) and chronic symptoms of fear, anxiety, and anhedonia. So it is possible that lower CRH levels are associated with lower vulnerability to stress and higher levels of resilience (Bremner et al. 1997; Charney 2004; Connor & Zhang 2006). Whether high CRH level is a cause or an effect of lower resilience to stress is not yet known. DHEA, an adrenal steroid, plays a protective role in increasing stress resistance by protecting against neural damage resulting from prolonged HPA axis activity. DHEA and its metabolites counteract corticosteroid-induced neurotoxicity in the hippocampus (Morfin & Starka 2001).

These neurobiological findings constitute promising new directions for mapping the neurophysiological substrates of resilient people, who are also likely to maintain high levels of psychological well-being in the face of life challenges (Charney & Manji 2004; Southwick & Charney 2012).

Aging, Allostatic Load, and Responsivity to Stress

Aging can modify responsivity to stress due to reduced resilience (Seeman et al. 2001). Individual differences in the aging process can be conceptualized as an accumulation of the wear and tear of daily experiences and major life stressors that interact with the individual's genetic constitution and predisposing early life experiences (Karlamangla, Singer, McEwen, Rowe, & Seeman 2002; McEwen 2004; Seeman, McEwen, Rowe, & Singer 2001).

An additional consideration regarding the comparison of risk in younger and older persons relates to underlying systems of older persons, which are likely to have been overexposed due to cumulative deleterious effects of modest, and often subtle, increases in potentially harmful physiologic factors, that is, blood pressure, glucose, insulin, cortisol, and so on. Thus, the "vascular tree" or brain of an older individual may reflect the cumulative effects of numerous deleterious insults or heavy allostatic loads (Karlamangla et al. 2002; McEwen & Stellar 1993; Seeman et al. 2001). As a result of impaired resilience with advancing age (McEwen & Stellar 1993), allostatic load accumulates and "safe operating range" narrows. Accordingly, the tolerance of an individual for out-of-range physiological stimuli may be constrained, and the risk of an adverse effect such as myocardial ischemia or cerebral vascular insufficiency may be increased. McEwen (2003) suggests that increased excursion of plasma cortisol may represent one example of the potential adverse effects of such an allostatic load. In some aged individuals, evening cortisol levels are consistently higher than is seen normally in middle-aged persons. Since cortisol in high levels is toxic for neurons, it is possible that daily exposure to modest "excess" cortisol might have a cumulative deleterious effect on the central nervous system, reducing neuronal resilience and the capacity to respond to stress (McEwen & Stellar 1993).

Stress Responsivity
IMMUNITY, INFLAMMATION, AND AGING

Normal aging is accompanied by dysregulated immune function with a two- to four-fold increase in the plasma/serum levels of inflammatory mediators such as cytokines and acute-phase proteins. A wide range of factors seems to contribute to this low-grade inflammation, including an increased amount of fat tissue, decreased production of sex steroids, smoking, subclinical infections (e.g., asymptomatic bacteriuria), and chronic disorders such as cardiovascular diseases and Alzheimer's disease.

Inflammatory response has been increasingly targeted as an integral part of the stress response (Black, Markides, & Ray 2003). In addition, chronic inflammatory processes are implicated in diverse health outcomes associated with aging, such as atherosclerosis, insulin resistance, diabetes, and metabolic syndrome. Furthermore, evidence suggests that aging is associated with a dysregulated cytokine response following stimulation. Several inflammatory mediators, such as tumor necrosis factor-alpha and interleukin-6 (IL-6), have the potential to induce and/or aggravate risk factors in age-associated pathology, providing a positive feedback mechanism. Thus it is possible that inflammatory mediators constitute a link between lifestyle factors, infection, and the physiological changes of aging on the one hand and risk factors for age-associated diseases on the other.

Consistent with this, inflammatory mediators are strong predictors of mortality in elderly cohorts, independent of other known risk factors and comorbidity. A direct pathogenetic role of inflammatory mediators would be highly likely if longevity were shown to be associated with cytokine polymorphisms regulating cytokine production. Indeed, several studies support this hypothesis—but, unfortunately, findings in this area are conflicting, which probably reflects the complexity of the effect of cytokine polymorphisms and their interaction with lifestyle and sex. For example, IL-6, a proinflammatory factor whose concentration generally increases in the blood with age (Ershler 1993), has been linked with Alzheimer's disease, osteoporosis, rheumatoid arthritis, cardiovascular disease, and some forms of cancer (Ershler 1993; Ferrucci et al. 1999; Harris et al. 1999; Kiecolt-Glaser et al. 2003; Krabbe, Pedersen, & Bruunsgaard 2004; Papanicolaou, Wilder, Manolagas, & Chrousos 1998), and it is prospectively associated with general disability and mortality in large population-based studies.

Interleukin-6 is characterized by pleiotropy and redundancy of action. Apart from its hematologic, immune, and hepatic effects, it has many endocrine and metabolic actions. Specifically, it is a potent stimulator of the hypothalamic-pituitary-adrenal axis and is under the tonic negative control of glucocorticoids. It acutely stimulates the secretion of growth hormone, inhibits thyroid-stimulating hormone secretion, and decreases serum lipid concentrations. Furthermore, it is secreted during stress and is positively controlled by catecholamines. Administration of IL-6 results in fever, anorexia, and fatigue. Potential links between social relationships and IL-6 are less well established, although one study reported that positive relations with others significantly predicted lower plasma levels of IL-6 in aging women (Friedman, Hayney, Love, Singer, & Ryff 2007).

Sickness behaviors, fatigue, and depressive symptoms that impair older adults' quality of life can be consequences of inflammation. Physically ill humans and animals exhibit sickness behaviors when they are exposed to infection. Sickness behaviors are functional in that they help sick individuals to restructure their perceptions and actions in order to conserve energy and resources (Dantzer, O'Connor, Freund, Johnson, & Kelley et al. 2008). Although feeling tired and lethargic is a normal and adaptive response to an acute infection, persistent low-grade inflammation has been linked to fatigue and depression (Dantzer et al. 2008), as well as to frailty and disability in older adults (Ershler & Keller 2000). Elevated inflammation is associated with cardiovascular disease, type 2 diabetes, Alzheimer's, osteoporosis, rheumatoid arthritis, periodontal disease, and cancer (Ershler &

Keller 2000). Given that inflammation is linked to diverse negative mental and physical health outcomes, it is important to understand the factors contributing to increased inflammation associated with stress and aging.

Study results on caregiver stress, as commonly tested among informal dementia caregivers, provide useful insights into stress responsivity in aging. Such caregiver stress has been linked with various biological outcomes, including inflammatory markers (Lavretsky, 2005). A six-year study of persons caring for a spouse with senile dementia showed increases in their inflammatory markers, which were not evident for matched controls who had no caregiving responsibilities (Kiecolt-Glaser et al. 2003). Caregivers had an average increase in levels of IL-6 that was four times greater than the increase seen for noncaregivers. These contrasting average profiles might be further illuminated by taking into account ratings of psychological well-being and ill-being, given that the caregiving role has been previously linked with both heightened distress and enhanced well-being (Marks 1998). Caregivers who experience a deep sense of purpose, meaning, and connection in their work may not show the same increments in IL-6 that are seen with those who find caregiving to be an adverse life stressor. Similarly, among noncaregivers, those with high levels of ill-being may also show marked increments in IL-6 across time. Older caregivers have poorer antibody response to vaccination, poorer control of latent herpes virus, slower wound healing, and higher systemic inflammation than their noncaregiver peers (Glaser & Kiecolt-Glaser 2005). The caregiver stress model may prove useful in uncovering gene–environment interactions in the regulation of stress response in older adults.

GENETIC VULNERABILITY AND ENVIRONMENTAL RISK

Our understanding of individual differences in stress responsivity and affect regulation is still very limited, particularly as it applies to aging. Emerging evidence suggests that the combination of genetics, early life stresses, and ongoing stress may ultimately determine individual responsiveness to stress and vulnerability to psychiatric disorders, such as depression. It is likely that genetic factors and life stress contribute not only to neurochemical alterations but also to impairments of cellular plasticity and resilience (Charney & Manji 2004). Gene–environment interactions seem to play a crucial role in determining the degree of adaptability of stress-response systems to acute or chronic stressors, both during human development and adulthood (McEwen 1998). Certain alleles might be associated with hypersensitivity to stress (DeRijk et al. 2006) and increased risk for psychiatric disorders.

Theories of depression indicate that individual responsivity to stress depends on genetic predisposition (Costello et al. 2002). Over the course of a century, findings from twin, adoption, and family studies have demonstrated that genes influence the etiology of most psychiatric disorders, but this genetic influence is complex. In most cases, the etiology is multifactorial and influenced by the gene–environment interaction (Costello et al. 2002). In support of this idea, Caspi and colleagues (2003) performed a prospective epidemiologic study investigating possible genetic vulnerability to depression with serotonin-promoter region (5-HTTLPR) polymorphism and a potential gene–environment interaction examining the 5-HTTLPR polymorphism moderation in the influence of life stress on depression. In a large birth cohort followed longitudinally for 26 years, childhood mistreatment predicted major depression only in subjects with the s-allele. These findings support the idea of gene–environment interaction in which an individual's response to environmental insults early in life is moderated by the genetic makeup.

Although genetic factors may be important contributors in stress coping and resilience, environmental factors are important as well. For example, over 50% of U.S. adults experience a trauma during their lifetime that could be associated with the development of PTSD, yet epidemiologic studies reveal that the lifetime prevalence of PTSD in the United States is only 7–8% (Kessler, Sonnega, Bromet, Hughes, & Nelson 1995). It is unclear why some persons develop PTSD and others do not. Furthermore, it is unclear why some individuals can cope and function well under stress while others are overwhelmed and function poorly.

The concept of vulnerability indicates predisposition to affective disorder, characterized by greater sensitivity to stress but with no added risk in its absence. Mastery, self-esteem, and attributional style may be involved, but exogenous factors can also act as markers of vulnerability. A follow-up study of a national cohort of 36-year-olds was used to identify endogenous and exogenous vulnerability factors (Rodgers 1991). Financial hardship and childhood trauma were implicated for women, and financial hardship and unemployment for men. However, low rates of symptoms for "stress-free" vulnerable individuals were only observed when chronic cases were excluded from analysis. Two alternative models are suggested: (1) a conditional vulnerability effect with an additional component to account for inception of long-term disorders and (2) an additive burden model with vulnerability represented as a continuum from "resilience" to "susceptibility." Differentiating these models will require greater attention to the measurement of vulnerability and a more comprehensive consideration of the significance of chronic disorders (Rodgers 1991).

Telomeres, Telomerase, and Cellular Aging

Stress may also facilitate cellular aging by reducing telomere length. A telomere is a group of nucleoprotein complexes that caps chromosomes to protect and stabilize their integrity across the life span (Epel et al. 2004). Each time a cell replicates, telomeres shorten. Telomere length is a proxy for a cell's biological age. Cells with shorter telomeres reach the critical minimum length more rapidly and subsequently die more quickly than cells with longer telomeres (Epel et al. 2004).

Telomere length has recently been proposed as a useful "psychobiomarker" linking chronic psychological stress and diseases in aging (Epel et al. 2006). The telomere is present in a region of repetitive DNA sequences at the end of a chromosome and protects the end of the chromosome from deterioration. Shortened telomere length and reduced telomerase (the cellular enzyme primarily responsible for telomere length and maintenance) are associated with premature mortality and predict a host of health risks and diseases (Lin, Epel, & Blackburn 2009), which may be regulated in part by psychological stress (Epel et al. 2004; Epel, Daubenmier, Moskowitz, Folkman, & Blackburn 2009; Ornish et al. 2008). Over the long term, high telomerase likely promotes improvement in telomere maintenance and immune cell longevity (Jacobs et al. 2011). However, the link between replicative senescence and exhaustion that controls T-cell proliferative activity and function is still not clear (Akbar & Henson 2011). Studies examining the effects of meditation on telomere length or telomerase activity report protective effects of stress reduction on the biomarkers of cellular aging (Jacobs et al. 2011; Lavretsky 2012), which raises the question of whether stress-reducing interventions can increase resilience and reverse the stress-related cellular aging process.

Neuroimaging, Neural Circuitry, and Resilience

Affective neuroscience provides insights into the brain's regulation of positive emotions and resilience (Davidson 2000). Animal studies and human neuroimaging studies have begun to identify interconnected brain circuits that mediate different aspects of mood and emotion under normal circumstances and in various pathological conditions associated with low resilience. The brain circuitry underlying emotion includes several territories of the prefrontal cortex (PFC), the amygdala, hippocampus, anterior cingulate, and related structures. In general, the PFC represents emotion in the absence of immediately present incentives. It plays a crucial role in the anticipation of the future affective consequences of action, as well as in the persistence of emotion following the offset of an elicitor (Davidson 2000). There are several different functional divisions of the PFC, including the dorsolateral, ventromedial, and orbital sectors. Each plays a role in processing affect in the absence of immediate rewards and punishments, as well as in regulating different aspects of emotion. The amygdala appears to be needed to learn new stimulus-threat contingencies and also appears to be important in the expression of cue-specific fear (Davidson 2002).

Individual differences in both tonic activation and phasic reactivity in this circuit are important in governing different aspects of anxiety. Emphasis is placed on affective chronometry, or the time-course of emotional responding, as a key attribute that accounts for individual differences in propensity for anxiety regulated by this circuitry. Individual differences such as asymmetries within the PFC and activation of the amygdala influence an individual's affective style (Davidson 2000, 2002).

The nucleus accumbens, part of the ventral striatum, is best understood as a key region of the brain that regulates an individual's response to natural rewards (e.g., food, sex, and social interaction). It is thought to function as a critical link between the motor responses needed to obtain rewards and avoid aversive stimuli (Hyman, Malenka, & Nestler 2006). These individual differences are related to behavioral and biological variables associated with affective style and the regulation of emotion. Plasticity in this circuitry has implications for transforming emotion and cultivating positive affect and resilience (Davidson 2000, 2002).

Stress, Sleep, and Aging

Quality of sleep is another important determinant of resilience to stress. According to folk wisdom, sleep is the best medicine, and scientific research has shown that there is much truth in this. Therefore, changes in the sleeping patterns associated with aging may affect resilience and coping. Sleep disruption in the laboratory, for example, is associated with alterations in HPA activity (Spath-Schwalbe, Gofferje, Kern, Born, & Fehm 1991), and age-related changes in sleep are linked to dysregulation of the HPA axis (Van Cauter, Leproult, & Kupfer 1996; Van Cauter, Leproult, & Plat 2000). Psychological stress and clinical depression, both of which are associated with HPA dysfunction (Plotsky, Owens, & Nemeroff 1998; McEwen 2000), are also linked to impaired regulation of IL-6 production, at least in immunocompetent persons (Zorrilla 2001). The ability of glucocorticoids to restrain IL-6 production in vitro, for example, is impaired in individuals experiencing chronic stress (G. E. Miller, Cohen, & Ritchey 2002). Importantly, however, support provided by social interactions partially restores sensitivity to regulation by glucocorticoids regulation (G. E. Miller et al. 2002).

Friedman and colleagues reported the interplay of social engagement, sleep quality, and plasma levels of IL-6 in a sample of aging women (Friedman et al. 2007). Regarding subjective assessment, poorer sleep was associated with lower positive social-relations scores. Improvement in sleep efficiency and by more positive social relations predicted lower levels of plasma IL-6. Women with the highest IL-6 levels were those with both poor sleep efficiency and poor social relations. However, when good social relationships compensated for low sleep efficiency or high sleep efficiency compensated for poor social relationships, levels of IL-6 levels were comparable to those with the protective influences of both good social ties and good sleep (Friedman et al. 2007). Hence, it is likely that improvement in the quality of sleep could promote individual resilience and coping.

As we have seen, neurobiological studies of resilience often stem from studies in older people. Older people seem to have an equivalent or even higher degree of psychological resilience than younger people in psychosocially oriented studies. From a biological standpoint, however, they have more sleep problems, lower capacity to recover from injury, and greater susceptibility to inflammation, infection, and toxins, all of which have the potential to reduce their physiological and psychological resistance to stress. A greater appreciation of life-course issues may help to reconcile this discrepancy and could help in developing preventive interventions that enhance resilience in older adults. Improved understanding of stress-related pathology expressed in insufficient glucocorticoid signaling will encourage development of novel drug targets and therapeutic strategies to enhance glucocorticoid signaling pathways (Raison & Miller 2001).

Cognitive Reserve as Evidence of Resilience in Brain Aging

The concept of cognitive reserve (CR) is relevant to the resilience of cognitive functions, especially in the presence of brain pathology that invokes processes that permit some individuals to remain cognitively intact despite substantial pathology (Stern 2002). The amyloid hypothesis of Alzheimer's disease suggests that we consider the concept of resilience in face of the documented in vivo brain amyloid burden (Jagust & Mormino 2011). While the amyloid cascade hypothesis of Alzheimer's disease posits an initiating role for the β-amyloid (Aβ) protein, our understanding of why Aβ is deposited is limited. A growing body of evidence based on in vitro, animal studies, and human imaging work suggests that synaptic activity increases Aβ, which is deposited preferentially in multimodal brain regions that show continuous levels of heightened activation and plasticity across the life span.

For example, individuals with larger temporal lobe volumes may better withstand the effects of Aβ deposition (Chetelat et al. 2010). Reserve, however, is likely a complex construct in epidemiological studies. It is related to education, occupation, socioeconomic status, social networks, and lifelong participation in cognitive and physical activity (Fratiglioni, Paillard-Borg, & Winblad 2004; Middleton & Yaffe 2010; Wilson et al. 2002). Such factors are difficult to disentangle and, taken together, are likely to have profound effects on an individual's brain across the life span, affecting cognition through multiple pathways.

Reserve can be considered as a reflection of lifelong patterns of behaviors, endogenous factors (including genetics), and exposure to environmental factors that have consequences for how the brain processes information. Furthermore, cognitive reserve may play different roles during pre- and postamyloid plaque stages. Once Aβ deposition begins, cognitive reserve may mitigate detrimental effects by allowing high CR individuals to cope with more downstream neuronal dysfunction and loss than individuals with low CR can. However, in pre-amyloid plaque stages, CR could act to diminish Aβ production through better "neural efficiency," a concept that is widely applied in interpreting fMRI data. For example, a polymorphism in the catechol-O-methyltransferase (COMT) gene affects the rate of dopamine metabolism: Individuals with less activity of this enzyme show greater neural efficiency, demonstrated as less brain activation required for executive tasks (Egan et al. 2001). Similar mechanisms of neural efficiency have been invoked to explain age-related differences in behavioral performance and fMRI activation on cognitive tasks (Park & Reuter-Lorenz 2009).

Bastin and colleagues (2012) reported the relationships between cognitive reserve, as measured by education, verbal intelligence, and cerebral metabolism at rest (FDG-PET) in a sample of 74 healthy older participants. Higher levels of education and verbal intelligence were associated with less metabolic activity in the right posterior temporoparietal cortex and the left anterior intraparietal sulcus. Functional connectivity analyses of resting-state fMRI images indicated that these regions belong to the default mode network and the dorsal attention network respectively. Lower metabolism in the temporoparietal cortex was also associated with better memory abilities. The findings provide evidence of an inverse relationship between cognitive reserve and resting-state activity in key regions of two functional networks respectively that are involved in internal mentation and goal-directed attention.

Even during development, low CR (in this case, linked to socioeconomic status) is associated with greater bilateral prefrontal recruitment during phonological processing (Raizada et al. 2008). Evidence of the link between increased neuronal efficiency and reduced Aβ was demonstrated in another study in which individuals who participated in more physical exercise, which has been independently associated with improvements in network efficiency (Voss et al. 2010), showed less evidence of brain Aβ (Liang et al. 2010). The Nun Study revealed that adolescent women with more complex autobiographical essays (and high CR) showed less cognitive decline and Aβ deposition in old age (Snowdon et al. 1996). Animal data showing that transgenic mice reared in enriched environments deposit less Aβ (Lazarov et al. 2005) are also consistent with this idea. Thus, cognitive reserve could act differently in pre- and postamyloid plaque stages, reducing Aβ deposition early and mitigating its effects later (Negash et al. 2012).

Wisdom and Cognitive Reserve

Fortunately, some areas of cognition show improvement with age. Depp and colleagues (2012) noted that improvement in cognitive abilities related to wisdom may increase with age, and such increases may contribute just as much, if not more, to the maintenance of independence. Wisdom remains a fledgling area for neurobiological research, and it suffers from the same definitional issues as successful cognitive aging. Nevertheless, newer measures such as the three-dimensional wisdom scale (3D-WS) have resulted in a clearer understanding of wisdom (Ardelt 1997; Jeste et al. 2010). Based on this definition and a review of related sources in the literature (Jeste & Vahia 2008; Meeks & Jeste 2009), a putative neurobiological basis for wisdom has been proposed. According to this proposed model, wisdom comprises six distinct domains: (1) prosocial attitudes and behavior; (2) social decision making or pragmatic knowledge of life; (3) emotional homeostasis; (4) reflection or self-understanding; (5) value relativism or tolerance; and (6) acknowledgment of, and effective dealing with, uncertainty and ambiguity. Based on a comprehensive review of the literature related to these domains, the authors suggest that multiple neurotransmitters have roles in acquiring and maintaining wisdom, including dopamine (in regulating impulsivity and selflessness), serotonin (in maintaining social cooperation), norepinephrine (in regulation and dampening stress-related performance and decision making), vasopressin (for affiliative behavior in animal models) and oxytocin (for social cognition and social decision making). The authors also identify several brain regions that may be part of a circuitry involved in the process of being "wise." These regions have been identified through multiple neuroimaging studies.

The neurobiological model proposed by the authors suggests that the lateral prefrontal cortex, in concert with the dorsal anterior cingulate cortex (ACC), orbitofrontal cortex (OFC), and the medial prefrontal cortex (MPFC), appears to have an important inhibitory effect on several brain areas associated with emotionality and immediate reward dependence (e.g., amygdala and ventral striatum). They also note a complementary emotion-based subcomponent, including prosaic attitudes and behaviors that involve MPFC, PFC, OFC, superior temporal sulcus, and reward neurocircuitry. Research on wisdom shows how more esoteric concepts associated with successful aging can be deconstructed, studied using laboratory experiments, and related to brain structure and function.

Lifestyle Factors and Resilience
SOCIAL SUPPORT

Evidence suggests that persons who report receiving more support from others enjoy healthy relationships with family and friends to a greater extent than those who lack this support, and they have lower rates of morbidity and mortality (Uchino, Cacioppo, & Kiecolt-Glaser 1996). Social support may be one possible explanation for these findings, as it can buffer the negative physical and mental effects of stress. It can also influence inflammation and buffer negative outcomes in caregiving (Esterling, Kiecolt-Glaser, Bodnar, & Glaser 1994) and in women with late-stage ovarian cancer (Kiecolt-Glaser, Dura, Speicher, Trask, & Glaser 1991).

Social support has been described as support accessible to an individual through social ties to other individuals, groups, and the larger community. Theoretical models of social support specify a *structural dimension*, which includes network size and frequency of social interactions, and a *functional dimension*, with emotional (such as receiving love and empathy) and instrumental (practical help such as gifts of money or assistance with child care) components. Most research has found that quality of relationships (functional dimension) is a better predictor of good health than quantity of relationships (structural dimension), although both are important (Ozbay et al. 2007; Southwick, Vythilingam, & Charney 2005).

Studies indicate that social support is essential for maintaining physical and psychological health. The harmful consequences of poor social support and the protective effects of good social support in mental illness have been well documented. Social support may moderate genetic and environmental vulnerabilities and confer resilience to stress, possibly via its effects on the hypothalamic-pituitary-adrenocortical (HPA) system, the noradrenergic system, and central oxytocin pathways (Ozbay et al. 2007).

Low levels of social support and social isolation have been shown to be associated with increased morbidity and mortality in a host of medical illnesses. For example, in the well-known Alameda County Studies, men and women without ties to others were 1.9 to 3 times more likely to die from ischemic heart disease, cerebral vascular disease, cancer, or a host of other diseases within a nine-year period compared to individuals with many more social contacts (Berkman 1995). The effect of social support on life expectancy appears to be as strong as the effects of obesity, cigarette smoking, hypertension, or level of physical activity (Sapolsky 2004).

Based on the significance of social support, there is a substantial need for additional research and development of specific interventions aiming to increase social support to enhance resilience to stress in at-risk populations of aging adults.

EXERCISE AND WEIGHT

In a randomized trial, older adults (aged 60–83) who participated in a cardiovascular exercise program for 10 months had lower C-reactive protein (CRP) and less total and central trunk adiposity than those who participated in noncardiovascular flexibility training (Vieira et al. 2009). Furthermore, reduced trunk fat was associated with reduced CRP (Vieira et al. 2009). Other studies have also found an association between higher levels of physical activity and lower levels of IL-6 and CRP (Ford 2002). Exercise may also reduce the physiological consequences of stress. Thus, exercise helps maintain homeostasis and increase protective immunity (IL-10, an anti-inflammatory cytokine) (Jankord & Jemiolo 2004). Studies of mindful exercise (tai chi, qigong, or yoga) have been shown to have a consistently positive influence on stress-related inflammation, mood, and mental health (Lavretsky 2012; Lavretsky et al. 2011).

Conclusion

Neurobiological research on resilience has contributed to understanding the neurobiology of protective factors associated with achieving long life spans and encouraging positive aging. A coherent pattern of characteristics associated with successful adaptation is emerging. These include sound intellectual functioning with protection of cognitive reserve, the ability to cope with emotions, and an engaged and active coping style in the face of adversity. Prospective neurobiological determinants of resilience for future investigations include neuroendocrine, immunological, neural, genetic, temperamental, and environmental influences. Multimodal assessment of the biological determinants of resilience will help identify targets for intervention that can enhance resilience individually and culturally.

It is vital to understand the interaction between increasing psychological resilience in the presence of decreasing physiological resilience with aging. Most likely this interaction occurs because of sufficient neuronal plasticity. Learning to enhance psychological resilience may help overcome health problems and resulting disability. Deeper understanding of the biological factors contributing to the altered stress response, including genetic and individual vulnerability, can lead to the development of more effective somatic and psychosocial treatments. Most importantly, it can lead to preventive interventions for depression and anxiety in older adults.

A comprehensive multidimensional model that combines psychological, social, genetic, and neurobiological factors based on previous research and theory is needed to guide future research in the area of stress responsivity and resilience. This added framework will allow the researcher to model not only the direct relationships between constructs of interest and their outcomes but also the indirect effects through intervening constructs.

References

Akbar, A. N., & Henson, S. M. (2011). Are senescence and exhaustion intertwined or unrelated processes that compromise immunity? *Nat Rev Immunol*, *11*(4), 289–95.

Ardelt, M. (1997). Wisdom and life satisfaction in old age. *J Gerontol B Psychol Sci Soc Sci*, *52*(1), P15–27.

Bastin, C., Yakushev, I., Bahri, M. A., Fellgiebel, A., Eustache, F., Landeau, B., . . . & Salmon, E. (2012). Cognitive reserve impacts on inter-individual variability in resting-state cerebral metabolism in normal aging. *Neuroimage*, *63*(2), 713–22.

Berkman, L. F. (1995). The role of social relations in health promotion. *Psychosom Med*, *57*(3), 245–54.

Black, S. A., Markides, K. S., & Ray, L. A. (2003). Depression predicts increased incidence of adverse health outcomes in older Mexican Americans with type 2 diabetes. *Diabetes Care*, *26*(10), 2822–28.

Bremner, J. D., Licinio, J., Darnell, A., Krystal, J. H., Owens, M. J., Southwick, S. M., . . . & Charney, D. S. (1997). Elevated CSF corticotropin-releasing factor concentrations in posttraumatic stress disorder. *Am J Psychiatry, 154*(5), 624–29.

Caspi, A., Sugden, K., Moffitt, T. E., Taylor, A., Craig, I. W., Harrington, H., . . . & Poulton, R. (2003). Influence of life stress on depression: Moderation by a polymorphism in the 5-HTT gene. *Science, 301*(5631), 386–89.

Charney, D. S. (2004). Psychobiological mechanisms of resilience and vulnerability: Implications for successful adaptation to extreme stress. *Am J Psychiatry, 161*(2), 195–216.

Charney, D. S., & Manji, H. K. (2004). Life stress, genes, and depression: Multiple pathways lead to increased risk and new opportunities for intervention. *Sci STKE, 2004*(225), re5.

Chetelat, G., Villemagne, V. L., Pike, K. E., Baron, J. C., Bourgeat, P., Jones, G., . . . & Rowe, C. C. (2010). Larger temporal volume in elderly with high versus low beta-amyloid deposition. *Brain, 133*(11), 3349–58.

Connor, K. M., & Zhang, W. (2006). Recent advances in the understanding and treatment of anxiety disorders. Resilience: determinants, measurement, and treatment responsiveness. *CNS Spectr, 11*(10 Suppl 12), 5–12.

Costello, E. J., Pine, D. S., Hammen, C., March, J. S., Plotsky, P. M., Weissman, M. M., . . . & Leckman, J. F. (2002). Development and natural history of mood disorders. *Biol Psychiatry, 52*(6), 529–42.

Dantzer, R., O'Connor, J. C., Freund, G. G., Johnson, R. W., & Kelley, K. W. (2008). From inflammation to sickness and depression: When the immune system subjugates the brain. *Nat Rev Neurosci, 9*(1), 46–56.

Davidson, R. J. (2000). Affective style, psychopathology, and resilience: Brain mechanisms and plasticity. *Am Psychol, 55*(11), 1196–214.

Davidson, R. J. (2002). Anxiety and affective style: role of prefrontal cortex and amygdala. *Biol Psychiatry, 51*(1), 68–80.

Depp, C. A., Harmell, A., & Vahia, I. V. (2012). Successful cognitive aging. *Curr Top Behav Neurosci, 10*, 35–50.

DeRijk, R. H., Wüst, S., Meijer, O. C., Zennaro, M. C., Federenko, I. S., Hellhammer, D. H., . . . & de Kloet, E. R. (2006). A common polymorphism in the mineralocorticoid receptor modulates stress responsiveness. *J Clin Endocrinol Metab, 91*(12), 5083–89.

Egan, M. F., Goldberg, T. E., Kolachana, B. S., Callicott, J. H., Mazzanti, C. M., Straub, R. E., . . . & Weinberger, D. R. (2001). Effect of COMT Val108/158 Met genotype on frontal lobe function and risk for schizophrenia. *Proc Natl Acad Sci U S A, 98*(12), 6917–22.

Epel, E. S., Blackburn, E. H., Lin, J., Dhabhar, F. S., Adler, N. E., Morrow, J. D., & Cawthon, R. M. (2004). Accelerated telomere shortening in response to life stress. *Proc Natl Acad Sci U S A, 101*(49), 17312–15.

Epel, E., Daubenmier, J., Moskowitz, J. T., Folkman, S., & Blackburn, E. (2009). Can meditation slow rate of cellular aging? Cognitive stress, mindfulness, and telomeres. *Ann N Y Acad Sci, 1172,* 34–53.

Epel, E. S., Lin, J., Wilhelm, F. H., Wolkowitz, O. M., Cawthon, R., Adler, N. E., . . . & Blackburn, E. H. (2006). Cell aging in relation to stress arousal and cardiovascular disease risk factors. *Psychoneuroendocrinology, 31*(3), 277–87.

Ershler, W. B. (1993). Interleukin-6: A cytokine for gerontologists. *J Am Geriatr Soc, 41*(2), 176–81.

Ershler, W. B., & Keller, E. T. (2000). Age-associated increased interleukin-6 gene expression, late-life diseases, and frailty. *Annu Rev Med, 51,* 245–70.

Esterling, B. A., Kiecolt-Glaser, J. K., Bodnar, J. C., & Glaser, R. (1994). Chronic stress, social support, and persistent alterations in the natural killer cell response to cytokines in older adults. *Health Psychol, 13*(4), 291–98.

Ferrucci, L., Harris, T. B., Guralnik, J. M., Tracy, R. P., Corti, M. C., Cohen, H. J., . . . & Havlik, R. J. (1999). Serum IL-6 level and the development of disability in older persons. *J Am Geriatr Soc, 47*(6), 639–46.

Ford, E. S. (2002). Does exercise reduce inflammation? Physical activity and C-reactive protein among U.S. adults. *Epidemiology, 13*(5), 561–68.

Fratiglioni, L., Paillard-Borg, S., & Winblad, B. (2004). An active and socially integrated lifestyle in late life might protect against dementia. *Lancet Neurol, 3*(6), 343–53.

Friedman, E. M., Hayney, M., Love, G. D., Singer, B. H., & Ryff, C. D. (2007). Plasma interleukin-6 and soluble IL-6 receptors are associated with psychological well-being in aging women. *Health Psychol, 26*(3), 305–13.

Glaser, R., & Kiecolt-Glaser, J. K. (2005). Stress-induced immune dysfunction: Implications for health. *Nat Rev Immunol, 5*(3), 243–51.

Goldstein, S., & Brooks, R. B. (2005). *Handbook of resilience in children.* New York: Kluwer Academic/Plenum.

Harris, T. B., Ferrucci, L., Tracy, R. P., Corti, M. C., Wacholder, S., Ettinger Jr., W. H., . . . & Wallace, R. (1999). Associations of elevated interleukin-6 and C-reactive protein levels with mortality in the elderly. *Am J Med, 106*(5), 506–12.

Hyman, S. E., Malenka, R. C., & Nestler, E. J. (2006). Neural mechanisms of addiction: The role of reward-related learning and memory. *Annu Rev Neurosci, 29,* 565–98.

Jacobs, T. L., Epel, E. S., Lin, J., Blackburn, E. H., Wolkowitz, O. M., Bridwell, D. A., . . . & Saron, C. D. (2011). Intensive meditation training, immune cell telomerase activity, and psychological mediators. *Psychoneuroendocrinology, 36*(5), 664–681.

Jagust, W. J., & Mormino, E. C. (2011). Lifespan brain activity, beta-amyloid, and Alzheimer's disease. *Trends Cogn Sci, 15*(11), 520–26.

Jankord, R., & Jemiolo, B. (2004). Influence of physical activity on serum IL-6 and IL-10 levels in healthy older men. *Med Sci Sports Exerc, 36*(6), 960–64.

Jeste, D. V., Ardelt, M., Blazer, D., Kraemer, H. C., Vaillant, G., & Meeks, T. W. (2010). Expert consensus on characteristics of wisdom: A Delphi method study. *Gerontologist, 50*(5), 668–80.

Jeste, D. V., & Vahia, I. V. (2008). Comparison of the conceptualization of wisdom in ancient Indian literature with modern views: Focus on the Bhagavad Gita. *Psychiatry, 71*(3), 197–209.

Juster, R. P., McEwen, B. S., & Lupien, S. J. (2010). Allostatic load biomarkers of chronic stress and impact on health and cognition. *Neurosci Biobehav Rev, 35*(1), 2–16.

Karlamangla, A. S., Singer, B. H., McEwen, B. S., Rowe, J. W., & Seeman, T. E. (2002). Allostatic load as a predictor of functional decline: MacArthur studies of successful aging. *J Clin Epidemiol, 55*(7), 696–710.

Kessler, R. C., Sonnega, A., Bromet, E., Hughes, M., & Nelson, C. B. (1995). Posttraumatic stress disorder in the National Comorbidity Survey. *Arch Gen Psychiatry, 52*(12), 1048–60.

Kiecolt-Glaser, J. K., Dura, J. R., Speicher, C. E., Trask, O. J., & Glaser, R. (1991). Spousal caregivers of dementia victims: Longitudinal changes in immunity and health. *Psychosom Med, 53*(4), 345–62.

Kiecolt-Glaser, J. K., Preacher, K. J., MacCallum, R. C., Atkinson, C., Malarkey, W. B., & Glaser, R. (2003). Chronic stress and age-related increases in the proinflammatory cytokine IL-6. *Proc Natl Acad Sci U S A, 100*(15), 9090–95.

Kim, J. J., & Diamond, D. M. (2002). The stressed hippocampus, synaptic plasticity and lost memories. *Nat Rev Neurosci, 3*(6), 453–62.

Koolhaas, J. M., Bartolomucci, A., Buwalda, B., De Boer, S. F., Flügge, G., Korte, S. M., . . . & Fuchs, E. (2011). Stress revisited: A critical evaluation of the stress concept. *Neurosci Biobehav Rev, 35*(5), 1291–1301.

Krabbe, K. S., Pedersen, M., & Bruunsgaard, H. (2004). Inflammatory mediators in the elderly. *Exp Gerontol, 39*(5), 687–99.

Lavretsky, H. (2005). Stress and depression in informal dementia caregivers. *Health and Aging, 1*(1), 117–33.

Lavretsky, H. (2012). Resilience, stress, and late life mood disorders. *Annu Rev Gerontol Geriatr, 32*, 49–72.

Lavretsky, H., Alstein, L. L. Olmstead, R. E., Ercoli, L. M., Riparetti-Brown, M., Cyr, N. S., & Irwin, M. R. (2011). Complementary use of tai chi chih augments escitalopram treatment of geriatric depression: A randomized controlled trial. *Am J Geriatr Psychiatry, 19*(10), 839–50.

Lavretsky, H., & Irwin, M. R. (2007). Resilience and aging. *Aging Health, 3*(3), 309–23.

Lazarov, O., Robinson, J., Tang, Y. P., Hairston, I. S., Korade-Mirnics, Z., Lee, V. M. Y., . . . & Sisodia, S. S. (2005). Environmental enrichment reduces Abeta levels and amyloid deposition in transgenic mice. *Cell, 120*(5), 701–13.

Liang, K. Y., Mintun, M. A., Fagan, A. M., Goate, A. M., Bugg, J. M., Holtzman, D. M., . . . & Head, D. (2010). Exercise and Alzheimer's disease biomarkers in cognitively normal older adults. *Ann Neurol, 68*(3), 311–18.

Lin, J., Epel, E. S., & Blackburn, E. H. (2009). Telomeres, telomerase stress and aging. In G. G. Bernston & J. T. Cacioppo (Eds.), *Handbook of neuroscience for the behavioral sciences* (chap. 65). Hoboken, NJ: Wiley.

Marks, N. F. (1998). Does it hurt to care? Caregiving, work-family conflict, and midlife well-being. *J Marriage Fam, 60*(4), 951–66.

McEwen, B. S. (1998). Stress, adaptation, and disease: Allostasis and allostatic load. *Ann N Y Acad Sci, 840*, 33–44.

McEwen, B. S. (2000). Allostasis, allostatic load, and the aging nervous system: Role of excitatory amino acids and excitotoxicity. *Neurochem Res, 25*(9–10), 1219–31.

McEwen, B. S. (2002). Sex, stress, and the hippocampus: Allostasis, allostatic load, and the aging process. *Neurobiol Aging, 23*(5), 921–39.

McEwen, B. S. (2003). Interacting mediators of allostasis and allostatic load: towards an understanding of resilience in aging. *Metabolism, 52*(10 suppl 2), 10–16.

McEwen, B. S. (2004). *The end of stress as we know it*. Washington, DC: Joseph Henry Press.

McEwen, B. S., & Stellar, E. (1993). Stress and the individual: Mechanisms leading to disease. *Arch Intern Med, 153*(18), 2093–2101.

Meeks, T. W., & Jeste, D. V. (2009). Neurobiology of wisdom: A literature overview. *Arch Gen Psychiatry, 66*(4), 355–65.

Middleton, L. E., & Yaffe, K. (2010). Targets for the prevention of dementia. *J Alzheimers Dis, 20*(3), 915–24.

Miller, G. E., Cohen, S., & Ritchey, A. K. (2002). Chronic psychological stress and the regulation of pro-inflammatory cytokines: A glucocorticoid-resistance model. *Health Psychol, 21*(6), 531–41.

Miller, M. M., & McEwen, B. S. (2006). Establishing an agenda for translational research on PTSD. *Ann N Y Acad Sci, 1071*, 294–312.

Morfin, R., & Starka, L. (2001). Neurosteroid 7-hydroxylation products in the brain. *Int Rev Neurobiol, 46*, 79–95.

Negash, S., Xie, S., Davatzikos, C., Clark, C. M., Trojanowski, J. Q., Shaw, L. M., . . . and Arnold, S. E. (2012). Cognitive and functional resilience despite molecular evidence of Alzheimer's disease pathology. *Alzheimers Dement, 9*(3), e89–95.

Nestler, E. J., & Hyman, S. E. (2010). Animal models of neuropsychiatric disorders. *Nat Neurosci, 13*(10), 1161–69.

Ong, A. D., Bergeman, C. S., & Boker, S. M. (2009). Resilience comes of age: Defining features in later adulthood. *J Pers, 77*(6), 1777–1804.

Ornish, D., Lin, J., Daubenmier, J., Weidner, G., Epel, E., Kemp, C., . . . & Blackburn, E. H. (2008). Increased telomerase activity and comprehensive lifestyle changes: A pilot study. *Lancet Oncol, 9*(11), 1048–57.

Ozbay, F., Johnson, D. C., Dimoulas, E., Morgan, C. A., Charney, D., & Southwick, S. (2007). Social support and resilience to stress: from neurobiology to clinical practice. *Psychiatry,* 4(5), 35–40.

Papanicolaou, D. A., Wilder, R. L., Manolagas, S. C., & Chrousos, G. P. (1998). The pathophysiologic roles of interleukin-6 in human disease. *Ann Intern Med,* 128(2), 127–37.

Park, D. C., & Reuter-Lorenz, P. (2009). The adaptive brain: Aging and neurocognitive scaffolding. *Annu Rev Psychol,* 60, 173–96.

Plotsky, P. M., Owens, M. J., & Nemeroff, C. B. (1998). Psychoneuroendocrinology of depression: Hypothalamic-pituitary-adrenal axis. *Psychiatr Clin North Am,* 21(2), 293–307.

Raison, C. L., & Miller, A. H. (2001). The neuroimmunology of stress and depression. *Semin Clin Neuropsychiatry,* 6(4), 277–94.

Raizada, R. D., Richards, T. L., Meltzoff, A., & Kuhl, P. K. (2008). Socioeconomic status predicts hemispheric specialisation of the left inferior frontal gyrus in young children. *Neuroimage,* 40(3), 1392–1401.

Rodgers, B. (1991). Models of stress, vulnerability, and affective disorder. *J Affect Disord,* 21(1), 1–13.

Rutter, M. (2007). Resilience, competence, and coping. *Child Abuse Neglect,* 31(3), 205–9.

Rutter, M. (2010). From individual differences to resilience: From traits to processes. Presented at the 118th Convention of the American Psychological Association (August, San Diego, CA).

Sapolsky R. M. *Why zebras don't get ulcers.* 3d ed. New York: Times Books.

Seeman, T. E., McEwen, B. S., Rowe, J. W., & Singer, B. H. (2001). Allostatic load as a marker of cumulative biological risk: MacArthur studies of successful aging. *Proc Natl Acad Sci U S A,* 98(8), 4770–75.

Snowdon, D. A., Kemper, S. J., Mortimer, J. A., Greiner, L. H., Wekstein, D. R., & Markesbery, W. R. (1996). Linguistic ability in early life and cognitive function and Alzheimer's disease in late life. Findings from the Nun study. *JAMA,* 275(7), 528–32.

Southwick, S. M., & Charney, D. S. (2012). *Resilience: The science of mastering life's greatest challenges.* New York: Cambridge University Press.

Southwick, S. M., Vythilingam, M., Charney, D. S. (2005). The psychobiology of depression and resilience to stress: Implications for prevention and treatment. *Annu Rev Clin Psychol,* 1, 255–91

Spath-Schwalbe, E., Gofferje, M., Kern, W., Born, J., & Fehm, H. L. (1991). Sleep disruption alters nocturnal ACTH and cortisol secretory patterns. *Biol Psychiatry,* 29(6), 575–84.

Sterling, P., & Eyer, J. (1988). Allostasis: A new paradigm to explain arousal pathology. In S. Fisher & J. T. Reason (Eds.), *Handbook of life stress, cognition, and health.* New York: Wiley.

Stern, Y. (2002). What is cognitive reserve? Theory and research application of the reserve concept. *J Int Neuropsychol Soc, 8*(3), 448–60.

Uchino, B. N., Cacioppo, J. T., & Kiecolt-Glaser, J. K. (1996). The relationship between social support and physiological processes: A review with emphasis on underlying mechanisms and implications for health. *Psychol Bull, 119*(3), 488–531.

Van Cauter, E., Leproult, R., & Kupfer, D. J. (1996). Effects of gender and age on the levels and circadian rhythmicity of plasma cortisol. *J Clin Endocrinol Metab, 81*(7), 2468–73.

Van Cauter, E., Leproult, R., & Plat, L. (2000). Age-related changes in slow wave sleep and REM sleep and relationship with growth hormone and cortisol levels in healthy men. *JAMA, 284*(7), 861–68.

Vieira, V. J., Hu, L., Valentine, R. J., McAuley, E., Evans, E. M., Baynard, T., & Woods, J. A. (2009). Reduction in trunk fat predicts cardiovascular exercise training-related reductions in C-reactive protein. *Brain Behav Immun, 23*(4), 485–91.

Voss, M. W., Prakash, R. S., Erickson, K. I., Basak, C., Chaddock, L., Kim, J. S., . . . & Kramer A. F. (2010). Plasticity of brain networks in a randomized intervention trial of exercise training in older adults. *Front Aging Neurosci, 2.* doi: 10.3389/fnagi.2010.00032.

Wilson, R. S., De Leon, C. F. M., Barnes, L. L., Schneider, J. A., Bienias, J. L., Evans, D. A., & Bennett, D. A. (2002). Participation in cognitively stimulating activities and risk of incident Alzheimer disease. *JAMA, 287*(6), 742–48.

Wright, M. O., & Masten, A. S. (2006). Resilience processes in development: Fostering positive adaptation in the context of adversity. In S. Goldstein & R. B. Brooks (Eds.), *Handbook of resilience in children* (pp. 17–37). New York: Springer.

Zorrilla, E. P., Luborsky, L., McKay, J. R., Rosenthal, R., Houldin, A., Tax, A., . . . & Schmidt, K. (2001). The relationship of depression and stressors to immunological assays: A meta-analytic review. *Brain Behav Immun, 15*(3), 199–226.

CHAPTER 5

Gene–Environment Interaction
and Resilience

THE CONCEPT OF RESILIENCE ENCOMPASSES the recognition that individuals vary in their response to adversities, even to adversities of the same severity. The concept also considers the neurobiological mechanisms underlying variations in individual response that can cast light on the causal processes that have implications for developing preventive strategies and treatments. The best way to demonstrate the process of gene–environment interactions with resilience is to examine the effects of early traumatic experiences, with an eye to the future development of vulnerabilities to mental disorders in which genetics and environment play important roles in individual resilience or vulnerability to mental disorders. Early adversity is a strong and enduring predictor of future vulnerability to mental illness, including mood disorders, anxiety disorders, substance abuse or dependence, and post-traumatic stress disorder (PTSD). However, the mechanisms through which these effects manifest are not well understood, mostly because of the difficulties involved in tracking effects of early traumatic experiences in older adults.

In this chapter, I provide an overview of the current research pertaining to the long-term effects of early and later adversity on psychiatric disorders in later life, as well the role of potential biological and environmental mediators and moderators of the relationship between early adversity and psychiatric disorders. I also examine the role of resilience as a protective construct that carries clinical implications and presents methodological challenges and include suggestions for future research.

The Role of Early Trauma in Developing Vulnerability to Later Life Mental Disorders

Large-scale community-based studies with adults have documented that exposure to adversity early in life is a robust predictor of adult-onset mood disorders, anxiety disorders, eating disorders, substance abuse or dependence, and PTSD (Bifulco, Brown, & Adler 1991; Green et al. 2010; Kendler et al. 2000, 2002, 2006; Kessler & Magee 1994; Kessler, Davis, & Kendler 1997; MacMillan et al. 2001; Molnar, Buka, & Kessler 2001; Nelson et al. 2002; Widom 1999), as well as personality disorders (Afifi et al. 2011; Gershon et al. 2013).

Moreover, the risk for psychiatric outcomes following early adversity appears to persist into old age (Clark, Caldwell, Power, & Stansfeld 2010; Comijs et al. 2007; Kivela, Luukinen, Koski, Viramo, & Pahkala 1998; Wilson et al. 2006). Some evidence indicates that specific types of early adversity, such as child abuse, may increase the risk of developing disorders compared to other types of adversity. However, not everyone who experiences an early adversity will subsequently develop a psychiatric disorder, and data are limited with respect to the pathways by which adversity effects persist in late life, especially considering personal resilience factors. Thus, there has been an increase in research aimed at improving understanding of the mechanisms by which adversity leads to mental disorders and identifying the factors that may modify these long-term effects, such as resilience or genetic vulnerability.

Early Trauma: Definitions, Severity, and Critical Periods of Development

The term *early trauma* refers to a wide array of early adversities, including abuse or assault, neglect, poverty, death of a parent, parental chronic physical or mental illness, alcohol or substance problems, incarceration, parental divorce, physical illness or injury during childhood, domestic violence, peer victimization (bullying), violence, and exposure to a war or a natural disaster. Early trauma includes single or multiple incidences and acute or chronic stressful events that may be biological or psychological in nature, which have occurred during childhood and have precipitated a biological and/or psychological stress response. In addition to consideration of the above distinctions, the impact of early adversity on psychiatric risk also likely depends on the type, severity, and critical timing of traumatic experience relative to an individual's development.

Although establishing or verifying sources and severity of trauma in older adults is typically difficult (due to recall bias, etc.), some studies are available to provide evidence linking later psychopathology to early trauma. In a sample of over 22,000 adults 60 years of age or older, the effects of experiencing both physical and sexual abuse in childhood was associated with worse outcomes than experiencing either form of abuse alone (Draper, Pfaff, et al. 2008). Thus, the initial data in older adults suggest that risk of developing a psychiatric disorder may, as at other stages of the life span, be proportionally related to the severity of adversity exposure.

Findings from the National Comorbidity Survey ($N = 5,692$, 18 and older) indicate that while exposure to early adversities is associated with psychiatric illness in adulthood, this relationship also appears to be nonspecific (Green et al. 2010; McLaughlin et al. 2010). Cross-national data from the WHO World Mental Health surveys conducted in 21 countries also lack substantial evidence of specificity in the association between adversity type and psychiatric disorder (Kessler et al. 2010). Thus, the risk for psychiatric disorders stemming from early trauma is nonspecific and may be shaped by other influences (e.g., genetic and environmental).

However, the severity of trauma appears to be important to the severity of psychopathology in adulthood. Several studies support a dose-response relationship in which the probability of developing a psychiatric disorder is proportional to the number of adversities experienced and their severity. in a study of community-dwelling women ($N = 732$, ages 36–45 years), those who experienced multiple categories of childhood abuse were found to be at highest relative risk for depression, compared to women who reported one form of abuse. The latter were, in turn, at higher risk for depression than women with no abuse history (Wise, Zierler, Krieger, & Harlow 2001).

Felitti et al. (1998) similarly identified a strong dose-response relationship between the number of childhood exposures and the risk for negative health outcomes, including alcohol or substance abuse, depression, and suicidality, in a large sample of HMO members ($N = 9,508$, mean age = 56.1 years). A dose-response effect between severity of childhood sexual abuse and risk for disorder was also found in a population-based sample of 1,411 female twins (ages 17–55 years) (Kendler et al. 2000). Similar patterns have been found for the effects of early adversity on neurocognitive impairment. Echoing the cumulative effect found for psychiatric outcomes, Evans and Schamberg (2009) showed that the greater the proportion of childhood spent in poverty, the poorer one's working memory as a young adult. The dose-response effect appears to persist into old age.

Exposure to traumatic experiences during the critical developmental periods of late childhood and early adolescence may lead to high vulnerability to particular forms of psychiatric disorders (Kaplow, Dodge, Amaya-Jackson, & Saxe 2005; Rudolph & Flynn 2007). Exposure to sexual abuse after age 12 has been associated with increased risk for PTSD in adulthood, whereas sexual abuse before age 12 has been associated with increased risk for depression (Schoedl et al. 2010). In a birth cohort sample of 496 cases of court-substantiated abuse (mean age = 39.5 years) the experience of abuse before age 12 was associated with increased risk for internalizing outcomes in adulthood while the experience of abuse after age 12 was associated with externalizing outcomes (Kaplow & Widom 2007). Thus, puberty may be a critical developmental period during which individuals are at increased risk for particular forms of mental disorders that may be carried into adulthood.

Trauma in Later Life and Increased Risk of Mental Disorders

The risk associated with adversity during stages of critical brain development may persist into late life. Yehuda and colleagues (2004) found that Holocaust survivors diagnosed with current PTSD ($n = 35$) showed impaired ability to learn new information compared to survivors without a current PTSD diagnosis ($n = 26$) versus controls ($n = 40$). Interestingly, the specific long-term cognitive impairments identified among Holocaust survivors differed from those identified among Vietnam veterans. The authors speculate that these differences may relate to the timing of the trauma exposure: While Vietnam veterans were exposed to trauma during early adulthood (military service), many Holocaust survivors were still children or adolescents during the exposure. Exposure to severe trauma even in resilient individuals may result in the development of PTSD because of an innate inability to self-regulate emotional homeostasis. In meta-analytic studies, individual risk factors in younger adults are shown to have consistent effects on the risk for PTSD and include familial psychopathology, child abuse, and preexisting psychopathology.

• In the elderly, poor health and nutrition, along with cognitive decline, might contribute to vulnerability to developing emotional problems under stress or extreme trauma. Yehuda et al. (2006) examined the concept of resilience as related to the development of post-traumatic stress syndrome following exposure to trauma in older veterans with and without chronic PTSD. Measures included the hippocampal size on MRI scan, as well as stress neuroendocrine assessment (e.g., 24-h urinary cortisol excretion) and cognitive performance. Although veterans with PTSD did not differ from those without PTSD in hippocampal volume, they did show significantly lower urinary cortisol levels, and poorer memory performance on the Wechsler Logical Memory test and the Digit Span test. The authors concluded that smaller hippocampal volumes in PTSD may be associated with specific risk and resilience factors. Grossman and colleagues (2006) reported that PTSD was associated with substantial impairments in cognition including learning, free and cued recall, and recognition memory in veterans and in Holocaust survivors as compared to respective nonexposed subjects.

Biological Predictors, Mediators, and Moderators of Resilience to Adversity

At least two broad pathways have been hypothesized to explain the impact of adversity on risk for later psychiatric disorders (figure 5.1). First, expo-

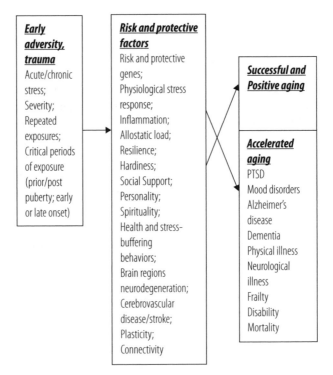

FIGURE 5.1 The relationship of early trauma to later-life mental disorders mediated by biological biomarkers and resilience

sure to early adversity may become "biologically embedded" (Miller et al. 2011), altering the development of key physiological systems (hypothalamic-pituitary-adrenal axis, HPA, and immune function). Second, exposure to early adversity is a psychosocial index of continued stress exposure; that is, those who experience adversity in childhood are more likely to suffer subsequent stress (Hazel, Hammen, Brennan, & Najman 2008).

HPA FUNCTION

Adversity in the form of acute stress activates an immediate response of the HPA and sympathetic adrenal medullary axes, beginning with the release of the hypothalamic corticotropin-releasing hormone (CRH) that initiates the endocrine response to stress. CRH then prompts the release of adrenocorticotropin (ACTH). ACTH promotes the release of glucocorticoids from the adrenal cortex. Glucocorticoids regulate the utilization of energy and provide negative feedback at the level of the hypothalamus and pituitary (Gunnar & Quevedo 2007; Heim et al. 2001; Kaufman Plotsky, Nemeroff, & Charney 2000).

Glucocorticoids also affect the morphology and functionality of central nervous system target tissues, including those responsible for mood and cognitive functions relevant to psychiatric disorders in later life (Abercrombie et al. 2011; de Quervain et al. 2003; Karst et al. 2002; Mitra & Sapolsky 2010). HPA-axis adaptations to a chronically highly adverse environment or to traumatic events may have short-term survival advantages for living in dangerous environments, but they also carry the risk of long-term effects on cognition and emotion in addition to risk for psychiatric disorders later in life.

Few prospective longitudinal studies have linked the HPA response to adversity in youth to mental disorders in late life. However, retrospective studies suggest that early stressors can have an enduring influence on HPA-axis activity. Adults with a history of early adversity, in the form of childhood abuse, exhibit signs of HPA-axis trauma adaptations, including flattened diurnal variability and lowered early morning cortisol secretion (Gerritsen et al. 2010), more robust dexamethasone suppression of cortisol (Stein, Yehuda, et al. 1997), increased ACTH release and lower cortisol responses to either CRH administration (Heim et al. 2001) or a laboratory stressor (Heim et al. 2000). Similarly, adult Holocaust survivors with PTSD demonstrate similar adaptations compared to adults who did not experience the Holocaust (Yehuda, Golier, & Kaufman 2005). In addition to trauma and PTSD, impaired HPA activity in later life has also been associated with depression (Sudheimer et al. 2013).

The HPA axis is not the only physiological system affected by stress. The immune system encompasses a complex set of pro-inflammatory mediators, specifically cytokines, chemokines, and growth factors, all of which have been proposed as mediators of the impact of adversity on psychiatric outcomes. It is very difficult to investigate long-term effects of early adversity on immune function in adulthood; animal models are often too simple with regard to the range of stressors and life episodes that can be tested. In animal models, stressors exerted to the mother (pre- or postnatally) and/or to the infant, in the form of nutritional imbalance, infectious agents and/or toxicants, physical restraint, or mother-infant separation, can lead to long-lasting immune imbalances or altered "immune set points" (Graham, Christian, & Kiecolt-Glaser 2006; Langley-Evans & McMullen 2010; Merlot, Couret, & Otten 2008). Altered immune set points may lead to the chronic secretion of pro-inflammatory signals and specifically heightened immune responsiveness. These altered set points are sometimes associated with changes in the HPA axis, notably glucocorticoid levels (Miller et al. 2009), emphasizing the functional link between the brain and the immune system.

Early stressors, such as abuse, can result in PTSD-like symptoms and manifest as changes in the immune set points (Bauer et al. 2010). One of the only large-scale prospective longitudinal studies of a birth cohort followed subjects to age 32. The results show that maltreatment in the first decade of life is associated with high-sensitivity C-reactive protein (hsCRP) levels, a biomarker of inflammation (Danese et al. 2007). This effect was independent of potential confounds (e.g., low SES, depression, high levels of stress in adulthood, smoking, unhealthy diet), and findings support a dose-response relationship between severity of early adversity and inflammation.

Among healthy older adults who were dementia caregivers and non-caregivers ($N = 132$, mean age = 70), those who experienced childhood adversity showed a greater proinflammatory cytokine level, including shorter telomeres, amplified interleukin-6 (IL-6), and tumor necrosis factor (TNF)-α levels, than those without such history. Effects were only partially attributable to caregiving, suggesting that early adversity influenced immune function beyond the effects of the stress associated with caregiving (Kiecolt-Glaser et al. 2011). In a follow-up study with this sample, Gouin and colleagues (2012) found that those exposed to abuse, in particular, exhibited elevated IL-6 responses to daily stressors. Similar to findings on HPA, altered immune set points have the potential to be normalized, or "buffered," by positive influences such as social support (Macphee et al. 2010). Although it stands to reason that these effects could persist through adulthood, studies have not yet examined the role of social support in general for moderating long-term effects of early adversity.

Psychosocial Mediators: Adult Stressors

Theorists have formulated a transactional model of stress continuity, in which exposure to early adversity alters psychosocial processes, generating further stress and leading to increased psychiatric risk. Using data from a longitudinal survey of adults, Kessler and Magee (1994) found that interpersonal stress and recurrence of depression in adulthood was linked to childhood family violence. The authors speculated that exposure to family violence in childhood may have disrupted interpersonal functioning, thereby increasing reactivity to future stressors and, in turn, depressive recurrence. Similarly, McLeod (1991) found an association between that marital strain and depression in adulthood and exposure to parental divorce in childhood.

At the same time, some studies indicate that adult stressors do not contribute to adult psychopathology over and above exposure to early adversity. Much research has attested to the role of hardiness, that is, personality traits that are protective and contribute to resilience to stress or to neuroticism that contributes to increased risk of psychopathology in adult life (Lavretsky 2012).

SEX DIFFERENCES IN VULNERABILITY TO STRESS AND ADVERSITY

Rates of exposure to childhood adversity vary between the sexes by type of adversity. Childhood sexual abuse is more prevalent in females while childhood physical abuse is more prevalent in males (Gorey & Leslie 1997; MacMillan et al. 1997, 2001; Molnar et al. 2001). A recent literature review of community-based samples in which sex differences were specifically analyzed found that nearly half of all studies report no sex differences in effects of childhood victimization on risk for psychiatric disorder across the life span. In studies that included a focus on sex differences, victimization tended to be associated with higher psychiatric risk in females in studies with adult samples, whereas in males victimization tended to be associated with higher psychiatric risk in youth samples (Gershon, Minor, et al. 2008). These results underscore the need to elucidate more precise sex- and age-specific trauma exposure patterns leading to mental disorders.

GENETIC SUSCEPTIBILITY

Genetic markers may moderate the effects of early adversity on later psychopathology. A functional insertion/deletion polymorphism in the serotonin gene linked to the promoter region (5-HTTLPR) has repeatedly been found to moderate the influence of early adversity and stressful events on the development of psychopathology (Caspi, Hariri, et al. 2010). The 5-HTT s-allele may thus affect depression and anxiety via an interaction with the fear circuits of the brain. Individuals with the s-allele variant and early adversity show hyper-reactivity of the autonomic system and of the amygdala and anterior cingulate circuits in response to fear signals. Among adults with psychotic disorders ($N = 118$), homozygotic s-allele carriers who experienced childhood trauma showed greater cognitive impairment (Aas et al. 2012).

Most research in this area is limited to younger-age samples. Caspi and colleagues' seminal study, which showed that the 5-HTT s-allele moderates the effect of risk for depression stemming from childhood maltreatment, was limited to a relatively young sample of 26-year-old males ($N = 1,037$) (Caspi et al. 2003). The persistence of the interactive effect of 5-HTT and early adversity on psychiatric risk across the life span is less clear. O'Hara and colleagues (2007) found no interactive effects of stress and the 5-HTT s-allele on cognitive function in older adults ($N = 154$, mean age $= 71.1$ years) in their analysis of cumulative life stress or early trauma. However, significant interactions of 5-HTT with elevated levels of waking cortisol did predict lower memory performance and hippocampal volume. Further, a direct association was found between 5-HTT genotype status and increased levels of waking cortisol, suggesting that biological measures of stress may be more important in advanced age than self-reports of early life adversity and stress.

However, not all studies agree with these conclusions. In the large meta-analysis of published data by Risch et al. (2009), no association was found between 5-HTTLPR genotype and depression in any of the individual studies or in the weighted average (OR, 1.05; 95% CI, 0.98–1.13), and no interaction effect between genotype and stressful life events on depression was observed (OR, 1.01; 95% CI, 0.94–1.10). This meta-analysis yielded no evidence that the serotonin transporter genotype alone or in interaction with stressful life events is associated with an elevated risk of depression in men alone, women alone, or in both sexes combined.

In another investigation, which included older adults, Gillespie and colleagues (2005) found no interactive effect of stressful events and 5-HTT genotype on levels of depressive symptoms. However, in another large population-based study of older men and women ($N = 906$, aged 65 years or older), a link was found between childhood adversity and depression that was significantly stronger for those with the 22/23EK or the 9beta variant (Bet, Penninx, et al. 2009). Additional polymorphisms, such as the FK506 binding protein 5 (FKBP5), have been identified as moderators of the effect of early adversity on later psychopathology (Binder et al. 2008). This suggests that several different pathways and mechanisms may underlie the interaction of early adversity and late-life neuropsychiatric disorders, including dementias.

Assessment of Early Adversity in Later Life

Recall of early trauma may be influenced by later life events. Therefore, it is critical for future research to assess adversity history comprehensively so that more precise delineations of the relationships among adversities and their contributions to psychiatric outcomes in late life can be obtained (Finkelhor, Ormrod, et al. 2007). Second, reporting bias continues to present a challenge, particularly in samples with older adults (O'Hara et al. 2007). It is possible that the retrospective self-report measures underestimate the level of life stress and early adversity and trauma experienced by older adults. Older individuals often have recall difficulties, and evidence suggests that older adults are less likely to pay attention to and recall events they associate with negative emotional valence (Steinmetz, Muscatell, & Kensinger 2010).

In addition, traumatic events that occurred decades in the past may be important but less relevant to older adults than the chronic daily stress of multiple losses. While recall of lifetime events has been found to be fairly reliable in research on depression (Brewin, Andrews, & Gotlib 1993), reliability is vastly improved by use of interview measures (Brown & Harris 1998) designed to enhance recall and minimize reporting bias. However, interview measures are lengthy and present challenges in cost, manpower, and participant burden.

Most of the studies reporting the gene–environment interaction ($G \times E$) effect on psychopathology are based on retrospective design. Prospective studies, following participants from childhood into late adulthood with frequent assessments of adversity and symptoms, could improve the validity of the longitudinal trajectories of risk or protective factors for disease outcomes. However, it would take decades to provide results for the older adult stages of life covering 60–100 years. Structured, multi-cohort designs, such as accelerated longitudinal designs, offer significant advantages for examining differential effects of early adversity by age of exposure, and thus for identifying critical periods in development that represent heightened risk/protective factors for late-life neuropsychiatric disorders (Thompson, Hallmayer, & O'Hara 2011).

The few studies that have had the ability to look at mediators in a longitudinal design indicate that some of the risk associations between childhood adversity and psychiatric outcomes in older adulthood may be associated with psychopathology developed in early adulthood (Clark et al. 2010). Such findings further highlight the need for longitudinal designs that allow psychopathology to be assessed continually over time to identify the points of emerging illness.

Clinical Implications

The reviewed findings indicate that exposure to adversity early in life is capable of increasing long-term risk for a range of later-life neuropsychiatric disorders. Assessment of traumatic experiences needs to be comprehensive and to include measures of key dimensions of the experience such as severity, chronicity, and the timing of critical periods of development. As our understanding of the effects of adversity develops, treatment and preventive interventions may be individually tailored to the type and timing of exposure.

Four main lessons are evident from the body of research on gene–environment interaction. First, as in Dunedin's three examples of $G \times E$ in defining adult psychopathology (Rutter 2006), the influence of the genes was only shown through demonstration of the interaction with the environmental hazard. Second, in each case, the $G \times E$ was specific to a particular psychopathological outcome. The finding underlines the fact that resilience is not identified with only one universally applicable trait. Third, the implication of the $G \times E$ is that both the G and the E share the same causal pathophysiological pathway. Fourth, the genetic variant is neither a risk nor a protective factor in itself. That is, little or no effect occurs on psychopathology in the absence of the environmental risk factor (Rutter 2006). In addition, resilience may derive from physiological or psychological coping processes rather than from external risk or protective factors. Delayed recovery from exposure to adversity may derive from "turning point" experiences in adult life. However, resilience may be limited by certain biological epi-genetic mechanisms of stress/adversity on neural structures that impede recovery or accelerate improvement due to interventions (Rutter 2006).

Studies of gene–environment interaction in defining individual resilience to adversity are limited by the lack of prospective longitudinal designs, particularly with samples of older persons. Efforts to identify mediators of the relationship between adversity and psychopathology have largely focused on HPA function, which is just one marker of the stress function. Although emergent evidence points to the immune function as a potential mediator, relatively few studies have been conducted in this domain (Bauer et al. 2010; Groer & Morgan 2007; Pace et al. 2006).

Evidence of genetic moderators similarly suggests the need for greater focus on gene–environment interactions on psychopathology, as well as further implementing neuroimaging endophenotypes to document brain effects of exposure to trauma and treatment interventions. Nevertheless, one of the most important lessons from this literature, particularly in samples of older adults (O'Hara et al. 2007), is that improved and routine assessment of early adversity is needed before we can elucidate the mechanisms by which genetic susceptibility interacts with adversity, leading to increased risk for psychopathology in older adults.

Conclusion

This chapter complements chapter 4 in presenting the interaction of genetic, neurobiological variables with environmental influences, particularly early trauma. To better understand the pathways to competent functioning in the presence of significant adversity, we need multiple levels of analysis. This new perspective would incorporate biological measures into the predominantly psychosocial and environmental-contextual measurement batteries for research on the determinants of resilience (Cicchetti & Blender 2004). The concurrent examination of environmental-contextual, psychological, and biological processes along with their interplay at varying developmental periods will provide a more integrative conceptualization of the developmental course (Cicchetti 2002).

Although it would be impractical for most investigators to include all levels of analysis within the same experimental design, the growing movement toward collaborative interdisciplinary research within the disciplines of neuroscience and developmental psychopathology suggests that a multiple-levels approach will become increasingly prevalent (Grinspoon & Bakalar 1998). The incorporation of this augmented perspective will result in a more sophisticated and comprehensive portrayal of resilience, thus advancing the scientific knowledge of resilience as well as informing efforts to translate research on positive adaptation in the face of adversity into the development of interventions that will promote higher levels of resilient functioning.

References

Aas, M., Djurovic, S., Athanasiu, L., Steen, N. E., Agartz, I., Lorentzen, S., . . . & Melle, I. (2012). Serotonin transporter gene polymorphism, childhood trauma, and cognition in patients with psychotic disorders. *Schizophr Bull, 38*(1), 15–22.

Abercrombie, H. C., Jahn, A. L., Davidson, R. J., Kern, S., Kirschbaum, C., & Halverson, J. (2011). Cortisol's effects on hippocampal activation in depressed patients are related to alterations in memory formation. *J Psychiatr Res, 45*(1), 15–23.

Afifi, T. O., Mather, A., Boman, J., Fleisher, W., Enns, M. W., MacMillan, H., & Sareen, J. (2011). Childhood adversity and personality disorders: Results from a nationally representative population-based study. *J Psychiatr Res, 45*(6), 814–22.

Bauer, M. E., Wieck, A., Lopes, R. P., Teixeira, A. L., & Grassi-Oliveira, R. (2010). Interplay between neuroimmunoendocrine systems during post-traumatic stress disorder: A minireview. *Neuroimmunomodulation, 17*(3), 192–95.

Bellinger, D. L., Lubahn, C., & Lorton, D. (2008). Maternal and early life stress effects on immune function: Relevance to immunotoxicology. *J Immunotoxicol, 5*(4), 419–44.

Bet, P. M., Penninx, B. W., Bochdanovits, Z., Uitterlinden, A. G., Beekman, A. T., van Schoor, N. M., . . . & Hoogendijk, W. J. (2009). Glucocorticoid receptor gene polymorphisms and childhood adversity are associated with depression: New evidence for a gene–environment interaction. *Am J Med Genet B Neuropsychiatr Genet, 150B*(5), 660–69.

Bifulco, A., Brown, G. W., & Adler, Z. (1991). Early sexual abuse and clinical depression in adult life. *Br J Psychiatry, 159*, 115–22.

Binder, E. B., Bradley, R. G., Liu, W., Epstein, M. P., Deveau, T. C., Mercer, K. B., . . . & Ressler, K. J. (2008). Association of FKBP5 polymorphisms and childhood abuse with risk of posttraumatic stress disorder symptoms in adults. *JAMA, 299*(11), 1291–305.

Brewin, C. R., Andrews, B., & Gotlib, I. H. (1993). Psychopathology and early experience: A reappraisal of retrospective reports. *Psychol Bull, 113*(1), 82–98.

Brown, G. W., & Harris, T. O. (1998). *Social origins of depression: A study of psychiatric disorder in women.* New York: Free Press.

Caspi, A., Hariri, A. R., Holmes, A., Uher, R., & Moffitt, T. E. (2010). Genetic sensitivity to the environment: The case of the serotonin transporter gene and its implications for studying complex diseases and traits. *Am J Psychiatry, 167*(5), 509–27.

Caspi, A., Sugden, K., Moffitt, T. E., Taylor, A., Craig, I. W., Harrington, H., . . . & Poulton, R. (2003). Influence of life stress on depression: Moderation by a polymorphism in the 5-HTT gene. *Science, 301*(5631), 386–89.

Cicchetti, D. (2002). How a child builds a brain: Insights from normality and psychopathology. In W. H. Weinberg & and R. Weinberg (Eds.), *Minnesota symposia on child psychology: Child psychology in retrospect and prospect.* Mahwah, NJ: Lawrence Erlbaum Associates.

Cicchetti, D., & Blender, J. A. (2004). A multiple-levels-of-analysis approach to the study of developmental processes in maltreated children. *Proc Natl Acad Sci U S A, 101*(50), 17325–26.

Clark, C., Caldwell, T., Power, C., & Stansfeld, S. A. (2010). Does the influence of childhood adversity on psychopathology persist across the lifecourse? A 45-year prospective epidemiologic study. *Ann Epidemiol, 20*(5), 385–94.

Comijs, H. C., Beekman, A. T., Smit, F., Bremmer, M., Tilburg, T. V., & Deeg, D. (2007). Childhood adversity, recent life events, and depression in late life. *J Affect Disord, 103*(1–3), 243–46.

Danese, A., Pariante, C. M., Caspi, A., Taylor, A., & Poulton, R. (2007). Childhood maltreatment predicts adult inflammation in a life-course study. *Proc Natl Acad Sci U S A, 104*(4), 1319–24.

de Quervain, D. J., Henke, K., Aerni, A., Treyer, V., McGaugh, J. L., Berthold, T., . . . & Hock, C. (2003). Glucocorticoid-induced impairment of declarative memory retrieval is associated with reduced blood flow in the medial temporal lobe. *Eur J Neurosci, 17*(6), 1296–302.

Draper, B., Pfaff, J. J., Pirkis, J., Snowdon, J., Lautenschlager, N. T., Wilson, I., & Almeida, O. P. (2008). Long-term effects of childhood abuse on the quality of life and health of older people: Results from the Depression and Early Prevention of Suicide in General Practice Project. *J Am Geriatr Soc, 56*(2), 262–71.

Evans, G. W., & Schamberg, M. A. (2009). "Childhood poverty, chronic stress, and adult working memory. *Proc Natl Acad Sci U S A, 106*(16), 6545–49.

Felitti, V. J., Vincent, J., Anda, M. D., Robert, F., Nordenberg, M. D., Williamson, M. S., . . . & James, S. (1998). Relationship of childhood abuse and household dysfunction to many of the leading causes of death in adults. The Adverse Childhood Experiences (ACE) study. *Am J Prev Med, 14*(4), 245–58.

Finkelhor, D., Ormrod, R. K., & Turner, H. A. (2007). Re-victimization patterns in a national longitudinal sample of children and youth. *Child Abuse Negl, 31*(5), 479–502.

Gerritsen, L., Geerlings, M. I., Beekman, A. T. F., Deeg, D. J. H., Penninx, B. W. J. H., & Comijs, H. C. (2010). Early and late life events and salivary cortisol in older persons. *Psychol Med, 40*(9), 1569–78.

Gershon, A., Minor, K., & Hayward, C. (2008). Gender, victimization, and psychiatric outcomes. *Psychol Med, 38*(10), 1377–91.

Gershon, A., Sudheimer, K., Tirouvanziam, R., Williams, L. M., & O'Hara, R. (2013). The long-term impact of early adversity on late-life psychiatric disorders. *Curr Psychiatry Rep, 15*(4), 352.

Gillespie, N. A., Whitfield, J. B., Williams, B. E. N., Heath, A. C., & Martin, N. G. (2005). The relationship between stressful life events, the serotonin transporter (5-HTTLPR) genotype, and major depression. *Psychol Med, 35*(1), 101–11.

Gorey, K. M., & Leslie, D. R. (1997). The prevalence of child sexual abuse: Integrative review adjustment for potential response and measurement biases. *Child Abuse Negl, 21*(4), 391–98.

Gouin, J. P., Glaser, R., Malarkey, W. B., Beversdorf, D., & Kiecolt-Glaser, J. K. (2012). Childhood abuse and inflammatory responses to daily stressors. *Ann Behav Med, 44*(2), 287–92.

Graham, J. E., Christian, L. M., & Kiecolt-Glaser, J. K. (2006). Stress, age, and immune function: Toward a lifespan approach. *J Behav Med, 29*(4), 389–400.

Green, J. G., McLaughlin, K. A., Berglund, P. A., Gruber, M. J., Sampson, N. A., Zaslavsky, A. M., & Kessler, R. C. (2010). Childhood adversities and adult psychiatric disorders in the national comorbidity survey replication I: Associations with first onset of DSM-IV disorders. *Arch Gen Psychiatry, 67*(2), 113–23.

Grinspoon, L., & Bakalar, J. B. (1998). The use of cannabis as a mood stabilizer in bipolar disorder: Anecdotal evidence and the need for clinical research. *J Psychoactive Drugs, 30*(2), 171–77.

Groer, M. W., & Morgan, K. (2007). Immune, health, and endocrine characteristics of depressed postpartum mothers. *Psychoneuroendocrinology, 32*(2), 133–39.

Grossman, R., Yehuda, R., Golier, J., McEwen, B., Harvey, P., & Maria, N. S. (2006). Cognitive effects of intravenous hydrocortisone in subjects with PTSD and healthy control subjects. *Ann N Y Acad Sci, 1071*, 410–21.

Gunnar, M., & Quevedo, K. (2007). The neurobiology of stress and development. *Annu Rev Psychol, 58*, 145–73.

Hazel, N. A., Hammen, C., Brennan, P. A., & Najman, J. (2008). Early childhood adversity and adolescent depression: The mediating role of continued stress. *Psychol Med, 38*(4), 581–89.

Heim, C., Newport, D. J., Bonsall, R., Miller, A. H., & Nemeroff, C. B. (2001). Altered pituitary-adrenal axis responses to provocative challenge tests in adult survivors of childhood abuse. *Am J Psychiatry, 158*(4), 575–81.

Heim, C., Newport, D. J., Heit, S., Graham, Y. P., Wilcox, M., Bonsall, R., . . . & Nemeroff, C. B. (2000). Pituitary-adrenal and autonomic responses to stress in women after sexual and physical abuse in childhood. *JAMA, 284*(5), 592–97.

Kaplow, J. B., Dodge, K. A., Amaya-Jackson, L., & Saxe, G. N. (2005). Pathways to PTSD, part II: Sexually abused children. *Am J Psychiatry, 162*(7), 1305–10.

Kaplow, J. B., & Widom, C. S. (2007). Age of onset of child maltreatment predicts long-term mental health outcomes. *J Abnorm Psychol, 116*(1), 176–87.

Karst, H., Nair, S., Velzing, E., Rumpff-van Essen, L., Slagter, E., Shinnick-Gallagher, P., & Joëls, M. (2002). Glucocorticoids alter calcium conductances and calcium channel subunit expression in basolateral amygdala neurons. *Eur J Neurosci, 16*(6), 1083–89.

Kaufman, J., Plotsky, P. M., Nemeroff, C. B., & Charney, D. S. (2000). Effects of early adverse experiences on brain structure and function: Clinical implications. *Biol Psychiatry, 48*(8), 778–90.

Kendler, K. S., Bulik, C. M., Silberg, J., Hettema, J. M., Myers, J., & Prescott, C. (2000). Childhood sexual abuse and adult psychiatric and substance use disorders in women: An epidemiological and cotwin control analysis. *Arch Gen Psychiatry, 57*(10), 953–59.

Kendler, K. S., Gardner, C. O., & Prescott, C. A. (2002). Toward a comprehensive developmental model for major depression in women. *Am J Psychiatry, 159*(7), 1133–45.

Kendler, K. S., Gardner, C. O., & Prescott, C. A. (2006). Toward a comprehensive developmental model for major depression in men. *Am J Psychiatry, 163*(1), 115–24.

Kessler, R. C., Davis, C. G., & Kendler, K. S. (1997). Childhood adversity and adult psychiatric disorder in the U.S. National Comorbidity Survey. *Psychol Med, 27*(5), 1101–19.

Kessler, R. C., & Magee, W. J. (1994). Childhood family violence and adult recurrent depression. *J Health Soc Behav, 35*(1), 13–27.

Kessler, R. C., McLaughlin, K. A., Green, J. G., Gruber, M. J., Sampson, N. A., Zaslavsky, A. M., . . . & Williams, D. R. (2010). Childhood adversities and adult psychopathology in the WHO World Mental Health Surveys. *Br J Psychiatry, 197*(5), 378–85.

Kiecolt-Glaser, J. K., Gouin, J. P., Weng, N. P., Malarkey, W. B., Beversdorf, D. Q., & Glaser, R. (2011). Childhood adversity heightens the impact of later-life caregiving stress on telomere length and inflammation. *Psychosom Med, 73*(1), 16–22.

Kivela, S. L., Luukinen, H., Koski, K., Viramo, P., & Pahkala, K. (1998). Early loss of mother or father predicts depression in old age. *Int J Geriatr Psychiatry, 13*(8), 527–30.

Langley-Evans, S. C., & McMullen, S. (2010). Developmental origins of adult disease. *Med Princ Pract, 19*(2), 87–98.

Lavretsky, H. (2012). Resilience, stress, and late life mood disorders. *Annu Rev Gerontol Geriatr, 32*, 49–72.

MacMillan, H. L., Fleming, J. E., Streiner, D. L., Lin, E., Boyle, M. H., Jamieson, E., . . . & Beardslee, W. R. (2001). Childhood abuse and lifetime psychopathology in a community sample. *Am J Psychiatry, 158*(11), 1878–83.

MacMillan, H. L., Fleming, J. E., Trocme, N., Boyle, M. H., Wong, M., Racine, Y. A., . . . & Offord, D. (1997). Prevalence of child physical and sexual abuse in the community: Results from the Ontario Health Supplement. *JAMA, 278*(2), 131–35.

Macphee, A. G., Divol, L., Kemp, A. J., Akli, K. U., Beg, F. N., Chen, C. D., . . . & Wilks, S. C. (2010). Limitation on prepulse level for cone-guided fast-ignition inertial confinement fusion. *Phys Rev Lett, 104*(5), 055002.

McLaughlin, K. A., Green, J. G., Gruber, M. J., Sampson, N. A., Zaslavsky, A. M., & Kessler, R. C. (2010). Childhood adversities and adult psychiatric disorders in the National Comorbidity Survey Replication II: Associations with persistence of DSM-IV disorders. *Arch Gen Psychiatry, 67*(2), 124–32.

McLeod, J. D. (1991). Childhood parental loss and adult depression. *J Health Soc Behav, 32*(3), 205–20.

Merlot, E., Couret, D., & Otten, W. (2008). Prenatal stress, fetal imprinting, and immunity. *Brain Behav Immun, 22*(1), 42–51.

Miller, G. E., Chen, E., Fok, A. K., Walker, H., Lim, A., Nicholls, E. F., . . . & Kobor, M. S. (2009). Low early-life social class leaves a biological residue manifested by decreased glucocorticoid and increased proinflammatory signaling. *Proc Natl Acad Sci U S A, 106*(34), 14716–21.

Miller, G. E., Chen, E., & Parker, K. J. (2011). Psychological stress in childhood and susceptibility to the chronic diseases of aging: Moving toward a model of behavioral and biological mechanisms. *Psychol Bull, 137*(6), 959–97.

Mitra, R., & Sapolsky, R. M. (2010). Gene therapy in rodent amygdala against fear disorders. *Expert Opin Biol Ther, 10*(9), 1289–303.

Molnar, B. E., Buka, S. L., & Kessler, R. C. (2001). Child sexual abuse and subsequent psychopathology: Results from the National Comorbidity Survey. *Am J Public Health, 91*(5), 753–60.

Nelson, E. C., Heath, A. C., Madden, P. A., Cooper, M. L., Dinwiddie, S. H., Bucholz, K. K., . . . & Martin, N. G. (2002). Association between self-reported childhood sexual abuse and adverse psychosocial outcomes: Results from a twin study. *Arch Gen Psychiatry, 59*(2), 139–45.

O'Hara, R., Schröder, C. M., Mahadevan, R., Schatzberg, A. F., Lindley, S., Fox, S., . . . & Hallmayer, J. F. (2007). Serotonin transporter polymorphism, memory, and hippocampal volume in the elderly: Association and interaction with cortisol. *Mol Psychiatry, 12*(6), 544–55.

Ozbay, F., Fitterling, H., Charney, D., & Southwick, S. (2008). Social support and resilience to stress across the life span: A neurobiologic framework. *Curr Psychiatry Rep, 10*(4), 304–10.

Pace, T. W., Mletzko, T., Alagbe, O., Musselman, D., Nemeroff, C., Miller, A., & Heim, C. (2006). Increased stress-induced inflammatory responses in male patients with major depression and increased early life stress. *Am J Psychiatry, 163*(9), 1630–33.

Risch, N., Herrell, R., Lehner, T., Liang, K. Y., Eaves, L., Hoh, J., . . . & Merikangas, K. R. (2009). Interaction between the serotonin transporter gene

(5-HTTLPR), stressful life events, and risk of depression: A meta-analysis. *JAMA, 301*(23), 2462–71.

Rudolph, K. D., & Flynn, M. (2007). Childhood adversity and youth depression: Influence of gender and pubertal status. *Dev Psychopathol, 19*(2), 497–521.

Rutter, M. (2006). Implications of resilience concepts for scientific understanding. *Ann N Y Acad Sci, 1094*, 1–12.

Schoedl, A. F., Costa, M. C. P., Mari, J. J., Mello, M. F., Tyrka, A. R., Carpenter, L. L., & Price, L. H. (2010). The clinical correlates of reported childhood sexual abuse: An association between age at trauma onset and severity of depression and PTSD in adults. *J Child Sex Abus, 19*(2), 156–70.

Stein, M. B., Yehuda, R., Koverola, C., & Hanna, C. (1997). Enhanced dexamethasone suppression of plasma cortisol in adult women traumatized by childhood sexual abuse. *Biol Psychiatry, 42*(8), 680–86.

Steinmetz, K. R., Muscatell, K. A., & Kensinger, E. A. (2010). The effect of valence on young and older adults' attention in a rapid serial visual presentation task. *Psychol Aging, 25*(1), 239–45.

Sudheimer, K., Flournoy, J., Gershon, A., Demuth, B., Schatzberg, A., & O'Hara, R. (2013). HPA axis and late-life depression. In H. Lavretsky, M. Sajatovic, & C. F. Reynolds (Eds.), *Late-life mood disorders.* New York: Oxford University Press.

Thompson, W. K., Hallmayer, J., & O'Hara, R. (2011). Design considerations for characterizing psychiatric trajectories across the lifespan: Application to effects of APOE-epsilon4 on cerebral cortical thickness in Alzheimer's disease. *Am J Psychiatry, 168*(9), 894–903.

Widom, C. S. (1999). Posttraumatic stress disorder in abused and neglected children grown up. *Am J Psychiatry, 156*(8), 1223–29.

Wilson, R. S., Krueger, K. R., Arnold, S. E., Barnes, L. L., de Leon, C. F. M., Bienias, J. L., & Bennett, D. A. (2006). Childhood adversity and psychosocial adjustment in old age. *Am J Geriatr Psychiatry, 14*(4), 307–15.

Wise, L. A., Zierler, S., Krieger, N., & Harlow, B. L. (2001). Adult onset of major depressive disorder in relation to early life violent victimisation: A case-control study. *Lancet, 358*(9285), 881–87.

Yehuda, R., Golier, J. A., Halligan, S. L., & Harvey, P. D. (2004). Learning and memory in Holocaust survivors with posttraumatic stress disorder. *Biol Psychiatry, 55*(3), 291–95.

Yehuda, R., Golier, J. A., & Kaufman, S. (2005). Circadian rhythm of salivary cortisol in Holocaust survivors with and without PTSD. *Am J Psychiatry, 162*(5), 998–1000.

Yehuda, R., Tischler, L., Golier, J. A., Grossman, R., Brand, S. R., Kaufman, S., & Harvey, P. D. (2006). Longitudinal assessment of cognitive performance in Holocaust survivors with and without PTSD. *Biol Psychiatry, 60*(7), 714–21.

CHAPTER 6

Common Stressors of Old Age
and Their Effect on Resilience

THROUGHOUT THEIR LIVES, all people are destined to experience adversities that have the potential to affect their health and quality of life. However, the effects of adversity on health and function in later life can vary significantly depending on the individual. Typical adversities experienced in the context of aging include chronic illnesses, cognitive impairment, the psychosocial stress of caregiving, grief or bereavement, and personal losses of independence and financial security. Although some individuals succumb to depression and early death as a result of such adversities, others continue to lead lives of personal fulfillment despite these challenges. These individuals' protective factors lead to successful aging, even in the face of the conditions that increase the risk of disease and mortality.

The common psychological mechanisms that underlie coping with many stressors in the end of life can be affected by loss or crisis of attachment in significant relationships. Although John Bowlby conceptualized attachment theory as applicable across the life span, researchers have been relatively slow to examine attachment phenomena specifically among older adults. Three common areas of focus emerge: (1) the role of attachment bonds in caregiving and chronic illness; (2) the influence of attachment in coping with bereavement and loss; and (3) the relationship of attachment to adjustment and well-being in old age (Fricchione 2011). Bowlby believed that "reorganization" of one's working models was necessary for successful adaptation to the loss of an attachment. To the extent that individuals possessed insecure (i.e., rigid and defensive) models of attachment, such "grief work" was unlikely to occur, leading to maladaptive or pathological bereavement (Bradley & Cafferty 2001).

Can we reverse negative outcomes of exposure to adversity by boosting individual resilience? Is it possible to estimate rates of resilience in the population of older adults? Or can resilience only be appreciated in a context of one individual? Clearly, the answer is far from simple. In addition to the nature of stressors and their potential impact on an individual's future, a host of genetic, family, social, and cultural elements influence individual differences in resilience. However, the rate of depression in at-risk populations serves as a tentative estimate of the incidence of individuals who experience reduced psychological resilience. Models of chronic exposure to stress as a forerunner of mental illness in older adults have been studied in several populations, including the chronically medically ill, those with spousal bereavement, and family dementia caregivers. This evidence supports the stress-health relationships associated with stress, coping, and mental illnesses.

Resilience in Chronic Illness

With the benefit of contemporary advances in treating chronic illnesses related to increasing age spans, resilient individuals are more likely to recover and adapt after illnesses such as heart disease and cancer. The rate of depression in victims of stroke, heart disease, and certain cancers can approach 40–50%; this provides an estimate of the proportion of individuals with reduced psychological resilience.

Friedman and Booth-Kewey (1987) analyzed the health outcomes of the disease-prone personality, in which negative emotions (depression and anxiety) were associated with an increased risk of chronic disease. Increasing evidence suggests that neuroticism predicts increased distress and disease. However, it is unclear whether positive traits such as optimism predict a lack of disease or, rather, reflect a more positive perception of health status. The World Health Organization (2002) defined health as a general sense of well-being, accompanied by physical well-being, mental, social, and functional improvement. Thus, health is more than achieving a singular outcome; it involves a process of challenge, negotiation, and adaptation that unfolds over the course of life. Together, healthy aging and longevity can serve as markers of personal resilience, whereas rates of mortality and morbidity (e.g., rates of depression associated with physical illness) can serve as proxies for deriving estimates of less resilient individuals. Kern and Friedman (2010) describe personality features, such as conscientiousness, that relate to greater productivity, good physical health, and longevity, which also involve better health habits, involvement in life, and better relationships.

Therefore, in the context of adaptation to chronic illness, resilience involves flexibility and adaptability to stress rather than just hardiness or the absence of disease. Further, psychological and physical resilience are not necessarily separate entities; instead, they are two sides of the same coin. Temperamental predisposition, internal stress and coping, social relationships, and health behaviors may all be relevant in predicting whether an individual will thrive in the face of challenge or succumb to depression and disease.

Resilience in Bereavement

Another common stressor in older adults is bereavement. According to the U.S. Census Bureau, in 2003 approximately 14% of men and 45% of women 65 years and older were widowed. Among those age 85 and older, this increased to 43% of men and 80% of women. About 33% of surviving older-adult spouses experience a "complicated bereavement," placing them at significant risk for major depression, high morbidity, and mortality (Fry & Debats 2010). Previous research has identified psychosocial resources that serve as protections against stress and promote health, well-being, and resilience. A good example is community or familial support that involves affect-type ties and social engagement.

Additional factors that positively influence morbidity and mortality are beliefs in self-efficacy, self-control, and self-esteem. Moreover, spirituality and religious beliefs can compensate for a lack of close relationships following trauma and loss (Granqvist & Hagekull 2000) and can protect against early mortality and morbidity. The association of psychosocial resources—such as spiritual development, family stability, social engagement, and commitment to life tasks—with increased longevity may represent important resource domains, and these may contribute significantly to a surviving spouse's resilience and healthy longevity by assisting with psychological adjustment following his or her loss. It is plausible that a life span may be lengthened when a person possesses personal and psychosocial resources like the ones just mentioned. Thus, it may be that those with more psychosocial resource networks are better protected against early mortality. Intervention programs for older surviving spouses can concentrate on coping with grief and mobilizing psychosocial resources to promote resilience and preserve longevity.

Resilience in Death and Dying: Is There a "Good Death"?

End-of-life care for older adults frequently presents challenges because the pervasive suffering of those who die from incurable illnesses is often characterized by profound psychosocial and spiritual crises that may manifest as depression, heightened anxiety, and hopelessness (Grassi, Malacarne, Maestri, & Ramelli 1997; Hopwood & Stephens 2000; Loge, Abrahamsen, Ekeberg, & Kaasa 2000; Mraz & Runco 1994; Pollock & Williams 1998). Terminal care, as it is conceived and practiced, emerged as a visible social issue in the final quarter of the last century. For the majority of Western-trained providers in healthcare settings, the suffering and pain of dying older adults drives a problem-focused approach to death and dying. Elisabeth Kübler-Ross's (1969) development of a stage theory about people's adjustment to dying, described in her renowned book *On Death and Dying*, made a great contribution and raised awareness about this issue. Her theory laid the groundwork for the idea that human development and insight can grow as people work through difficult feelings and situational challenges associated with dying, although several studies have since indicated that the details of her stage theory were not supported by empirical evidence.

Despite the benefits of medical approaches to life prolongation and symptom relief, addressing psychosocial and spiritual care at the end of life solely from a medical point of view limits the potential for helping. The limitation is due to the traditional focus on human shortcomings instead of on trying to discover what people can achieve. Recently, researchers in gerontology have begun to coalesce around the need to adopt a more holistic conceptual framework (Sulmasy 2002). This interest expands the current prevailing negative conceptualization of aging, death, and dying that is centered on coping and adapting to losses and grief in old age.

This recent research synthesizes emerging trends in terminal care and gerontology that view human beings as capable of more than coping and adaptation. In death and dying studies, some writers have found that people can find profound support in spirituality to heal and grow during serious and terminal illnesses (Canda & Furman 1999; Reese 2001; Smith 1995, 2001; Wilber 1991). To advance the cause of optimal aging, some gerontologists have moved away from a stance of pathology and prevention through the development of enhancement research (Mackenzie, Rajagopal, Meibohm, & Lavizzo-Mourey 2000; Miller 1991; Ryff & Essex 1992; Ryff & Singer 1996; Seeman, McEwen, Rowe, & Singer 2001; Wong & Watt 1991). These scholars and clinicians honor people's resiliency and urge us embrace a more affirming and hopeful notion of dying in old age. This stance represents a major shift in intensity, away from the current paradigm that is preoccupied with deficits and pathology.

Nakashima and Canda (2005) reported that resilient older adults in a hospice setting did not deny or unrealistically portray their suffering or dying. They experienced many losses and grief issues of differing natures and magnitudes, suggesting that good quality of life at the end of life is not necessarily dependent on the absence of problems. Individual resilience co-existed with the ability to proactively approach death and the dying process. A close association was found between a high level of quality of life in the psychosocial and spiritual dimensions and personal growth and healing. Preparation for such a positive end-of-life experience cannot be accomplished without fostering resilience factors over the years.

Among the barriers to better coping with death and dying include a lack of resources for care, conflicts in relationships, long-standing mental illnesses, and similar stumbling blocks. In contrast, protective factors in facing mortality include an open awareness of the universality of death and an affirmative outlook on dying. Such positive qualities are often attained through personal experiences with death and dying, as well as through spiritual beliefs (Nakashima & Canda 2005).

Resilience in Caregiver Stress and Depression

Studies of caregiver stress have supported the dominant view of the diathesis stress model emphasizing stress-induced mental illness, particularly in the presence of a neurobiological or genetic vulnerability. Stressful life events are robust predictors of the onset or recurrence of a variety of neuropsychiatric disorders. Different types of stress—acute stress, chronic stress, early childhood trauma—may differentially influence the type and severity of a neurocognitive or neuropsychiatric disorder. A disorder may develop with age, or the stress may increase the risk of developing comorbid medical and psychiatric conditions.

The relationship of adverse experiences to the onset of illnesses in special populations (e.g., caregivers) has provided epidemiological estimates of the rates of subsequent psychiatric disorders following exposure to stress. In the case of family dementia caregivers, the prevalence and incidence of depression are estimated to be 50%, which means that at any given time, 50% of dementia caregivers can be diagnosed with clinical depression but another 50% are not depressed (Lavretsky 2005). Both acute and chronic stressors increase the risk that older adults will experience depression, declining resilience, and compromised quality of life.

Stress among family caregivers taking care of their relatives with dementia has been a recognized chronic-stress model resulting in high levels of depression, anxiety, and mortality (Lavretsky 2005). The majority of dementia caregivers are elderly women. These caregivers are twice as likely to report physical strain and high levels of emotional stress as a direct result of their caregiving responsibilities. Caregiver burden and depression are related to the severity of the patient's dementia, disability, and behavioral disturbances. As a result of impaired resilience to stress with advancing age, an increased allostatic load and reduced tolerance to stress may result in cardiovascular disease and declines in health and quality of life. In a longitudinal cohort study of 400 older spousal caregivers, caregivers who experienced mental or emotional strain related to caregiving had mortality risks 63% higher than noncaregiving controls (Lavretsky 2005).

Pinquart and Sorensen (2006) integrated findings from 84 articles on differences between caregivers and noncaregivers on perceived stress, depression, self-efficacy, general subjective well-being, and physical health. The largest differences were found with regard to the first four of these, whereas differences in the levels of physical health in favor of noncaregivers were statistically significant but relatively small. However, larger differences were found between dementia caregivers and noncaregivers than between heterogeneous samples of caregivers and noncaregivers.

Bereavement can further fuel caregiver depression. Aneshensel, Botticello, and Yamamoto-Mitani (2004) describe trajectories of evolving depressive symptoms among caregivers following bereavement. Aneshensel, Pearlin, and Schuler (1993) connect these trajectories to earlier features of caregiving using life-course and stress-process theory in a six-wave longitudinal survey of spouses and adult children caring for patients with Alzheimer's disease. Of the four trajectories identified, three represent stable symptom levels over time, with two-thirds of the surveyed caregivers being repeatedly symptomatic (medium symptom levels), compared to two smaller groups of repeatedly asymptomatic (effectively absent of symptoms) and repeatedly distressed (severe symptoms) caregivers. According to the findings, caregivers with few symptoms before bereavement tended to maintain these states afterward, but emotionally distressed caregivers tended to become more distressed. Role overload before bereavement substantially increased the odds of following an unfavorable trajectory afterward, whereas self-esteem and socioemotional support played protective roles. These findings suggest that an intervention during caregiving may facilitate more positive adaptation following the death of a loved one.

The nature of psychiatric symptoms that develop as a result of stress exposure most often depends on the individual predisposition, severity and nature of stressors, and duration of exposure. However, knowledge concerning the temporal relationship between adverse experiences and the onset of anxiety and depressive disorders remains sparse despite the awareness that life stress forms a pivotal component to social, neurological, and cognitive scientific models of their etiology. Analyses show clear evidence of progressive decay in the adverse effects of life events over time. The time until recovery depends on other vulnerability and resilience factors, such as coping and personality styles, prior history of depression, and anxiety (Surtees & Wainwright 1999). Developing preventive interventions for mood and anxiety disorders in these high-risk groups should take into account relevant vulnerability and resilience factors in developing interventions that would boost their resilience to stress.

Major and Nonmajor Depression: A Continuum of Vulnerability

Older adults commonly experience depressive disorders in the form of major and minor depression, as well as transient depressive reactions to stress. Despite a lower severity of depressive symptoms, from a population perspective the overall burden is greater for those with minor depression than it is for those with major depression. Although minor depression represents a time-limited condition in some people, others experience it on a continuum toward more severe and persistent states. However, individuals with minor depression may become "at risk" for chronic or major depression, particularly around adverse life events such as bereavement or caregiving.

In the absence of intervention studies, clinicians are limited in the availability of guidelines to support their decisions about using antidepressants rather than psychosocial treatments, or using "watchful waiting" strategies in the treatment of minor depression. Age-appropriate psychotherapeutic approaches (e.g., cognitive-behavioral, interpersonal, or problem-solving) involving major and nonmajor types of depression have been developed since the early 2000s. In clinical practice, antidepressants are being prescribed for patients with significant levels of depression and functional impairment regardless of the *Diagnostic and Statistical Manual of Mental Disorders* (DSM) categorical diagnosis. For individuals with major or nonmajor depression, the question of predicting who is more likely to require active psychotherapeutic or pharmacological intervention is especially important.

In our recent studies involving caregiver depression, my colleagues and I established both that antidepressant drugs can be helpful in building resilience to stress and depression and that yoga and meditation can reduce caregiver burden and improve coping. Accordingly, psychotherapeutic and mind-body approaches (e.g., meditation, yoga, tai chi) can be tried prior to instituting pharmacological therapies (Lavretsky et al. 2011). It would be beneficial to develop preventive interventions for high-risk groups based on the available empirical knowledge of these and other protective factors (e.g., increased social support, resilience training, and so on).

Optimism as a Protective Factor in Late Life

As mentioned in chapter 2, research now supports the long-held folk belief that positive emotions are good for health. Robust evidence demonstrates that the stress process includes positive and negative emotions (Edwards & Cooper 1988). Previously, a revision of stress and coping theory incorporated these positive aspects of stress. "Coping" can be defined as efforts to prevent or reduce the negative impact of stress on individual well-being (Edwards & Cooper 1988). The paradigm offered by the broaden-and-build theory of positive emotions outlines the part positive emotions can play in coping and in related psychological and physical well-being, even during stressful times. Lazarus, Kanner, and Folkam (1980) long ago described hope and optimism as contributors to overall successful coping. Now we are also finding that successful aging is associated with a positive psychological outlook in later years, along with general well-being and happiness (Depp & Jeste 2006; Peel, McClure, & Bartlett 2005; Vaillant 2002).

So we see that the drive to seek personal happiness and fulfillment is inherent regardless of age (Lazarus et al. 1980). With populations aging globally, many nations are developing and implementing healthy aging policies designed to promote *quality* of life in addition to extending the number of years of health (Peel et al. 2005). One such approach is to implement interventions that boost resilience to stress in older adults.

A recognizable pattern has emerged of individual characteristics associated with resilience and successful adaptation. Salient characteristics include commitment, dynamism, humor in the face of adversity, patience, optimism, faith, and altruism (Lavretsky & Irwin 2007). Certain emotional and cognitive aspects of resilience are innate or can be learned. The innate affective or emotional styles of an individual that are likely to influence resilience refer to styles of affect regulation, which are usually a part of personality structure (e.g., optimism, pessimism, social intelligence). Protective factors relating to an individual's temperament include sociability, intelligence, social competence, internal locus of control, warmth and closeness of emotional ties, and active emotional support within the family network or within religious groups. As such, resilience may represent an important target of treatment and prevention for anxiety, depression, and abnormal stress reactions in aging. The question remains whether or not resilience can be taught to older individuals coping with daily stress to boost their coping response to stress and life's adversities.

Resilient Outcomes and Preventive Interventions

What would be the outcome of developing preventive interventions in the earlier-discussed specific stressful situations? For those still free of chronic disease, the continued absence (i.e., prevention) of any disease should be considered an ideal outcome in the general population, as well as in the at-risk population (e.g., caregivers at risk for depression). In populations with established disease, an example of a resilient outcome would be successful coping with the disease. Of course, it is impossible to prevent death and dying in the elderly, as these represent a universal phase of the life cycle. Therefore, the emphasis in older-age populations, especially in hospice and palliative care settings, should be on developing successful coping and resilience. In particular, hospice and palliative care settings could involve spiritual care, life review, and acceptance as therapeutic approaches. Some of these interventions may cause tension in the defiance-surrender attitudes toward death by creating meaningful narratives of living and dying (Nakashima & Canda 2005). Finally, secondary and tertiary preventive interventions in those with mood disorders should focus on preventing relapses and recurrences of mood disorders.

Prevention of late-life depression affects the entire population of older people. Public awareness campaigns have been launched in many countries. Cuijpers (2003) has asserted that even in a disorder like depression, which has quite a high incidence, studies testing the effects of universal prevention are unlikely to be feasible. One way to prepare the public would be to mount educational campaigns to teach that depression is a disorder that can be successfully treated and, if left untreated, can lead to chronic mental and medical illness and premature mortality. Given the rapid technological advances and widespread access to electronic media among older people, "e-health" preventive interventions for older people are being developed. These may shift action toward much more widespread prevention. While it is feasible to launch universal preventive programs aiming to prevent depression, current methods of research do not allow rigorous testing of their effects.

An interesting example of public health significance of building public resilience is the global need to cope with climate change and extreme weather events, including heat waves, drought, wildfire, cyclones, and heavy precipitation that could cause floods and landslides. Such events create significant public health needs that can exceed local and individual capacity to respond, resulting in excess morbidity or mortality and in the declaration of disasters. Human vulnerability to any disaster is a complex phenomenon with social, economic, health, and cultural dimensions. Enhancing individual capacity to cope with or recover from disaster consequences has become an obvious imperative for local governments and healthcare providers. Vulnerability reduction programs reduce susceptibility and increase resilience. Susceptibility to disasters is reduced largely by prevention and mitigation of emergencies. Emergency preparedness and response and recovery activities—including those that address climate change—increase disaster resilience. Because adaptation must occur at the community level, local public health agencies are uniquely placed to build human resilience to climate-related disasters (Keim 2008), and the use of social media can facilitate this process (Keim & Noji 2011).

Conclusion

I have reviewed the common stressors of later life that typically test individual vulnerability and resilience and may lead to depression or disability. Examples of high risk groups are older people with chronic disease, those who have lost spouses, caregivers, and those who have a prior history of depression. Selective prevention aims to reach older people who are exposed to known risk factors for depression. Several tested interventions are available. They usually involve identifying those at risk and engaging them in the intervention. However, engaging older people who are currently not depressed in an intervention is not easy. Prevention on the societal level would involve education of the general population about mental health and risks for illness. Some helpful preventive interventions in cases of natural disasters or mass-traumatic experiences would resemble self-help versions of cognitive therapy, interpersonal therapy, reminiscence, and problem-solving. Often these are modified to cater to people exposed to specific risk factors and circumstances. Other intervention components involve engaging in pleasant activities, physical activity, and using nutritional supplements. Although these do not target resilience itself, the prevention of disease is an important example of a resilient outcome. Future research should include measures of psychological and cognitive resilience in older adults along with other lifestyle factors subject to examination.

Clinical Case

Mrs. A. first came to see me following the suicide of her eldest son, an aspiring jazz musician who killed himself at the age of 45. She was 84 years old and also dealing with losing her vision to macular degeneration, increasing arthritis, and becoming more dependent on her husband of 50 years. She was legally blind and attended Braille Institute in Los Angeles. She was depressed and grieving her loss, and she contemplated whether to keep her son's musical instruments because they reminded her so much of him.

Over the course of the following year, she responded nicely to a low-dose antidepressant and bereavement counseling. Some closure to her grief occurred during a jazz concert in her son's memory that his friends put together at a New York jazz club. It gave her some solace to know that his presence was cherished by so many. She decided to donate his musical instruments to his alma mater school of music. At the same time, she found more relief in her own creative endeavors, which included gardening and, of all things, silk painting. To my surprise, this almost blind woman was able to create the most colorful and poetic silk scarfs and paintings. She either exhibited them, including at the Braille Institute, or sold them online or gave them to friends. Although the lines of the drawings were not well defined, the colors of her creations were vibrant and alive.

She overcame the worst within two years of counseling and treatment, and tapered off her antidepressant. She continued to draw pleasure from her paintings, despite her increasing vision loss, and from gardening, limited by her worsening arthritis. I always admired her gentle, sensitive, but resilient soul that refused to succumb to any of the challenges and was constantly beating the odds. Her spirituality also played a role in her recovery; she received some counseling from her rabbi and used Bible reading as a tool to maintain balance in life by maintaining gratitude for what she had been given. Her example was truly inspiring, and I frequently use it in lecturing about resilience.

. . .

References

Aneshensel, C. S., Botticello, A. L., Yamamoto-Mitani, N. (2004) When caregiving ends: The course of depressive symptoms after bereavement. *J Health Soc Behav*, 45(4), 422–40.

Aneshensel, C. S., Pearlin, L. I., & Schuler, R. H. (1993). Stress, role captivity, and the cessation of caregiving. *J Health Soc Behav, 34*(1), 54–70.

Bradley, J. M., & Cafferty, T. P. (2001). Attachment among older adults: Current issues and directions for future research. *Attach Hum Dev, 3*(2), 200–221.

Canda, E. R., & Furman, L. D. (1999). *Spiritual diversity in social work practice: The heart of helping.* New York: Free Press.

Cuijpers, P. (2003). Examining the effects of prevention programs on the incidence of new cases of mental disorders: the lack of statistical power. *Am J Psychiatry, 160*(8), 1385–91.

Depp, C. A., & Jeste, D. V. (2006). Definitions and predictors of successful aging: A comprehensive review of larger quantitative studies. *Am J Geriatr Psychiatry, 14*(1), 6–20.

Edwards, J. R., & Cooper, C. L. (1988). The impacts of positive psychological states on physical health: A review and theoretical framework. *Soc Sci Med, 27*(12), 1447–59.

Fricchione, G. L. (2011). *Compassion and healing in medicine and society: On the nature and use of attachment solutions to separation challenges.* Baltimore: John Hopkins University Press.

Friedman, H. S., & Booth-Kewley, S. (1987). The "disease-prone personality." A meta-analytic view of the construct. *Am Psychol, 42*(6), 539–55.

Fry, P. S., & Debats, D. L. (2010). Sources of human life strength, resilience, and health. In P. S. Fry & C. L. Keyes (Eds.), *New frontiers in resilient aging* (pp. 15–59). New York: Cambridge University Press.

Granqvist, P., & Hagekull, B. (2000). Religiosity, adult attachment, and "why singles are more religious." *Int J Psychol Relig, 10,* 111–23.

Grassi, L., Malacarne, P., Maestri, A., & Ramelli, E. (1997). Depression, psychosocial variables, and occurrence of life events among patients with cancer. *J Affect Disord, 44*(1), 21–30.

Hopwood, P., & Stephens, R. J. (2000). Depression in patients with lung cancer: Prevalence and risk factors derived from quality-of-life data. *J Clin Oncol, 18*(4), 893–903.

Keim, M. E. (2008). Building human resilience: The role of public health preparedness and response as an adaptation to climate change. *Am J Prev Med, 35*(5), 508–16.

Keim, M. E., & Noji, E. (2011). Emergent use of social media: A new age of opportunity for disaster resilience. *Am J Disaster Med, 6*(1), 47–54.

Kern, M. L., & Freidman, H. S. (2010). Why do some people thrive while others succumb to disease and stagnation? Personality, social relations, and resilience. In P. S. Fry & C. L. Keyes (Eds.), *New Frontiers in Resilient Aging* (pp. 162–84). New York: Cambridge University Press.

Kübler-Ross, E. (1969). *On death and dying.* New York: Macmillan.

Lavretsky, H. (2005). Stress and depression in informal dementia caregivers. *Health and Aging, 1*(1), 117–33.

Lavretsky, H., Alstein, L. L., Olmstead, R. E., Ercoli, L. M., Riparetti-Brown, M., St Cyr, N., & Irwin, M. R. (2011). Complementary use of tai chi chih augments escitalopram treatment of geriatric depression: A randomized controlled trial. *Am J Geriatr Psychiatry, 19*(10), 839–50.

Lavretsky, H., & Irwin, M. R. (2007). Resilience and aging. *Aging Health, 3*(3) 309–23.

Lazarus, R. S., Kanner, A. D., & Folkam, S. (1980). Emotions: A cognitive phenomenological analysis. In R. Plutchik and H. Kellerman (Eds.), *Emotion theory, research, and experience* (pp. 189–217). New York: Academic Press.

Loge, J. H., Abrahamsen, A. F., Ekeberg, & Kaasa, S. (2000). Fatigue and psychiatric morbidity among Hodgkin's disease survivors. *J Pain Symptom Manage, 19*(2), 91–99.

Mackenzie, E. R., Rajagopal, D. E., Meibohm, M., & Lavizzo-Mourey, R. (2000). Spiritual support and psychological well-being: Older adults' perceptions of the religion and health connection. *Altern Ther Health Med, 6*(6), 37–45.

Miller, M. P. (1991). Factors promoting wellness in the aged person: An ethnographic study. *ANS Adv Nurs Sci, 13*(4), 38–51.

Mraz, W., & Runco, M. A. (1994). Suicide ideation and creative problem solving. *Suicide Life Threat Behav, 24*(1), 38–47.

Nakashima, M., & Canda, E. R. (2005). Positive dying and resiliency in later life: A qualitative study. *J Aging Stud, 19*(1), 109–25.

Peel, N. M., McClure, R. J., & Bartlett, H. P. (2005). Behavioral determinants of healthy aging. *Am J Prev Med, 28*(3), 298–304.

Pinquart, M., & Sorensen, S. (2006). Helping caregivers of persons with dementia: Which interventions work and how large are their effects? *Int Psychogeriatr, 18*(4), 577–95.

Pollock, L. R., & Williams, J. M. (1998). Problem solving and suicidal behavior. *Suicide Life Threat Behav, 28*(4), 375–87.

Reese, D. J. (2001). Addressing spirituality in hospice: Current practices and a proposed role for transpersonal social work. *Journal of Religion & Spirituality in Social Work: Social Thought, 20*(1–2), 135–61. doi: 10.1080/15426432.2001.9960285

Ryff, C. D., & Essex, M. J. (1992). The interpretation of life experience and well-being: The sample case of relocation. *Psychol Aging, 7*(4), 507–17.

Ryff, C. D., & Singer, B. (1996). Psychological well-being: Meaning, measurement, and implications for psychotherapy research. *Psychother Psychosom, 65*(1), 14–23.

Seeman, T. E., McEwen, B. S., Rowe, J. W., & Singer, B. H. (2001). Allostatic load as a marker of cumulative biological risk: MacArthur studies of successful aging. *Proc Natl Acad Sci U S A, 98*(8), 4770–75.

Smith, E. D. (1995). Addressing the psychospiritual distress of death as reality: A transpersonal approach. *Soc Work, 40*(3), 402–13.

Smith, E. D. (2001). Alleviating suffering in the face of death. *Social Thought, 20*(1–2), 45–61. doi: 10.1300/J131v20n01_04.

Sulmasy, D. P. (2002). A biopsychosocial-spiritual model for the care of patients at the end of life. *Gerontologist, 42*(suppl 3), 24–33. doi: 10.1093/geront/42.suppl_3.24.

Surtees, P. G., & Wainwright, N. W. (1999). Surviving adversity: Event decay, vulnerability, and the onset of anxiety and depressive disorder. *Eur Arch Psychiatry Clin Neurosci, 249*(2), 86–95.

Vaillant, G. E. (2002). Aging well: Surprising guideposts to a happier life from the landmark Harvard study of adult development. Boston: Little, Brown.

Wilber, K. (1991). *Grace and grit.* Boston: Shambhala.

Wong, P. T., & Watt, L. M. (1991). What types of reminiscence are associated with successful aging? *Psychol Aging, 6*(2), 272–79.

World Health Organization (2002). The world health report 2002: Reducing risks, promoting healthy life. www.who.int/whr/2002.

CHAPTER 7

Spirituality and Aging

INTEREST IN SPIRITUALITY AND AGING has increased recently as empirical research has overwhelmingly demonstrated various health benefits attributable to spirituality and religious participation (Dalby 2006; Koenig, McCullough, & Larson 2001). Moreover, study results have shown that spirituality tends to increase during later adulthood (Koenig 1995; Moberg 1997, 2005). Interestingly, this trend of increased spiritual growth and religious activity in older age persists despite the significant secularization of society over the past 50 years. Spirituality is associated with positive relationships and measures of life satisfaction, psychosocial well-being, and physical and mental health, and it has a helping role in the quest for meaning and purpose in life (Moberg 2001). Understanding an individual's spiritual perspective becomes increasingly important for practitioners, given the loss, physical illness, disability, and mortality patients may confront in old age (Dalby 2006).

In this chapter I consider individual spirituality as a way of developing personalized, patient-centered healthcare according to societal priorities. I also present the trends toward spiritual development in older age in contemporary society and the existing evidence of close relationships between spirituality, mental and physical health, and successful aging. Finally, I provide an overview of research findings in the neurobiology of spirituality and the efficacy of spiritual interventions in aging adults.

Spirituality and Aging in Modern Society

The trend for increasing longevity in modern society moves the spiritual needs of older adults to the forefront of societal priorities. Yet Western society continues to struggle with anti-aging attitudes that tend to ignore the talents and creative contributions of older adults, as can be seen in a lack of opportunities for vocational retraining, employment, or community service. Additionally, retirement communities catering to older adults often emphasize physical or mental activities rather than spirituality (Moberg 2001).

Historically, the elders of a society functioned as transmitters of sacred knowledge and rituals. They established an awareness of the culture and its roots that is necessary for the health and growth of the community (Moberg 2001). With the growing population of older adults, the role of elders in society should now be expanded, in order to provide meaning to the lives of its aging citizens.

In the U.S. general population, religious participation has always been prominent, with over 90% of Americans believing in God or a higher power; 90% praying; 67%-75% praying daily; 69% holding membership in a church or a synagogue; 60% considering religion to be very important in their lives; and 82% acknowledging the need for spiritual growth (Gallup 1999; Gallup & Bezilla 1992; Miller & Thoresen 2003; Moberg 2001). Evidence from research suggests that patients want to be seen and treated as whole persons, not as disease states (Astrow, Puchalski, & Sulmasy 2001; Koenig, McCullough, & Larson 2001). Being a whole person implies having physical, emotional, social, and spiritual dimensions. Ignoring any of these aspects can interfere with healing (Koenig et al. 2001; Mohr 2006). In healthcare systems, more than 75% of patients want their physicians to integrate religion with their healthcare (Daaleman & Nease 1994; King & Bushwick 1994; Matthews & Clark 1998). Yet frequently, families and healthcare providers of older adults are ill-prepared to deal with incorporating spirituality into decisions affecting life and healthcare. According to surveyed physicians, lack of time, inadequate training, and discomfort in addressing spiritual topics are responsible for the relative inattention to a patient's spirituality (Armbruster Chibnall, & Legett 2003; Ellis, Vinson, & Ewigman 1999). However, overcoming barriers to proper assessment and understanding, as well as respecting an individual's spirituality, can help shape personalized medical care for older adults and improve health outcomes.

Maintaining a nonsectarian approach to research on spirituality is a thorny matter. Intensely heated religious preferences of various authors (Sapp 2010) polarize gerontological literature on spirituality, religiosity, and aging. Although the concept of spirituality—like that of resilience—is multifaceted and does not lend itself to easy definition, further progress in research mandates the use of stronger, nonambiguous definitions and measures that will unify research efforts and determine success (Moberg 2005). Atchley addresses this issue explicitly, asserting, "I avoid religious language as much as possible because I have found that, although it may be helpful for the in-group, it often activates a sense of intergroup division and difference" (Atchley 1997). Many would assert that finding common ground in pursuing knowledge about the benefits of spirituality outweighs the relatively minor differences among religious practices. The benefits of spiritual interventions for the field and within the population at large include easing psychological distress and fear of death, as well as reducing the stresses of caring for loved ones with chronic illnesses. As in all other domains of clinical research, spiritual interventions have limits and must be applied with caution for both technical and ethical reasons. As scientific knowledge of spirituality expands, so does awareness of the need for further research, including the refinement of methodological procedures, inclusion of new topics, and extension to international cultures and diverse religions (Moberg 2005).

Psychological and Gerontological Theories of Resurgence of Spirituality with Aging

Psychological and gerontological theorists have attempted to explain the increase in spiritual activities in later life from a range of perspectives. For example, socioemotional selectivity theory (Carstensen, Isaacowitz, & Charles 1999) proposes a greater emphasis on emotion-related goals as individuals become aware of the brevity of life. Jung (1959) proposed that increasing spiritual goals and pursuits accompanied by introspection from mid- to later life are a natural part of the maturational process. The disengagement theory (Cummings & Henry 1961) assumes that a societal benefit occurs when older adults withdraw from all roles and activities. Considered as a universal and inevitable process prior to death, this withdrawal prompts a mutually satisfying exchange in society when the youth begin to fill the void, taking on new roles as the older adults retire from them.

The Duke Longitudinal Study of Aging (Blazer & Palmore 1976) found that religious attitudes and satisfactions remain the same with aging, but the correlations with happiness, feelings of usefulness, and personal adjustment increase. Contrary to the disengagement theory, the activity theory emphasizes increased activities (e.g., volunteering) and taking more active roles in society (Bianchi 1984; Kalish 1979). Atchley (2009) developed the continuity theory, which assumes that individuals develop preferences as a part of their personalities; as they grow older, they continue in their spiritual traditions. Atchley also tried to use a nonreligious approach by describing spirituality as "deep inner silence," "insight," "compassion," "connection with the ground of being," "transcendence of personal self," "wonder," "transformation," and a "concept that sensitizes us to a region of human experience and tells us generally what to look for in that region." He also considered the role that spiritual beliefs and practices play in coping with the problems of later life, especially in the experience of time, dying, and death, before concluding with his own reflections and some implications of his work.

A related concept of gerotranscendence, introduced by Tornstam (1989, 1996), defined a transition from a materialistic and rationalistic perspective to a more cosmic and transcendent view of life that accompanies the process of aging (Adams 2001; Atchley 1997; Ruth & Coleman 1996; Wadensten & Carlsson 2003). The Cosmic Transcendence subscale of the Tornstam's Gerotranscendence Scale (available in Dutch) has proven to be the most consistent and relevant to the meaning of life and the degree of religious involvement (Atchley 1999; Braam, Bramsen, van Tilburg, van der Ploeg, & Deeg 2006).

Relationship of Spirituality to Successful Aging

The notion that a spiritual perspective becomes increasingly important with aging adds a "positive spin" to the end-of-life quest for a "positive death" or a "spiritual journey" (MacKinlay & Trevitt 2007). The concept of successful aging, which emerged in the 1990s from the MacArthur Foundation Research Network on Successful Aging, led to an interest in positive aging. Spirituality and religious participation are highly correlated with positive successful aging—just as much as diet, exercise, mental stimulation, self-efficacy, and social connectedness. This recognition has stimulated an interest in understanding why spirituality has such positive effects on quality of life and end of life. Crowther et al. (2002) proposed that "positive spirituality" is defined by developing an internalized relationship with the sacred and transcendent world that is not bound by race, ethnicity, economics, or class and that promotes the wellness and welfare of self and others. This positive attitude promotes self-enhancing behaviors and beliefs. Rogers (1976) claims the universality of religion is based upon its social function during later years of life, such as helping individuals to face inevitable losses and impending death while also discovering and maintaining meaningfulness in life.

Older adults who are more religious tend to demonstrate greater well-being than those who are less religious (McFadden 1995). However, Seifert (2002) warns against the "sentiment" of assuming that spirituality automatically increases with age. Additionally, MacKinlay implicitly addresses this concern when she observes that successful aging is essentially a wellness model of aging and, as defined, isolates older people with disabilities, physical or mental, outside the model (2001). In those individuals, the "success" of their aging should be measured according to spiritual traditions of humankind that respect the role of an elder in the society (Moberg 2001). In summary, spirituality appears to play an important and adaptive role in aging that seems to lead to a better quality of life, enhanced satisfaction with life, and longevity in the older adults.

Definitions of Spirituality: Spirituality versus Religiosity

The definitions of spirituality, as they have changed over time, are increasingly considered a construct related to mental and physical health. Despite centuries of debate, a consensus has not emerged on the meanings and definitions of spirituality and religion. Hill and Pargament (2003) suggest that spirituality can be understood as a search for the sacred, that is, a process of self-discovery in relation to the sacred. Many writers emphasize a search for life meaning as a central aspect of spirituality (Aponte 2002; MacKinlay 2001; McFadden 1996; Ortiz & Langer 2002). Spirituality traditionally has been used to describe the deeply religious person, but it has now expanded to include the seeker of religion, the seeker of well-being and happiness, and the completely secular person. The definitions of religion generally include an organized system of beliefs, practices, rituals, and symbols designed to facilitate closeness to the sacred and transcendent and to foster religious communities. Spirituality encompasses religion but spreads beyond to promote an understanding of the meaning of life and one's relationship to the transcendent.

Individuals involved in New Age spirituality frequently proclaim that they are "spiritual" but not "religious." In this context, spirituality is human awareness of a relationship or connection that goes beyond sensory perceptions. This relationship is perceived by each individual and is an expanded or heightened knowledge beyond or outside of his or her personal being. Holmes eloquently defined spirituality as "a human capacity for relationship with that which transcends sense phenomena" (1982). A person perceives it as a heightened or expanded consciousness that is independent of one's efforts and that deepens one's awareness of self, others, and the world.

In the landmark spiritual well-being section of the 1971 White House Conference on Aging, the definition of spirituality centers around people's inner resources, especially their ultimate concern for the basic value around which all other values are focused. The core philosophy of life, whether religious, antireligious, or nonreligious, guides a person's conduct to the supernatural and nonmaterial dimensions of human nature (Moberg 1971). The National Interfaith Coalition on Aging (NICA), organized in 1971, defined spiritual well-being as the affirmation of life in a relationship with God, self, community, and environment that nurtures and celebrates wholeness, permeates and gives meaning to all life. The term *spiritual well-being* indicates wholeness in contrast to fragmentation and isolation (Brennan & Missinne 1980). The evidence of spiritual well-being includes positive self-concepts, unselfish giving, moral character, beliefs in an all-encompassing God, personal transcendence, and so on.

In a study by Zinnbauer and colleagues of 346 individuals who were asked to define religiousness and spirituality, religiousness included both personal beliefs in God and organizational practices such as church attendance, as well as higher levels of authoritarianism, orthodoxy, parental religious attendance, and self-righteousness (Zinnbauer & Pargament 2002; Zinnbauer et al. 1997). Spirituality is most often described in experiential terms, such as faith in God or a higher power or integrating one's values and beliefs with behavior in daily life. It can be associated with mystical experiences and New Age beliefs and practices.

Although religiousness and spirituality describe different concepts, they are significantly correlated. Most people consider themselves to be both religious and spiritual. Their self-rated religiousness and spirituality are associated with frequency of prayer, church attendance, religious orthodoxy, and use of religion as a guiding point for everyday decisions. Although 93% identify themselves as spiritual, some rate themselves high on spirituality and low on religion, while others are moderate on both (Moberg 2001). Most believers approach the sacred through the personal, subjective, and experiential path of spirituality, even though they differ as to whether they should include organizational or institutional beliefs and practices in their self-identity. It is the responsibility of mental health professionals and general practitioners to understand what "being spiritual" means to an individual in order to provide complete "holistic" care of that person's psychological and spiritual needs.

Spiritual Development and Aging

Spirituality serves various purposes at different stages of life. Erikson (1963) offers the concept of eight stages of human development that reflect different needs and conflicts associated with different ages. In addition, Fowler (1981, 1991) recognizes six stages of faith, acknowledging that individual development may stop at any stage:

1. *Intuitive-projective faith* (ages 2–7), when a child becomes aware of the concept of God.
2. *Mythic-literal faith* (ages 7–12), when family-specified perspectives and meanings of morals and God are internalized.
3. *Synthetic-conventional faith* (adolescence onward), when faith is accepted without critical evaluation.
4. *Individuative-reflective stage*, when faith is critically examined and one's own belief-system is reconstructed.
5. *Conjunctive faith* (midlife and beyond), when disillusionment with that belief system sets in, and one is caught between it and openness to other religious traditions.
6. *Universalizing faith* (late life), which brings oneness with the power of being or divinity, willingness to promote justice in the world, and fellowship with others regardless of their faith stage or religious tradition.

Koenig (1994) questioned Fowler's approach of applying cognitive stages of faith development to older adults with low levels of education or with physical/cognitive dysfunction. Regardless of differences in the theories of faith development, however, most authors emphasize faith development in late life after completion of all developmental cognitive stages. Spirituality is a lifelong developmental task until death (Moberg 2001).

Spirituality and Physical Health

Empirical research clarifies the health benefits of spiritual and religious practices. Many large community surveys, such as the Established Populations for Epidemiological Studies of the Elderly, have included items assessing religious and spiritual practices (Koenig 2001). Despite racial, religious, and cultural variations, the main common finding emerged as diminished attendance at religious services among the elderly who have problems of health and mobility. Their reduced participation in attendance, however, is often accompanied by high levels of nonorganizational religiosity: praying, listening to religious radio programs and music, and gaining help from religion to understand their own lives (Mindel & Vaughan 1978).

The differential survival hypothesis suggests that persons who are more spiritual and religiously committed have lifestyles that lead to reduced mortality. Over their lifetimes they are less likely than others to use tobacco, abuse alcohol and drugs, engage in premarital sex, or become divorced. They are more likely to belong to supportive social networks and to experience serenity and peace with themselves, other people, and God. Lower age-specific mortality throughout adulthood could explain the high average spirituality in each older generation. A study of over 20,000 U.S. adults estimates that religious involvement prolongs life by about seven years (Hummer, Rogers, Nam, & Ellison 1999).

Various systematic reviews and meta-analyses have demonstrated that religious involvement correlates with decreased morbidity and mortality (Ball, Armistead, & Austin 2003; Berntson, Norman, Hawkley, & Cacioppo 2008; Braam, Beekman, Deeg, Smit, & van Tilburg 1997; Brown 2000; Kune, Kune, & Watson 1993; McCullough, Hoyt, Larson, Koenig, & Thoresen 2000; Oman, Kurata, Strawbridge, & Cohen 2002; Oxman, Freeman, & Manheimer 1995). Contrada and colleagues (2004) found that in patients after heart surgery, stronger religious beliefs were associated with shorter hospital stays and fewer complications. However, Hodges, Humphreys, and Eck (2002) did not find that spiritual beliefs affected recovery from spinal surgery. Some studies suggest that members of different religions may have different mortality and morbidity statistics, even when adjusting for major biological, behavioral, and socioeconomic differences (Rasanen, Kauhanen, Lakka, Kaplan, & Salonen 1996; Van Poppel, Schellekens, & Liefbroer 2002).

Both religious affiliation and regular attendance at religious services appear to buffer the need for and length of hospitalization (Koenig, Larson, & Matthews 1996). Most studies find positive correlations between religious beliefs, behaviors, and mental and physical health (Koenig 1995). For example, various studies have revealed an inverse relationship between people with religious commitment and hypertension, strokes, and pain from cancer and other illnesses compared with similar persons with low religious commitment (Armstrong, van Merwyk, & Coates 1977; Koenig 1995, 1997; Koenig, Smiley, & Gonzales 1988; Walsh 1998). In Comstock and Partridge's 1972 analysis of 91,000 people in Maryland, those who attended church had a lower prevalence of cirrhosis, emphysema, suicide, and death from ischemic heart disease.

The surge in the popularity of spiritual interventions such as yoga or meditation stems largely from motivations to improve and maintain health (Comstock & Partridge 1972; Corliss 2001; Van Montfrans, Karemaker, Wieling, & Dunning 1990). In three studies of prayer, large groups were invited to participate in a group prayer for patients with acute cardiovascular problems. Those who were prayed for did overall better than the control group in terms of the number of cardiovascular arrests, congestive heart failure, pneumonia, intubation, and antibiotic use (Ai, Dunkle, Peterson, & Boiling 1998; Byrd 1988; Harris et al. 1999).

Studies have compared people of high and low religiosity to people rated healthier with less risky lifestyle practices to account for the association with better health. Religion may provide structure, teaching, positive role models, and support to individuals, factors that lead to fewer risky behaviors. Compared to the general population, Mormons and Seventh Day Adventists have been found to have lower incidences of cancer and mortality rates from cancers that can be linked to tobacco and alcohol use (Fraser 1999; Grundmann 1992). However, other studies have not supported this relationship (Hasnain 2005; Poulson, Eppler, Satterwhite, Wuensch, & Bass 1998).

Although many patients consider religion and spirituality to be important in their healthcare, it is rarely explicitly included in the healing process—although spiritual activities such as yoga and meditation may be practiced (Corliss 2001; Van Montfrans et al. 1990). Religious beliefs may help patients cope and aid them in attaching meaning to their diseases (Autiero 1987; Foley 1988; Patel, Shah, Peterson, & Kimmel 2002). In addition, along with encouraging healthy lifestyles, religious groups may promote access to better healthcare by sponsoring preventive programs (e.g., blood pressure and diabetes screenings, soup kitchens, and food drives) (Heath et al. 1999; Koenig, George, & Peterson 1998).

Although most studies have shown positive effects of religion and spirituality on health, a few systematic studies have shown that religious involvement and spirituality are associated with negative physical and mental health outcomes. Religious beliefs can negatively affect a person's health by discouraging traditional treatments or contributing to discontinuing, delaying, or failing to seek timely medical care, such as transfusions or contraception, thereby leading to higher mortality (Donahue 1985). In addition, religions can stigmatize those with certain diseases and prevent them from seeking proper medical care (Lichtenstein 2003; Madru 2003). Religious practices such as exorcism can be dangerous and even lead to death (Ofran, Lavi, Opher, Weiss, & Elinav 2004). Finally, fanatical religious beliefs can affect physical and mental health adversely (Mueller, Plevak, & Rummans 2001).

Spirituality and Mental Health: Coping and Adaptation

Much of the research on spirituality and aging has looked at the relationship between spiritual or religious coping and health, though the impact of religion and spirituality on mental health has been studied more extensively than its impact on physical health. Musick and coauthors (2000) identified approximately 370 studies dealing with the association between religion and physical and mental health.

Many writers advocate for a greater understanding of spirituality and meaning in old age (Kimble 2001) or of religious coping and life outcomes (Seifert 2002). Spiritual health is closely related to mental health and psychological coping (Anderson 1998; Malony 1983). Providers of clinical services have a responsibility to take account of the "whole" person in their work with clients (Langer 2000) and integrate spiritual issues into the psychological or medical care of older adults (Dalby 2006; Koenig et al. 1996).

Substantial evidence has accumulated associating spirituality and religious participation with positive mental health outcomes. Koenig and coauthors reviewed 325 studies and found a strong relationship between religious involvement and mental health, physical health, and the use of health services (Koenig et al. 2001). Williams and colleagues (1991) concluded that religious attendance buffers the effects of stress on mental health. In a study of 107 women with advanced breast cancer, spirituality appeared to improve emotional well-being (Coward 1991). Other studies have demonstrated religiosity to be related to well-being in white Americans, Mexican Americans (Markides, Levin, & Ray 1987), African Americans (Coke 1992), and in different age groups (Yoon & Lee 2007). Some findings show that intrinsically religious people internalize their faith and have higher self-esteem, better personality functioning, less paranoia, and lower rates of depression or anxiety, while extrinsically religious people use religion to obtain status, security, sociability, or health (Koenig 1997; Richards & Bergin 1997). Other findings are mixed about whether religion increases or decreases anxiety (Koenig 1994). Religious coping is inversely related to the severity of depressive symptoms in veterans (Badawi, Eaton, Myllyluoma, Weimer, & Gallo 1999; Idler 1994). However, only two-thirds of the U.S. population consider religion to be an important or the *most* important influence in their lives (Richards & Bergin 1997).

Nevertheless, most studies have indeed found that higher religiousness and spirituality are associated with lower levels of mortality, anxiety, and alcoholism, along with better marriages, reduced loneliness, lessened distress among dementia caregivers, and better mental health (Koenig 1995). Data drawn from waves one and two of the Duke Established Populations for Epidemiologic Studies of the Elderly demonstrated that religious attendance may offer mental stimulation that helps maintain cognitive functioning in later life, particularly among older depressed women (Corsentino, Collins, Sachs-Ericsson, & Blazer 2009). A few studies have addressed differences between religions. One study of older women in Hong Kong showed that Catholics and Buddhists enjoyed better mental health status than Protestants (Boey 2003).

Studies also have examined the association of religion with depression. Prospective cohort studies have shown religious activity to be associated with remission of depression in Protestants, Catholic Netherlanders (Braam et al. 1997), and in ill older adults (Koenig et al. 1998). Twenty-four studies in the research literature have found that religiously involved people had fewer depressive symptoms and less depression (Mueller et al. 2001) or less anxiety (Koenig 2001). About 80% of research studies have also shown an inverse correlation between religiosity and suicide (Gartner, Larson, & Vacher-Mayberry 1990; Neeleman & Lewis 1999; Nisbet, Duberstein, Conwell, & Seidlitz 2000). Suicide may be less acceptable to people with strong religious devotion and beliefs. Several randomized clinical trials (RCTs) demonstrated benefits of religion-based cognitive therapy on Christian patients with clinical depression (Propst, Ostrom, Watkins, Dean, & Mashburn 1992). Three RCTs suggest that Islamic-based religious psychotherapy accelerates recovery from anxiety and depression in Muslim Malays, but these studies did not control for the use of antidepressants and benzodiazepines (Azhar, Varma, & Dharap 1994; Azhar & Varma 1995; Razali, Hasanah, Aminah, & Subramaniam 1998). Religious commitment also has been found to moderate the relationship between functional disability and depression (Koenig, Cohen, Blazer, & Pieper 1992).

Religious and spiritual themes can be present in the context of mental illness such as schizophrenia or bipolar disorder. Also, highly stressful life events can transform normative religious beliefs into excessive preoccupations that involve delusional guilt. Richards and Bergin advise restricting spiritual interventions and explorations to less-disturbed patients, such as outpatients without psychotic or severe mood disorders (Richards & Bergin 1997; Mohr 2006).

Spirituality and Attitudes toward Death and Dying

Continuing advances in medical technology have altered our attitudes toward dying. Dying is no longer a part of human daily consciousness, and many formerly terminal illnesses are no longer fatal. Kübler-Ross (1973) insisted that the dying stage in a life can be experienced as the most profound of life's experiences. Dying begins when the facts of life and death are finally recognized, communicated, and accepted (Kastenbaum 1986).

Most of the research on dying and death is recent and falls into two categories: studies that have probed emotions or attitudes surrounding death and investigations that have explored the experience of dying. Most elderly persons recognize when their own death is close. Older people tend to think about dying and death more than any other age group (Blesky 1990). Most researchers consider the fear of dying to be the most prevalent emotion. However, findings about the relationship of age and fear of dying are mixed (Feifel & Branscomb 1973; Templer 1971). Other emotions linked to death and dying are hope and the continuity of hope (Kalish 1985); the feeling of loss (of control, competence, independence, people, dreams for the future) (Bianchi 1984); loneliness (Feifel 1977); dignity or integrity (Johnson 1992); forgiveness (Thibault 1993); and love (Fischer 1998).

As a society, we shy away from death and the idea of termination. In recent years, research has kindled interest in death and has led people toward greater awareness of the dying process. Spirituality and storytelling can be used as resources in successful aging and in dying, but these need to be tempered to the constraints of current Western culture (Schenck & Roscoe 2009).

Interventions can raise awareness of the dying process and ultimately result in a more peaceful experience. These interventions are likely to improve the experience of death and dying for the patient and their families in various medical settings, such as palliative care, hospice, long-term care, and primary care (Balboni et al. 2007; Puchalski et al. 2009).

Spiritual Care by Healthcare Providers

Despite the complexity of the controversy, the role of religion in healthcare is growing; medical literature on religion and spirituality increased by 600% from 1993 to 2002 (Stefanek, McDonald, & Hess 2004). The guidelines of the Joint Commission on Accreditation of Healthcare Organizations (JCAHO) require hospitals to meet the spiritual needs of patients (La

Pierre 2003). The fourth edition of the *Diagnostic and Statistical Manual of Mental Disorders* (DSM) recognizes religion and spirituality as relevant sources of emotional distress or support (Kutz 2002; Turner, Lukoff, Barnhouse, & Lu 1995). The DSM-5 research agenda specifically addressed this interest in *Religious and Spiritual Issues in Psychiatric Diagnosis* (Peteet, Lu, & Narrow 2010), whose recommendations remain in the DSM-5, published in 2013.

Some authors in the field have recommended that physicians take into account their patients' religious and spiritual histories to better understand their backgrounds and beliefs (Kuhn, 1988; Lo et al. 2002). They may emphasize integrating various religious resources and professionals into patient care, especially when the patient is approaching the end of life (Lo et al. 2002). Or they may highlight efforts to train healthcare providers to better understand spiritual practices, listen to patients' religious concerns, and perform clergy-like duties when religious professionals are not available (Morse & Proctor 1998).

Assessment of Spirituality in Clinical Practice

Acknowledging the spiritual lives of patients may involve asking about their spirituality when recording their histories during clinical interviews, which may not be appropriate for every patient. Some practitioners suggest four simple questions that might be asked of seriously ill patients (Mohr 2006):

1. Is faith (religion, spirituality) important to you in this illness?
2. Has faith been important to you at other times in your life?
3. Do you have someone to talk to about religious matters?
4. Would you like to discuss religious matters with someone?

In addition, open-ended questions allow patients to tell healthcare providers about their view of relationships, the meaning of their illness, and the coping mechanisms that have helped them in the past. Patient responses to these questions can yield information about spiritual concerns and practices that may help healthcare providers better understand their patients' worldly perspectives. This understanding can help practitioners determine whether patients' religious and spiritual beliefs and community involvement can be useful resources to assist with their coping and healing processes.

Obtaining a spiritual history from the patient can be aided by using spiritual history tools, including (1) FICA (*F*aith, belief, meaning; *I*mportance/influence in healthcare decision making; Community; and *Address/ action in treatment plan*) (Puchalski & Romer 2000); (2) HOPE (sources of *Hope; Organized religion; Personal spirituality;* and *Effect on medical care and end-of-life issues*) (Anandarajah & Hight 2001); and (3) SPIRIT (*Spiritual beliefs; Personal beliefs; Integration with spiritual community; Rituals; Implications for care;* and *Terminal care*) (Maugans 1996; Puchalski 2006, 2007–2008).

Measuring Spirituality in Clinical Practice and Research

Measuring spirituality in clinical practice and research has been a challenge because of the intricacy of contributing elements and definitions. No widely accepted measure of spirituality has gained acceptance (Koenig, George, & Titus 2004). Components such as spiritual wellness and spiritual maturity receive more attention because scientific research depends upon measurement, while human services require assessments (Moberg 2002). Hill and Hood (1999) reviewed 125 measures of religion and spirituality from 17 categories (including beliefs, attitudes, religious orientation, faith development, fundamentalism, attitudes toward death, congregational involvement, and satisfaction). Others have identified similar dimensions of religion and spirituality (Fetzer Institute/National Institute on Aging Working Group 1999). Measurements of religion and spirituality rely almost exclusively on paper-and-pencil self-report measures with all the limitations of subjective reporting. Accurate assessments can extend knowledge about spiritual wellness, as well as helping to diagnose spiritual ailments and indicating the spiritual care needed to restore spiritual health. Instruments used to measure spirituality tend to emphasize questions about positive character traits or mental health: optimism, forgiveness, gratitude, meaning and purpose in life, peacefulness, harmony, and general well-being (Koenig 2008).

The more popular instruments are described in table 7.1, along with less well-known instruments proposed for future research. These instruments were selected to demonstrate the breadth of the aspects of spirituality that can contribute to improving health outcomes in the elderly. The prominent Spiritual Well-Being Scale (SWB) has proven an excellent way to assess spiritual and religious commitment in a person's life (Paloutzian & Ellison 1982). The Spiritual Perspective Scale (SPS) similarly assesses the importance of spirituality in a person's life but does not subdivide the religious and spiritual domains as the SWB does (Belcher, Dettmore, & Holzemer 1989; Reed 1987). The SPS was used in a terminal population; in order to

Rating scales	Conceptual model	Reliability		Validity
		Cronbach's alpha	Test-retest	
Spiritual Well-Being Scale (SWB) (Paloutzian & Ellison 1982)	20 items: 10 Religious well-being (RWB) 10 Existential well-being (EWB)	0.89(SWB) 0.87(RWB) 0.78(EWB)	0.93(SWB) 0.96(RWB) 0.86(EWB)	SWB, RWB, and EWB all correlated positively with the Purpose in Life Test
Multidimensional Measurement of Religiousness/ Spirituality Instrument (MMRS) (Fetzer Institute/National Institute on Aging Working Group 1999)	88 items divided into sections: Daily spiritual experiences (16); Meaning (20); Beliefs (7); Forgiveness (10); Religious practices (4); Religious coping (11); Religious spiritual history (5); Organizational religiousness (7); Commitment (2); Religious preference (1); Values (3); Overall Ranking (2)	0.72–0.96 range for all subsections	0.61–0.84 range for all subsections	Positively correlated with the SWB
Daily Spiritual Experience scale (DSES) (Underwood & Teresi 2002)	16 items full scale divided into 2 factors: Spiritual growth (SG); Spiritual decline (SD)	0.98 (SG) 0.86 (SD)	0.85 (SG)	Correlations with Positive Affect subscale of (PANSS)
Spiritual Perspective Scale (SPS) (Belcher, Dettmore, & Holzemer. 1989; Reed 1987)	10 items: Rates frequency of using a spiritual perspective on a 1 to 6 Likert scale (6 = most frequent use of spiritual perspective)	0.93 hospitalized 0.95 hospitalized terminal patients	0.57–0.68	Evidence for construct validity; having a religious back-ground indicated higher scores on SPS; open-ended questions indicated the validity of the SPS for participants in the study

Responsiveness	Interpretability	Properties		
		Burden	Alternative forms	Cultural adaptations
Higher scores indicate SWB	Higher scores indicate SWB and correlated with less loneliness	No difficulty	None	None
In most subsets, higher scores indicate higher religiosity/spirituality, except guilt (Stewart & Koeske 2006)	Correlated with physical and mental health	Long self-report scale	Brief version has been validated	None
Higher scores indicate Higher Spirituality	Positive correlations with decreased alcohol use, quality of life, social status	No difficulties	Short version (6 items) used in the MMRS	None
Adequate for terminally ill, healthy, and nonseriously ill adults; terminally ill adults indicated greater spirituality than both hospitalized nonterminally ill adults and healthy adults	Terminally ill adults indicated change toward increased spirituality (p 0.01); change in spiritual views correlated positively with SPS scores	20–26 minutes to complete	None	None

(continued)

TABLE 7.1 (continued)

Rating scales	Conceptual model	Reliability		Validity
		Cronbach's alpha	Test-retest	
Scales proposed for future research				
Death Attitude Profile (DAP) (Gesser, Wong, & Reker. 1987)	21-items: self-administered; Likert-type scale with four dimensions: Fear of death, Escape-oriented death acceptance, Approach-oriented death acceptance, Neutral death acceptance	Not addressed	Not addressed	Negatively related to happiness (p 0.001) and positively related to hopelessness (p 0.05); failed to support the predicted relationship between Approach-oriented Death Acceptance, happiness, and hopelessness; Escape-oriented Death Acceptance was positively related to hopelessness but unrelated to happiness; Neutral Acceptance was unrelated to hopelessness but positively related to happiness; not used in a terminally ill population
Herth Hope Index (HHI) (VandeCreek, Frankowski, & Ayres 1994)	12-items: 1 to 4 Likert scale with three dimensions: Temporality and future, Positive readiness and expectancy, Interconnectedness	0.88	Not addressed	Negative correlation with depression and positive relationship to self-esteem, both significant (p 0.001); statistically significantly affected the hope scores, education, and patterns of worship educated and attending worship more frequently scored higher on the HHI; has not been used in a terminally ill population to date

Responsiveness	Interpretability	Properties		
		Burden	Alternative forms	Cultural adaptations
Not used as an outcome measure to date; used to assess differences in death attitudes across the life span	Not used in clinical settings; young and middle-aged may have a harder time accepting the reality of death	Not addressed	None	None
Hope scores decreased in the hospital group that had increase depression; higher self-esteem scores scored higher on HHI; pastoral caregivers may increase hopefulness by encouraging self-esteem	Clinical setting not in a terminally ill population; no significant variation in scores based on age, gender, marital stature, or religious background	Useful in chronically ill and terminally ill populations; short and easy to administer; good for respondents with limited stamina or concentration	None	None

compare the use of the SWB, it would need to be tested in this same population. The 59-item Multidimensional Measurement of Religiousness/ Spirituality (MMRS) has been used in religion and spirituality research and has demonstrated good reliability and validity in assessing three primary factors—meaning, spirituality, and religious practices—and two secondary factors—guilt versus God's grace and loving or forgiving God. Stewart and Koeske (2006) and Underwood and Teresi (2002) reported on the reliability and validity of the Daily Spiritual Experience Scale with internal consistency greater than 0.9.

Three scales are of particular interest for future research because of the importance of the domains they address for the aging population coping with death and dying. The Death Attitude Profile (Gesser, Wong, & Reker 1987) analyzes the fear of death. The Death Transcendence Scale looks at how people transcend death; it can be used by healthcare professionals in guiding patients through their last days (VandeCreek, Benes, & Nye 1993; VandeCreek, Frankowski, & Ayres 1994). The Herth Hope Index (HHI) is an excellent scale used to assess the patient's hopefulness (VandeCreek et al. 1994). Knowing that a person is hopeful guides the provider in determining ways to sustain that hope. If a person lacks hope, the providers may need to determine which aspects of the patient's life could be drawn upon in order to ignite hope within the dying patient. Given the correlation of low scores on the HHI with depression and low self-esteem, the clinician would be well advised to assess the patient for these two factors. In addition, it would be beneficial to add specific questions regarding how well the patient's spiritual needs are being met.

For future research, new instruments will be needed to assess spiritual needs in the dying population. These would incorporate the concepts of death transcendence, spiritual and religious well-being, and hopefulness, and they would assess how well those needs are being met. We need to use these instruments to test whether specific interventions can improve patients' spiritual well-being, increase their hopefulness, and enhance their sense of the meaning of their lives.

Training in Spirituality for Healthcare Professionals

A growing number of medical schools are offering courses in spirituality in medicine (Fortin & Barnett 2004). Some programs focus solely on spirituality and medicine while others include components on cultural competency and end-of-life care. Most curricula use several educational methods, such as lectures, small group discussions, standardized patient interviews, and readings. Spirituality may be taught within course subjects, including courses on holistic medicine and complementary and alternative medicine. Brokaw and colleagues (Fortin & Barnett 2004) surveyed complementary and alternative medicine course directors at 53 medical schools and found that 64% included teaching about spirituality, faith, and prayer.

Puchalski (2006) recommended integration of the medical school curricula into a step-wise progression from basic to more sophisticated and specialty material. Extending into the residency years, interdisciplinary courses would include nursing, social work, allied health, and clinical pastoral education programs with faculty representation from theology, chaplaincy, and the humanities (Puchalski 2006). Spirituality can be taught in the context of compassionate communication skills, especially in end-of-life care in the chronic disease care model. Spirituality also can be integrated into courses on ethics or medical humanities and longitudinal courses in doctor-patient relationships. Use of standardized patient spirituality case scenarios for teaching, evaluation, and testing of the students and residents is also recommended (Puchalski 2006). Evaluation of programs that have covered religion and spirituality has been challenging, as schools have different curricula. Most schools evaluate program effectiveness with standard surveys assessing course satisfaction and changes in knowledge, skills, and attitudes, but they do not evaluate the entire curriculum.

Research on Spirituality

The challenges facing research on spirituality and religion include logistical and funding limitations and also the complication of ambiguous definitions and measurements of spirituality and religiosity. Very few well-designed, large-scale studies have been conducted. Much of the published information has been purely anecdotal or editorial, which serves to stimulate discussion but does not establish causality or scientifically justify the use of specific interventions (Lee & Newberg 2009). In addition, the majority of existing studies are correlational and may be plagued by spurious findings. For example, in a systematic review of studies from 1996 to 1999, Townsend and colleagues counted nine RCTs. Hopefully, with increasing interest in spirituality and mind, the number and sophistication of scientific studies should continue to improve (Townsend, Kladder, Ayele, & Mulligan 2002).

An inherent challenge in defining and measuring spirituality resides in the need to separate religiosity and spirituality (Tanyi 2002; Powell, Shahabi, & Thoresen 2003). This is particularly important in studying participants who consider themselves spiritual but not religious. Another consideration is that subjects may be unwilling to alter their religious beliefs or practices for a study with a design that uses a particular spiritual practice. Monitoring of practice adherence or correct performance by a subject may also become a problem. In these cases, a subject may inadvertently be noncompliant.

The need for accurate and valid measures of religiosity and spirituality is critical. Different rating scales need to identify subjective and objective measures. The use of daily diaries can be helpful to track compliance with daily practices. When considering the direct effects of religious or spiritual activities on a person's health, it is also important to consider secondary effects, such as an increase in social support, social activities leading to improved chances of finding life partners, or possibilities for better healthcare.

Establishing the direction of causality can be another challenge. For example, health status can influence whether a person can participate in a religious activity. Practices and doctrines can vary among different religions and denominations. Local environments can influence the status of a religious movement and add stress if a particular religion is an object of persecution.

The proper duration of a spiritual intervention such as prayer, yoga, or meditation is not entirely clear, and all of these practices may have immediate or delayed effects on physiological measures such as blood pressure or markers of inflammation. Multidisciplinary research, although necessary, can be daunting because of the differences in definitions and motivations. Scientific-approach limitations include failure to control for confounding variables and other covariates, as well as difficulties in controlling for multiple comparisons using multiple statistical procedures. These limitations can lead to biased estimations of associations (Berry 2005).

Spiritual Interventions

Religious or spiritual activities can assist in the treatment and prevention of illnesses. Richards and Bergin (1997) differentiate between religious and spiritual interventions on the basis of structure. Religious interventions are more structured, denominational, external, cognitive, ritualistic, and public, whereas spiritual interventions are more cross-cultural, affective, transcendent, and experiential. To be effective in helping during an illness or a crisis, patients should be accepting of the form of intervention, and it should be tailored to their perspectives. Spiritual interventions are contraindicated in cases of psychotic illnesses, when dealing with poor "ego boundaries," or when patients do not want to participate. Not all of the studies cited in the following paragraphs were performed strictly with the elderly, but they may inform future research on spirituality and aging.

PRAYER AND RELIGIOUS RITUALS

Prayer is a powerful form of coping that helps people physically and mentally. Nearly 60% of Americans report praying daily (Boehnlein 2000). Prayer is a communication or conversation with a divine power or a "higher self." Prayer is practiced by all Western theistic religions and several of the Eastern traditions (e.g., Hinduism, Sikkhism, Buddhism, Taoism). Group prayer is associated with greater well-being and happiness, while solitary prayer is associated with depression and loneliness (Poloma & Pendleton 1991). However, scientific validation of the efficacy of prayer, in terms of health outcomes, remains in its infancy when dealing with positive and negative biases (Jantos & Kiat 2007). Studies report negative findings on the therapeutic effects of intercessory prayer, which illustrates the need for nonbiased experimental designs. Critics of prayer research have proposed that the benefits of prayer may be similar to the results of a placebo effect (Jantos & Kiat 2007). In future studies of the health benefits of prayer, opening the dialogue and refining the research methodologies can help discern potential health effects.

Worship and rituals are integral to most religions. Benson suggests that potentially therapeutic elements of worship include music, aesthetic surroundings, rituals, prayer and contemplation, and opportunities to socialize with others (Benson 1997). Bibliotherapy involves the use of literature to help gain insight into feelings and behaviors and to assist with positive coping. All major world religions have a text that their followers view as holy and use as a source of comfort, wisdom, and guidance (Nigosian 1994). All major theistic world religions teach that people should accept and forgive those who have harmed them and seek forgiveness from those they have harmed (Richards & Bergin 1997). Spiritual reading and practicing forgiveness and repentance are significant parts of twelve-step programs (Finnegan & McNally 1995; Galanter 2008; Mohr 2006; Pearce, Rivinoja, & Koenig 2008). Steps four and five in Alcoholics Anonymous involve public "confessions" and recounting of one's wrongdoing. In medical settings, forgiveness and repentance are within the purview of a pastoral counselor and clergyperson (Latovich 1995). Both prayer and bibliotherapy with sacred writings must be consistent with patients' needs and requests.

MEDITATION

Meditation is essentially a physiological state of reduced metabolic activity that elicits physical and mental relaxation and is reported to enhance psychological balance and emotional stability (Young & Taylor 2001). Meditation produces a sense of calm, limited thought, and attention; it is widely used as an alternative therapy for physical ailments (Eisenberg et al. 1998). Meditation involves either the narrowing or focusing of attention on internal events such as breathing, a mental object, one point in space, or a mantra (in Buddhist or yoga practices), or the expanding of attention without judgment on moment-to-moment experience, observing thoughts and feelings from a metacognitive awareness state (Mindful Meditation, Vipassana, and Zen Buddhist practices) (Ivanovski & Malhi 2007).

Many physicians now routinely recommend meditation or yoga techniques to their patients and include them as a part of an integrated health program, although Christian patients may view some forms of Eastern mediation unfavorably (McLemore 1982). Although evidence is not yet definitive, preliminary studies suggest that individuals experience health benefits from practicing meditation, including improved reaction time, creativity, and comprehension (Domino 1977; Solberg, Berglund, Engen, Ekeberg, & Loeb 1996).

Ethical considerations should be taken into account for spiritual interventions practiced or recommended by healthcare professionals to avoid self-promotion or imposition of personal beliefs on patients by linking religious practices to better health outcomes (Mohr 2006). Ethical considerations also extend to acknowledging the limitations of current research on the effects of spirituality on health, and, most importantly, they extend to respecting patients' boundaries and beliefs. It is crucial to obtain patients' informed consent to share their spiritual histories and to provide them with choices regarding spiritual interventions (Mohr 2006).

MINDFULNESS MEDITATION
The effort to develop a cohesive understanding of mindfulness is useful for both clinicians and researchers, but it has proven to be difficult to define (Allen, Chambers, & Knight 2006; Rothwell 2006). Kabat-Zinn defines mindfulness as a conscious discipline of paying attention to the present moment in a particular way and in a nonjudgmental state (Kabat-Zinn 1994, 1996). Three key elements of the definition include intentionality, present-centeredness, and absence of judgment; or, as Shapiro described, the processes of intention, attention, and attitude engaged simultaneously in the process of mindfulness (Shapiro, Carlson, Astin, & Freedman 2006). The Mindfulness-Based Stress Reduction Program (MBSR) has been used with people who have physical or psychological symptoms to alleviate "stress" that tends to be inherently holistic and nonpathologizing (Rothwell 2006).

The structure of the MBSR program involves a limited number of sessions over the course of eight weeks. Scheduled class time each week is divided between a formal meditation practice, a small and large group discussion, and inquiry of individuals into their present-moment experiences. Formal MBSR practices may include mindfulness body scans; a sitting meditation while focusing on controlled breathing; mindfulness hatha yoga; a sitting meditation with expanded awareness of several objects of attention; a walking meditation; and an eating meditation. The participant outcomes include discovering embodiment (interoception and proprioception); experiencing new possibilities or new ways of perceiving; observing experience; moving toward acceptance; and increasing compassion for self and others.

Several studies and meta-analyses document the usefulness of the MBSR approach for mental health and psychosocial adjustment of cancer patients (Ledesma & Kumano 2009). The studies indicate that this approach resulted in decreased anxiety and distress in cancer patients and an overall improvement in immunity (Fang et al. 2010; Koszycki, Benger, Shlik, & Bradwejn 2007), chronic pain (Plews-Ogan, Owens, Goodman, Wolfe, & Schorling 2005), and health-related quality of life in community-dwelling and nursing-home populations of older adults (Ernst et al. 2008; Roth & Robbins 2004).

Conclusion

Interest in spirituality and aging has been on the increase since at least the 1990s; however, proper assessment of spirituality in clinical practice and research faces multiple barriers, including the lack of professional training for healthcare professionals, shortage of time, and discomfort of patients and healthcare providers in discussing spiritual issues and needs. On the whole, the Western society and healthcare professionals have not yet accepted death and dying as a part of life. Healthcare providers are trained to do everything to save dying patients, and some of it is driven by the fear of litigation from patients' families. Overcoming these barriers through training for healthcare professionals can improve care and its effectiveness in older adults. Improvement of research tools and assessment methods, as well as the development of spiritual interventions, can offer more choices of healthcare that are consistent with the belief systems of individuals and their families. An improved understanding and respect for individual spiritual practices can help shape personalized medical care for older adults and improve health outcomes.

The public health significance of spirituality, resilience, and positive aging is growing rapidly as the number of elderly persons increases. The cost of care for the victims of mental and physical illnesses will increase exponentially in the next several decades, which will make understanding the interaction between spirituality and physical and mental health in older adults all the more important. Learning to use and enhance spirituality may help improve health outcomes and reduce disability, while speeding the healing process. In addition, employing spiritual beliefs in coping with death and dying, especially in palliative and long-term healthcare settings and in hospice care, may help us understand these phemonena even better.

Training of healthcare professionals in assessing and integrating spirituality into healthcare should be elevated in importance in interdisciplinary training programs via the development of comprehensive curriculum in conjunction with medical schools, schools of nursing and social work, and allied health and clinical pastoral programs. A comprehensive multidimensional model that combines psychological, social, genetic, and neurobiological factors based on previous research and theory is needed to guide future research in the area of spirituality.

Future spiritual interventions that aim at enhancing coping and reducing stress in various populations must consider spiritual diversity and develop targeted programs. These should offer choices of healthcare based on individual spiritual beliefs, thus creating a basis for more personalized care. Moreover, future research should test culturally appropriate interventions that may be adapted to the needs of different populations. Interventions that combine methods demonstrated to be effective in reducing stress and improving well-being and coping could be applied with benefit. In addition, future studies of the neurobiology of spiritual interventions and individualized spiritual treatment should include neuroimaging as well as assessment of individual genetic, psychosocial, and biological vulnerability factors. More rigorously developed information can lead to more effective preventive interventions for depression, anxiety, and stress in older adults. Integrated use of spiritual interventions that enhance individual resilience to stress, plus the mind-body approaches to stress-reduction (e.g., meditation, yoga, mindfulness, tai chi), show great promise for improving overall functioning and well-being in older adults.

Clinical Case

Mr. D., who resided in a hospice facility, shared his experience of dealing with severe heart and lung disease, which forced him to give up activities he had enjoyed throughout his life. "I love to ski and hike, and I can't do those anymore. I gave up everything that I had. What you see is what you get. This is all I have left: breathing, eating, and sleeping, and sleep is not so good anymore either. Prayer is about the only thing that gets me inspired, because you have to get going. And if it wasn't for God, I would be in bed all day long, but it is just wonderful to talk to him. I feel he is there, you know. I feel like when I am in the bed there and I pray in the bed, you know that he is right on the corner of it sitting there."

Mr. D.'s efforts to connect with his concept of the divine gave him the confidence to transcend the ordinary limitations of his aging self; in that closeness to a divine power, he found meaning in both existence and death. Prayers, meditation, and rituals were used as ways to experience communion with the divine. In so doing, Mr. D. relied on a meaningful spiritual resource that contributed greatly to his resilience and quality of life.

· · ·

References

Adams, K. B. (2001). Depressive symptoms, depletion, or developmental change? Withdrawal, apathy, and lack of vigor in the Geriatric Depression Scale. *Gerontologist, 41*(6), 768–77.

Ai, A. L., Dunkle, R. E., Peterson, C., & Boiling, S. F. (1998). The role of private prayer in psychological recovery among midlife and aged patients following cardiac surgery. *Gerontologist, 38*(5), 591–601.

Allen, N. B., Chambers, R., & Knight, W. (2006). Mindfulness-based psychotherapies: A review of conceptual foundations, empirical evidence, and practical considerations. *Aust N Z J Psychiatry, 40*(4), 285–94.

Anandarajah, G., & Hight, E. (2001). Spirituality and medical practice: Using the HOPE questions as a practical tool for spiritual assessment. *Am Fam Physician, 63*(1), 81–89.

Anderson, R. S. (1998). On being human: The spiritual saga of a creaturely soul. In W. S. Brown, N. Murphy, and H. N. Molonly (Eds.), *What ever happened to the soul? Scientific and theological portraits of human nature* (pp. 175–94). Minneapolis, MN: Fortress.

Aponte, H. (2002). Spirituality: The heart of therapy. *J Fam Psychother, 13*,13–27.

Armbruster, C. A., Chibnall, J. T., & Legett, S. (2003). Pediatrician beliefs about spirituality and religion in medicine: Associations with clinical practice. *Pediatrics, 111*(3), e227–35.

Armstrong, B., van Merwyk, A. J., & Coates, H. (1977). Blood pressure in Seventh-day Adventist vegetarians. *Am J Epidemiol, 105*(5), 444–49.

Astrow, A. B., Puchalski, C. M., & Sulmasy, D. P. (2001). Religion, spirituality, and health care: Social, ethical, and practical considerations. *Am J Med, 110*(4), 283–87.

Atchley, R. C. (1997). Everyday mysticism: Spiritual development in later adulthood. *J Adult Dev, 4*(2), 123–24.

Atchley, R. C. (1999). Incorporating spirituality into professional work in aging. *Aging Today, 20*(4), 17.

Atchley, R. C. (2009). *Spirituality and aging.* Baltimore, MD: Johns Hopkins University Press.

Autiero, A. (1987). The interpretation of pain: The point of view of Catholic theology. *Acta Neurochir Suppl (Wien) 38*, 123–26.

Azhar, M. Z., & Varma, S. L. (1995). Religious psychotherapy in depressive patients. *Psychother Psychosom, 63*(3–4), 165–68.

Azhar, M. Z., Varma, S. L., & Dharap, A. S. (1994). Religious psychotherapy in anxiety disorder patients. *Acta Psychiatr Scand, 90*(1), 1–3.

Badawi, M. A., Eaton, W. W., Myllyluoma, J., Weimer, L. G., & Gallo, J. (1999). Psychopathology and attrition in the Baltimore ECA 15-year follow-up 1981–1996. *Soc Psychiatry Psychiatr Epidemiol, 34*(2), 91–98.

Balboni, T. A., Vanderwerker, L. C., Block, S. D., Paulk, M. E., Lathan, C. S., Peteet, J. R., & Prigerson, H. G. (2007). Religiousness and spiritual support among advanced cancer patients and associations with end-of-life treatment preferences and quality of life. *J Clin Oncol, 25*(5), 555–60.

Ball, J., Armistead, L., & Austin, B. J. (2003). The relationship between religiosity and adjustment among African-American, female, urban adolescents. *J Adolesc, 26*(4), 431–46.

Belcher, A. E., Dettmore, D., & Holzemer, S. P. (1989). Spirituality and sense of well-being in persons with AIDS. *Holist Nurs Pract, 3*(4), 16–25.

Benson, H. (1997). *Timeless healing: The power and biology of belief.* New York: Gale.

Berntson, G. G., Norman, G. J., Hawkley, L. C., & Cacioppo, J. T. (2008). Spirituality and autonomic cardiac control. *Ann Behav Med, 35*(2), 198–208.

Berry, D. (2005). Methodological pitfalls in the study of religiosity and spirituality. *West J Nurs Res, 27*(5), 628–47.

Bianchi, E. C. (1984). *Aging as a spiritual journey.* New York: Crossroad.

Blazer, D., & Palmore, E. (1976). Religion and aging in a longitudinal panel. *Gerontologist, 16*(1 Pt1), 82–85.

Blesky, J. K. (1990). *The psychology of aging.* 2d ed. Pacific Grove, CA: Brooks/Cole.

Boehnlein, J. K. (2000). *Psychiatry and religion: The convergence of mind and spirit.* Washington, DC: American Psychiatric Press.

Boey, K. W. (2003). Religiosity and psychological well-being of older women in Hong Kong. *Int J Psychiatr Nurs Res, 8*(2), 921–35.

Braam, A. W., Beekman, A. T., Deeg, D. J., Smit, J. H., & van Tilburg, W. (1997). Religiosity as a protective or prognostic factor of depression in later life: Results from a community survey in the Netherlands. *Acta Psychiatr Scand, 96*(3), 199–205.

Braam, A. W., Bramsen, I., van Tilburg, T. G., van der Ploeg, H. M., & Deeg, D. J. (2006). Cosmic transcendence and framework of meaning in life: Patterns among older adults in the Netherlands. *J Gerontol B Psychol Sci Soc Sci, 61*(3), S121–28.

Brennan, C. L., & Missinne, L. E. (1980). Personal and institutionalized religiosity of the elderly. In J. A. Thorson & T. C. Cook Jr. (Eds.), *Spiritual well-being of the elderly* (pp. 92–99). Springfield, IL: Charles C. Thomas.

Brown, C. M. (2000). Exploring the role of religiosity in hypertension management among African Americans. *J Health Care Poor Underserved, 11*(1), 19–32.

Byrd, R. C. (1988). Positive therapeutic effects of intercessory prayer in a coronary care unit population. *South Med J, 81*(7), 826–29.

Carstensen, L. L., Isaacowitz, D. M., & Charles, S. T. (1999). Taking time seriously: A theory of socio-emotional selectivity. *Am Psychol, 54*(3), 165–81.

Coke, M. M. (1992). Correlates of life satisfaction among elderly African Americans. *J Gerontol, 47*(5), P316–20.

Comstock, G. W., & Partridge, K. B. (1972). Church attendance and health. *J Chronic Dis, 25*(12), 665–72.

Contrada, R. J., Goyal, T. M., Cather, C., Rafalson, L., Idler, E. L., & Krause, T. J. (2004). Psychosocial factors in outcomes of heart surgery: The impact of religious involvement and depressive symptoms. *Health Psychol, 23*(3), 227–38.

Corliss, R. (2001). The power of yoga. *Time, 157*(16), 54–63.

Corsentino, E. A., Collins, N., Sachs-Ericsson, N., & Blazer, D. G. (2009). Religious attendance reduces cognitive decline among older women with high levels of depressive symptoms. *J Gerontol A Biol Sci Med Sci, 64*(12), 1283–89.

Coward, D. D. (1991). Self-transcendence and emotional well-being in women with advanced breast cancer. *Oncol Nurs Forum, 18*(5), 857–63.

Crowther, M. R., Parker, M. W., Achenbaum, W. A., Larimore, W. L., & Koenig, H. G. (2002). Rowe and Kahn's model of successful aging revisited: Positive spirituality—the forgotten factor. *Gerontologist, 42*(5), 613–20.

Cummings, E., & Henry, W. E. (1961). *Growing old: The process of disengagement.* New York: Basic.

Daaleman, T. P., & Nease, D. E. Jr. (1994). Patient attitudes regarding physician inquiry into spiritual and religious issues. *J Fam Pract, 39*(6), 564–68.

Dalby, P. (2006). Is there a process of spiritual change or development associated with ageing? A critical review of research. *Aging Ment Health, 10*(1), 4–12.

Domino, G. (1977). Transcendental meditation and creativity: An empirical investigation. *J Appl Psychol, 62*(3), 358–62.

Donahue, M. J. (1985). Intrinsic and extrinsic religiousness: Review and meta-analysis. *J Pers Soc Psychol, 48*(2), 400–419.

Eisenberg, D. M., Davis, R. B., Ettner, S. L., Appel, S., Wilkey, S., Van Rompay, M., & Kessler, R. C. (1998). Trends in alternative medicine use in the United States, 1990–1997: Results of a follow-up national survey. *JAMA, 280*(18), 1569–75.

Ellis, M. R., Vinson, D. C., & Ewigman, B. (1999). Addressing spiritual concerns of patients: Family physicians' attitudes and practices. *J Fam Pract, 48*(2), 105–9.

Erikson, E. H. (1963). *Childhood and society.* 2d ed. New York, Norton.

Ernst, S., Welke, J., Heintze, C., Zöllner, A., Kiehne, S., Schwantes, U., & Esch, T. (2008). Effects of mindfulness-based stress reduction on quality of life in nursing home residents: A feasibility study. *Forsch Komplementmed, 15*(2), 74–81.

Fang, C. Y., Reibel, D. K., Longacre, M. L., Rosenzweig, S., Campbell, D. E., & Douglas, S. D. (2010). Enhanced psychosocial well-being following participation in a mindfulness-based stress reduction program is associated with increased natural killer cell activity. *J Altern Complement Med, 16*(5), 531–38.

Feifel, H. (1977). *New meanings of death.* New York: McGraw-Hill.

Feifel, H., & Branscomb, A. B. (1973). Who's afraid of death? *J Abnorm Psychol, 81*(3), 282–88.

Fetzer Institute/National Institute on Aging Working Group (1999). *Multidimensional measurement of religiousness/spirituality for use in health research.* Report of the Fetzer Institute/NIA Working Group. Kalamazoo, MI: Fetzer Insitute.

Finnegan, D. G., & McNally, E. B. (1995). Defining God or a higher power: The spiritual center of recover. In R. J. Kus (Ed.), *Spirituality and chemical dependency* (pp. 39–48. Binghamton, NY: Haworth.

Fischer, K. (1998). *Winter grace.* Nashville: Upper Room.

Foley, D. P. (1988). Eleven interpretations of personal suffering. *J Relig Health, 27*, 321–28.

Fortin, A. H., & Barnett, K. G. (2004). STUDENTJAMA. Medical school curricula in spirituality and medicine. *JAMA, 291*(23), 2883.

Fowler, J. W. (1981). *Stages of faith: The psychology of human development and the quest for meaning.* San Francisco: Harper & Row.

Fowler, J. W. (1991). *Weaving the new creation: Stages of faith and the public church.* San Francisco: Harper & Row.

Fraser, G. E. (1999). Associations between diet and cancer, ischemic heart disease, and all-cause mortality in non-Hispanic white California Seventh-Day Adventists. *Am J Clin Nutr, 70*(3 Suppl), 532S–38S.

Galanter, M. (2008). Spirituality, evidence-based medicine, and Alcoholics Anonymous. *Am J Psychiatry, 165*(12), 1514–17.

Gallup, G. (1999). Assessing religion in U.S. on three levels. *Emerging Trends, 21*(3), 2–4.

Gallup, G., & Bezilla, R. (1992). *The religious life of young Americans*. Princeton, NJ: Gallup International Institute.

Gartner, J., Larson, D. B., & Vacher-Mayberry, C. D. (1990). A systematic review of the quantity and quality of empirical research published in four pastoral counseling journals, 1975–1984. *J Pastoral Care, 44*(2), 115–29.

Gesser, G., Wong, P. T., & Reker, G. T. (1987). Death attitudes across the life span: Development and validation of the death attitude profile. *Omega, 18*(2), 113–28.

Grundmann, E. (1992). Cancer morbidity and mortality in USA Mormons and Seventh-Day Adventists. *Arch Anat Cytol Pathol, 40*(2–3), 73–78.

Harris, W. S., Gowda, M., Kolb, J. W., Strychacz, C. P., Vacek, J. L., Jones, P. G., . . . & McCallister, B. D. (1999). A randomized, controlled trial of the effects of remote, intercessory prayer on outcomes in patients admitted to the coronary care unit. *Arch Intern Med, 159*(19), 2273–78.

Hasnain, M. (2005). Cultural approach to HIV/AIDS harm reduction in Muslim countries. *Harm Reduct J, 2*(23), 1–9.

Heath, A. C., Madden, P. A. F., Grant, J. D., McLaughlin, T. L., Todorov, A. A., & Bucholz, K. K. (1999). Resiliency factors protecting against teenage alcohol use and smoking: Influences of religion, religious involvement and values, and ethnicity in the Missouri Adolescent Female Twin Study. *Twin Res, 2*(2), 145–55.

Hill, P. C., & Hood, R. W. (1999). *Measures of religiosity*. Birmingham, AL: Religious Education Press.

Hill, P. C., & Pargament, K. I. (2003). Advances in the conceptualization and measurement of religion and spirituality. Implications for physical and mental health research. *Am Psychol, 58*(1), 64–74.

Hodges, S. D., Humphreys, S. C., & Eck, J. C. (2002). Effect of spirituality on successful recovery from spinal surgery. *South Med J, 95*(12), 1381–84.

Holmes, U. T. (1982). *Spirituality for ministry*. San Francisco: Harper & Row.

Hummer, R. A., Rogers, R. G., Nam, C. B., & Ellison, C. G. (1999). Religious involvement and U.S. adult mortality. *Demography, 36*(2), 273–85.

Idler, E. L. (1994). *Cohesiveness and coherence: Religion and the health of the elderly*. New York: Garland.

Ivanovski, B., & Malhi, G. S. (2007). The psychological and neurophysiological concomitants of mindfulness forms of meditation. *Acta Neuropsychiatr, 19*(2), 76–91.

Jantos, M., & Kiat, H. (2007). Prayer as medicine: How much have we learned? *Med J Aust, 186*(10 Suppl), S51–53.

Johnson, R. (1992). Forgiveness: Our bridge to peace. *Liguorian, 80*(6), 44–45.

Jung, C. (1959). *The basic writings of Jung*. New York: Modern Library.

Kabat-Zinn, J. (1994). *Wherever you go, there you are*. New York: Hyperion.

Kabat-Zinn, J. (1996). Mindfulness meditation: What is, what it isn't, and its role in health care and medicine. In Y. Haruki, Y. Ishii, & M. Suzuki (Eds.), *Comparative and psychological study on meditation*. Delft, NL: Eubron.

Kalish, R. A. (1979). The new ageism and the failure models: A polemic. *Gerontologist, 19*(4), 398–402.

Kalish, R. A. (1985). *Death, grief, and caring relationships.* 2d ed. Monterey, CA: Brooks/Cole.

Kastenbaum, R. J. (1986). *Death, society, and human experience.* 3d ed. Columbus, OH: Charles E. Merrill.

Kimble, M. (2001). Beyond the biomedical paradigm: Generating a spiritual vision of ageing. *J Relig Gerontol, 12*(3–4), 31–41.

King, D. E., & Bushwick, B. (1994). Beliefs and attitudes of hospital inpatients about faith healing and prayer. *J Fam Pract, 39*(4), 349–52.

Koenig, H. G. (1994). *Aging & God.* New York: Haworth Pastoral Press.

Koenig, H. G. (1995). *Research on religion and aging: An annotated bibliography.* Westport, CT: Greenwood.

Koenig, H. G. (1997). *Is religion good for your health? the effects of religion on the physical and mental health.* Binghamton, NY: Haworth.

Koenig, H. G. (2001). Religion, spirituality, and medicine: How are they related and what does it mean? *Mayo Clin Proc, 76*(12), 1189–91.

Koenig, H. G. (2008). Concerns about measuring "spirituality" in research. *J Nerv Ment Dis, 196*(5), 349–55.

Koenig, H. G., Cohen, H. J., Blazer, D. G., & Pieper, C. (1992). Religious coping and depression among elderly, hospitalized medically ill men. *Am J Psychiatry, 149*(12), 1693–1700.

Koenig, H. G., George, L. K., & Peterson, B. L. (1998). Religiosity and remission of depression in medically ill older patients. *Am J Psychiatry, 155*(4), 536–42.

Koenig, H. G., George, L. K., & Titus, P. (2004). Religion, spirituality, and health in medically ill hospitalized older patients. *J Am Geriatr Soc, 52*(4), 554–62.

Koenig, H. G., Larson, D. B., & Matthews, D. A. (1996). Religion and psychotherapy with older adults. *J Geriatr Psychiatry, 29*(2), 155–84.

Koenig, H. G., McCullough, M. E., & Larson, D. B. (2001). *Handbook of religion and health.* New York: Oxford University Press.

Koenig, H. G., Smiley, M., & Gonzales, J. A. P. (1988). *Religion, health, and aging: A review and theoretical integration.* Westport, CT: Greenwood.

Koszycki, D., Benger, M., Shlik, J., & Bradwejn, J. (2007). Randomized trial of a meditation-based stress reduction program and cognitive behavior therapy in generalized social anxiety disorder. *Behav Res Ther, 45*(10), 2518–26.

Kübler-Ross, E. (1973). *On death and dying.* London: Routledge.

Kuhn, C. C. (1988). A spiritual inventory of the medically ill patient. *Psychiatr Med, 6*(2), 87–100.

Kune, G. A., Kune, S., & Watson, L. F. (1993). Perceived religiousness is protective for colorectal cancer: Data from the Melbourne Colorectal Cancer Study. *J R Soc Med, 86*(11), 645–47.

Kutz, I. (2002). Samson, the bible, and the DSM. *Arch Gen Psychiatry, 59*(6), 565; author reply, 565–66.

Langer, N. (2000). The importance of spirituality in later life. *Gerontol Geriatr Educ, 20*(3), 41–50.

La Pierre, L. L. (2003). JCAHO safeguards spiritual care. *Holist Nurs Pract, 17*(4), 219.

Latovich, M. A. (1995). The clergyperson and the fifth step. In R. J. Kus (Ed.), *Spirituality and chemical dependency* (pp. 79–89). Binghamton, NY: Haworth.

Ledesma, D., & Kumano, H. (2009). Mindfulness-based stress reduction and cancer: A meta-analysis. *Psychooncology, 18*(6), 571–79.

Lee, B. Y., & Newberg, A. B. (2009). The interaction of religion and health. In D. A. Monti & B. D. Beitman (Eds.), *Integrative Psychology* (pp. 408–44). New York, Oxford University Press.

Lichtenstein, B. (2003). Stigma as a barrier to treatment of sexually transmitted infection in the American deep south: Issues of race, gender, and poverty. *Soc Sci Med, 57*(12), 2435–45.

Lo, B., Ruston, D., Kates, L. W., Arnold, R. M., Cohen, C. B., Faber-Langendoen, K., . . . & Tulsky, J. A. (2002). Discussing religious and spiritual issues at the end of life: A practical guide for physicians. *JAMA, 287*(6), 749–54.

MacKinlay, E. (2001). The spiritual dimension of caring: Applying a model for spiritual tasks of ageing. *J Relig Gerontol, 12*(3–4), 151–66.

MacKinlay, E. B., & Trevitt, C. (2007). Spiritual care and ageing in a secular society. *Med J Aust, 186*(10 Suppl), S74–76.

Madru, N. (2003). Stigma and HIV: Does the social response affect the natural course of the epidemic? *J Assoc Nurses AIDS Care, 14*(5), 39–48.

Malony, H. N. (1983). *Wholeness and holiness: Reading in the psychology/theology of mental health*. Grand Rapids, MI: Baker Book House.

Markides, K. S., Levin, J. S., & Ray, L. A. (1987). Religion, aging, and life satisfaction: An eight-year, three-wave longitudinal study. *Gerontologist, 27*(5), 660–65.

Matthews, D. A., & Clark, C. (1998). *The faith factor: Proof of the healing power of prayer*. New York: Viking.

Maugans, T. A. (1996). The SPIRITual history. *Arch Fam Med, 5*(1), 11–16.

McCullough, M. E., Hoyt, W. T., Larson, D. B., Koenig, H. G., & Thoresen, C. (2000). Religious involvement and mortality: A meta-analytic review. *Health Psychol, 19*(3), 211–22.

McFadden, S. (1995). Religion and well-being in aging persons in an aging society. *J Soc Issues, 51*(2), 161–75.

McFadden, S. (1996). Religion, spirituality, and aging. In J. Birren & K. Schaie (Eds.), *Handbook of the Psychology of Aging*, 4th ed. (pp. 162–77). San Diego: Academic.

McLemore, C. (1982). *The scandal of psychotherapy*. Wheaton, IL: Tyndale House.

Miller, W. R., & Thoresen, C. E. (2003). Spirituality, religion, and health. An emerging research field. *Am Psychol, 58*(1), 24–35.

Mindel, C. H., & Vaughan, C. E. (1978). A multidimensional approach to religiosity and disengagement. *J Gerontol, 33*(1), 103–8.

Moberg, D. O. (1971). *Spiritual well-being: Background and issues.* White House Conference on Aging. Washington, DC: U.S. Government Printing Office.

Moberg, D. O. (1997). Religion and aging. In J. M. Wimoth & K. F. Ferraro (Eds.), *Gerontology: Perspectives and issues* (pp. 193–220). New York: Springer.

Moberg, D. O. (2001). *Aging & spirituality: Spiritual dimensions of aging theory, research, practice, and policy.* Binghamton, NY: Haworth.

Moberg, D. O. (2002). Assessing and measuring spirituality: Confronting dilemmas of universal and particular evaluative criteria. *J Adult Dev, 9*(1), 47–60.

Moberg, D. O. (2005). Research in spirituality, religion and aging. *J Gerontol Soc Work, 45*(1–2), 11–40.

Mohr, W. K. (2006). Spiritual issues in psychiatric care. *Perspect Psychiatr Care, 42*(3), 174–83.

Morse, J. M., Proctor, A. (1998). Maintaining patient endurance. The comfort work of trauma nurses. *Clin Nurs Res, 7*(3), 250–274.

Mueller, P. S., Plevak, D. J., & Rummans, T. A. (2001). Religious involvement, spirituality, and medicine: Implications for clinical practice. *Mayo Clin Proc, 76*(12), 1225–35.

Musick, M., Traphagan, J. W., Koeing, H. G., & Larson, D. B. (2000). Spirituality in physical health and aging. *J Adult Dev, 7*(2), 73–86.

Neeleman, J., & Lewis, G. (1999). Suicide, religion, and socioeconomic conditions. An ecological study in 26 countries, 1990. *J Epidemiol Community Health, 53*(4), 204–10.

NICA (1975). *Spiritual well-being.* National Interfaith Coalition on Aging, Athens, GA.

Nigosian, S. A. (1994). *World faiths.* 2d ed. New York: St. Martin's.

Nisbet, P. A., Duberstein, P. R., Conwell, Y., & Seidlitz, L. (2000). The effect of participation in religious activities on suicide versus natural death in adults 50 and older. *J Nerv Ment Dis, 188*(8), 543–46.

Ofran, Y., Lavi, D., Opher, D., Weiss, T. A., & Elinav, E. (2004). Fatal voluntary salt intake resulting in the highest ever documented sodium plasma level in adults (255 mmol L-1): A disorder linked to female gender and psychiatric disorders. *J Intern Med, 256*(6), 525–28.

Oman, D., Kurata, J. H., Strawbridge, W. J., & Cohen, R. D. (2002). Religious attendance and cause of death over 31 years. *Int J Psychiatry Med, 32*(1), 69–89.

Ortiz, L., & Langer, N. (2002). Assessment of spirituality and religion in later life: Acknowledging clients' needs and personal resources. *J Gerontol Soc Work, 37*(2), 5–21.

Oxman, T. E., Freeman, D. H., & Manheimer, E. D. (1995). Lack of social participation or religious strength and comfort as risk factors for death after cardiac surgery in the elderly. *Psychosom Med, 57*(1), 5–15.

Paloutzian, R. F., & Ellison, C. W. (1982). Loneliness, spiritual well-being, and the quality of life. In L. A. Peplau & D. E. Perlman (Eds.), *Loneliness: A sourcebook of current theory, research, and therapy* (pp. 224–37). New York: Wiley Interscience.

Patel, S. S., Shah, V. S., Peterson, R. A., & Kimmel, P. L. (2002). Psychosocial variables, quality of life, and religious beliefs in ESRD patients treated with hemodialysis. *Am J Kidney Dis, 40*(5), 1013–22.

Pearce, M. J., Rivinoja, C. M., & Koenig, H. G. (2008). Spirituality and health: Empirically based reflections on recovery. *Recent Dev Alcohol, 18*, 187–208.

Peteet, J. R., Lu, F. G., & Narrow, W. E. (2010). *Religious and spiritual issues in psychiatric diagnosis: A research agenda for DSM-V.* Arlington, VA: American Psychiatric Publishing.

Plews-Ogan, M., Owens, J. E., Goodman, M., Wolfe, P., & Schorling, J. (2005). A pilot study evaluating mindfulness-based stress reduction and massage for the management of chronic pain. *J Gen Intern Med, 20*(12), 1136–38.

Poloma, M. M., & Pendleton, B. F. (1991). The effects of prayer and prayer experience on measures of general well-being. *J Psychol Theol, 19*, 71–83.

Poulson, R. L., Eppler, M. A., Satterwhite, T. N., Wuensch, K. L., & Bass, L. A. (1998). Alcohol consumption, strength of religious beliefs, and risky sexual behavior in college students. *J Am Coll Health, 46*(5), 227–32.

Powell, L. H., Shahabi, L., & Thoresen, C. E. (2003). Religion and spirituality. Linkages to physical health. *Am Psychol, 58*(1), 36–52.

Propst, L. R., Ostrom, R., Watkins, P., Dean, T., & Mashburn, D. (1992). Comparative efficacy of religious and nonreligious cognitive-behavioral therapy for the treatment of clinical depression in religious individuals. *J Consult Clin Psychol, 60*(1), 94–103.

Puchalski, C., B. Ferrell, Ferrell, B., Virani, R., Otis-Green, S., Baird, P., Bull, J., . . . & Sulmasy, D. (2009). Improving the quality of spiritual care as a dimension of palliative care: The report of the Consensus Conference. *J Palliat Med, 12*(10), 885–904.

Puchalski, C., & Romer, A. L. (2000). Taking a spiritual history allows clinicians to understand patients more fully. *J Palliat Med, 3*(1), 129–37.

Puchalski, C. M. (2006). Spirituality and medicine: Curricula in medical education. *J Cancer Educ, 21*(1), 14–18.

Puchalski, C. M. (2007–2008). Spirituality and the care of patients at the end-of-life: An essential component of care. *Omega (Westport), 56*(1), 33–46.

Rasanen, J., Kauhanen, J., Lakka, T. A., Kaplan, G. A., & Salonen, J. T. (1996). Religious affiliation and all-cause mortality: A prospective population study in middle-aged men in eastern Finland. *Int J Epidemiol, 25*(6), 1244–49.

Razali, S. M., Hasanah, C. I., Aminah, K., & Subramaniam, M. (1998). Religious-sociocultural psychotherapy in patients with anxiety and depression. *Aust N Z J Psychiatry, 32*(6), 867–72.

Reed, P. G. (1987). Spirituality and well-being in terminally ill hospitalized adults. *Res Nurs Health* 10(5), 335–44.

Richards, P. S., & Bergin, A. E. (1997). *A spiritual strategy for counseling and psychotherapy.* Washington, DC: American Psychological Association Press.

Rogers, T. (1976). Manifestations of religiosity and the aging process. *Religious Education, 71*(4), 405–15.

Roth, B., & Robbins, D. (2004). Mindfulness-based stress reduction and health-related quality of life: Findings from a bilingual inner-city patient population. *Psychosom Med, 66*(1), 113–23.

Rothwell, N. (2006). The different facets of mindfulness. *J Ration Emot Cogn Behav Ther,* 24(1), 79–86.

Ruth, J. E., & Coleman, P. (1996). Personality and aging: Coping and management of the self in later life. In J. E. Birren and K. W. Schaie (Eds.), *Handbook of the psychology of aging,* 4th ed. (pp. 308–22). San Diego: Academic.

Sapp, S. (2010). What have religion and spirituality to do with aging? Three approaches. *Gerontologist, 50*(2), 271–79.

Schenck, D. P., & Roscoe, L. A. (2009). In search of a good death. *J Med Humanit, 30*(1), 61–72.

Seifert, L. (2002). Toward a psychology of religion, spirituality, meaning-search, and aging: Past research and a practical application. *J Adult Dev,* 9(1), 61–70.

Shapiro, S. L., Carlson, L. E., Astin, J. A., & Freedman, B. (2006). Mechanisms of mindfulness. *J Clin Psychol, 62*(3), 373–86.

Solberg, E. E., Berglund, K. A., Engen, O., Ekeberg, O., & Loeb, M. (1996). The effect of meditation on shooting performance. *Br J Sports Med, 30*(4), 342–46.

Stefanek, M., McDonald, P. G., & Hess, S. A. (2004). Religion, spirituality and cancer: Current status and methodological challenges. *Psychooncology, 14*(6), 450–63.

Stewart, C., & Koeske, G. F. (2006). A preliminary construct validation of the multidimensional measurement of religiousness/spirituality instrument: A study of southern USA samples. *Int J Psychol Relig, 16*(3), 181–96.

Tanyi, R. A. (2002). Towards clarification of the meaning of spirituality. *J Adv Nurs, 39*(5), 500–509.

Templer, D. I. (1971). Death anxiety as related to depression and health of retired persons. *J Gerontol, 26*(4), 521–23.

Thibault, J. M. (1993). *A deepening love affair: The gift of God in later life.* Nashville: Upper Room.

Tornstam, L. (1989). Gero-transcendence: A reformulation of the disengagement theory. *Aging (Milano), 1*(1), 55–63.

Tornstam, L. (1996). Gerotranscendence—a theory about maturing into old age. *Journal of Aging and Identity, 1,*37–50.

Townsend, M., Kladder, V., Ayele, H., & Mulligan, T. (2002). Systematic review of clinical trials examining the effects of religion on health. *South Med J, 95*(12), 1429–34.

Turner, R. P., Lukoff, D., Barnhouse, R. T., & Lu, F. G. (1995). Religious or spiritual problem. A culturally sensitive diagnostic category in the DSM-IV. *J Nerv Ment Dis, 183*(7), 435–44.

Underwood, L. G., & Teresi, J. A. (2002). The daily spiritual experience scale: Development, theoretical description, reliability, exploratory factor analysis, and preliminary construct validity using health-related data. *Ann Behav Med, 24*(1), 22–33.

VandeCreek, L., Benes, S., & Nye, C. (1993). Assessment of pastoral needs among medical outpatients. *J Pastoral Care, 47*(1), 44–53.

VandeCreek, L., Frankowski, D., & Ayres, S. (1994). Use of the Threat Index with family members waiting during surgery. *Death Stud, 18*(6), 641–48.

Van Montfrans, G. A., Karemaker, J. M., Wieling, W., & Dunning, A. J. (1990). Relaxation therapy and continuous ambulatory blood pressure in mild hypertension: A controlled study. *BMJ, 300*(6736), 1368–72.

Van Poppel, F., Schellekens, J., & Liefbroer, A. C. (2002). Religious differentials in infant and child mortality in Holland, 1855–1912. *Popul Studies (Camb), 56*(3), 277–89.

Wadensten, B., & Carlsson, M. (2003). Theory-driven guidelines for practical care of older people, based on the theory of gerotranscendence. *J Adv Nurs, 41*(5), 462–70.

Walsh, A. (1998). Religion and hypertension: Testing alternative explanations among immigrants. *Behav Med, 24*(3), 122–30.

Williams, D. R., Larson, D. B., Buckler, R. E., Heckmann, R. C., & Pyle, C. M. (1991). Religion and psychological distress in a community sample. *Soc Sci Med, 32*(11), 1257–62.

Yoon, D. P., & Lee, E. K. (2007). The impact of religiousness, spirituality, and social support on psychological well-being among older adults in rural areas. *J Gerontol Soc Work, 48*(3–4), 281–98.

Young, J. D., & Taylor, E. (2001). Meditation as a voluntary hypometabolic state of biological estivation. *News Physiol Sci, 13,*149–53.

Zinnbauer, B. J., & Pargament, K. I. (2002). Capturing the meanings of religiousness and spirituality: One way down from a definitional Tower of Babel. *Research in the Social Scientific Study of Religion, 13,* 23–54.

Zinnbauer, B. J., Pargament, K. I., Cole, B., Rye, M. S., Butter, E. M., Belavich, T. G., . . . & Kadar, J. L. (1997). Religion and spirituality: Unfuzzying the fuzzy. *J Sci Study Relig, 36*(4), 549–64.

CHAPTER 8

Social Models of Promoting Resilience

To date, studies of adult resilience have originated from two research traditions. The long-standing tradition is the coping and stress research of the 1970s; the more recent trend was spurred by the events of September 11, 2001, and shifted the mental health community toward focusing on resilience-building interventions. Emergency mental health hotlines, programs for free screenings, and short-term counseling spread across the country. Mental health workers became one coherent community highly motivated to take care of the after-effects of the attacks.

Even though changes in therapeutic techniques that emphasized coping and resilience coincided with the 9/11 attacks, they were preceded by work on dialectical behavior therapy (DBT). Linehan (1993a, 1993b) recognized that a treatment focused on change would not work with chronically suicidal patients, whose exceeding sensitivity to criticism easily resulted in emotional dysregulation. Therapy was simply not possible without addressing the emotional dysregulation (Cloitre, Koenen, Cohen, L. R., & Han 2002). Najavits and colleagues (1998) applied cognitive behavioral therapy (CBT) to patients with post-traumatic stress disorder (PTSD) and substance abuse, also utilizing mindfulness and skill-building approaches. Some resilience-building techniques used as part of psychotherapeutic approaches are described in table 8.1.

Resilience-Building Interventions in Older Adults

The newer trend of developing interventions for older adults emphasizes their strengths and coping skills. Civic engagement has received attention both among academics and in the press. As health and education of older

TABLE 8.1   Therapeutic approaches to building resilience

Personal resilience as target	Therapeutic approach
Positive emotions Optimism, hope, humor, flexibility	Decrease stress-related illness, mood, and arousal; increase well-being and health, hope, adaptation (Affleck & Tennen 1996; Carver, Scheier, & Weintraub 1989; Folkman & Moskowitz 2000; Fredrickson 2001; Snyder, Rand, & Sigmon 2002)
Sense of control Locus of control, self-esteem, commitment, challenges, spiritual beliefs	Increased sense of internal locus of control can improve hardiness and decrease risk for post-traumatic stress disorder (Florian, Mikulincer, & Taubman 1995; King et al. 1998; Soet, Brack, & DiIorio 2003)
Active coping Task-focused versus emotion-focused versus avoidant coping, passive coping, facing fear, adaptation	Task-oriented coping versus denial, victimhood; courage, emotional coping, mastery, self-efficacy (Beaton et al. 1999; Johnsen et al. 2002; Regehr, Hill, & Glancy 2000; Stanton, Parsa, & Austenfeld 2002)
Cognitive flexibility Cognitive reframing, shift in perception and explanations, acceptance	Improved tolerance of stress, redefining stresses as challenges, "lessons," rebuilding assumptive world, acceptance of hardship and illness; life is an ongoing lesson (Manne et al. 2003; Schaefer & Moos 1992, 1998; Seligman 2002; Seligman et al. 1988; Southwick, Vythilingam, & Charney 2005; Wade et al. 2001)
Finding meaning and purpose Post-traumatic growth, learning from crises and adversity	Discovering purpose in life at life transitions
Altruism Survivor mission, empathy and compassion	Successful adaptation, activism based on tragedy, guiding principles (Bleuler 1984; Midlarsky 1991; Rachman 1979)
Spirituality Moral compass, religious coping	Physical and emotional survival, health, less depression, core beliefs (Koenig, George, & Peterson 1998; Koenig, George, & Titus 2004; McCullough et al. 2000;)
Training Previous experience of trauma	Training in stoicism, stressors, torture, emergency work, foster adaptation, positive thinking, resilience (Alvarez & Hunt 2005)

SOURCE: Adapted from Kent & Davis 2010

adults continues to improve, the opportunities for civic engagement also grow. Given the ability to achieve, retain, or regain a level of emotional or physical health after a loss or an illness, civic engagement can help reestablish a balance between self and personal contributions to community.

Civic engagement has many definitions (see www.civicengagement.org), but the common meaning is taking part in activities that have consequences for communities or for policymaking. Two spheres of participation are the political and the social. Political engagement refers to behaviors influencing governmental processes on the local, state, national, and even international levels; social engagement refers to actions that connect individuals and relate to care or personal development (Wuthnow 1991). In both spheres, actions are freely chosen and include mutual aid, volunteerism, and civic service.

Older Americans have a long history of volunteering. In 2008, 61.3% of people over age 55 years (which represents about 27% of the U.S. population) volunteered in various ways, according to the Corporation for National and Community Service (2009). Health issues contribute to declining rates of volunteering after age 75 (AARP 2003). However, once in volunteer roles, older adults commit more time to their volunteer activities, reporting a median of 96 hours a year, while those 45 to 54 years old report 50 hours a year and those 55 to 64 years old report 56 hours (U.S. Bureau of Labor Statistics 2009).

Evidence suggests that volunteering improves physical health, mental health, and socialization, and that it is protective in the face of loss and other life challenges. Volunteering has been associated with many positive outcomes for older adults (Grimm, Spring, & Dietz 2007), including reduced mortality (Musick, Herzog, & House 1999), increased physical function (Moen, Dempster-Mclain, & Williams 1992; Lum & Lightfoot 2005), and increased levels of self-rated health. Morrow-Howell and colleagues (2003) found reduced depressive symptomatology (Musick et al. 1999; Musick & Wilson 2003), reduced pain (Arnstein, Vidal, Wells-Federman, Morgan, & Caudill 2002), higher self-esteem (Omoto, Snyder, & Martino 2000), and greater satisfaction with life in general (Van Willigen 2000), thus documenting greater well-being over time.

According to the AARP, in 2008 as many as 68% of older Americans reported having performed some type of service, formal or informal (Koppen 2009). Another estimate comes from the Health and Retirement Survey, where about 33% of respondents aged 55 years or older reported participation in formal volunteerism, while 52% reported engagement in informal volunteerism (Zedlewski & Schaner 2005). Indeed, a full accounting of the helping activities of older adults must look beyond the boundaries of formal volunteering (Rozario 2007).

Volunteering-focused experimental studies have been emerging since the early 2000s. Fried and colleagues (2004) at Johns Hopkins University completed a randomized trial to evaluate the effects of participating in the Experience Corps (EC), a high-commitment volunteer program in which older adults perform service in elementary schools. In this study, 149 new recruits to the program were assigned to EC or to a wait list. Compared to the wait-list controls, EC volunteers reported increased physical strength and an increase in the number of people they could turn to for help. They also showed less decline in walking speed (Fried et al. 2004) and a trend toward improved cognitive function (Carlson et al. 2008). EC participants also reported being more physically active (Tan, Xue, Li, Carlson, & Fried 2006). In another study of the health effects of participation in the EC program, EC participants were matched with a comparison group from the Health and Retirement Study sample. At baseline the two groups were equal on health status and volunteer history; two years later EC participants reported fewer depressive symptoms and fewer functional limitations—and the effect sizes were substantial (Morrow-Howell, Hong, & Tang 2009).

Role theory helps explain the beneficial effect of volunteering. By assuming the role of volunteer, individuals often gain access to resources, social contacts, status, and recognition (Moen et al. 1992). A study of volunteering in Israel suggested that volunteering has positive effects above and beyond those reaped from activities such as physical exercise and hobbies (Shmotkin, Blumstein, & Modan 2003). Volunteering may provide unique opportunities for older adults, who report more gains, satisfaction, and improvement in depression compared to younger volunteers (Omoto et al. 2000; Van Willigen 2000). Midlarsky (1991) suggested that volunteering may substitute for paid work; Moen (1995) indicated that it may contribute to social connections that might otherwise diminish after retirement.

Volunteering and Resilience

The literature on the positive effects of volunteering for the physical and mental health, self-esteem, social connections, and life satisfaction among older adults suggests that volunteering is related to resiliency in several ways. For one thing, volunteering increases the potential for an adult to be resilient when faced with adversity and may serve as a coping strategy in the recovery process. As summarized by Musick and Wilson (2003), volunteering increases the personal and social resources of an individual. These resources are part of an individual's capacity to make a "psychosocial comeback." Moreover, individuals with fewer personal and social resources may be at greater risk for difficulties in recovering from an adverse event. That is, they may be more vulnerable and less resilient. Research suggests these same individuals may benefit far more from volunteering than those with more social interaction. For example, Musick and colleagues (1999) found that older adults with less social interaction experienced a greater protective effect from volunteering than those with more social interaction. Morrow-Howell et al. (2003) found that older adults with functional limitations benefited more from volunteering than those who are more functional. Less-educated and lower-income older adults report more benefits from volunteering than their better-educated and higher-income counterparts, including better health, improved self-esteem, increased socialization, and greater intellectual and practical generativity (Morrow-Howell et al. 2009). In sum, it appears that volunteers who are vulnerable to poorer quality-of-life outcomes, especially in the face of loss and other challenges, benefit the most from volunteering. Thus, volunteering can be a strategy to bolster resources that better prepare one for losses or crises.

Finally, volunteering might serve as a specific coping technique that an adult can utilize in response to adversity or as a way to recover after a crisis or loss. Volunteering can provide a means to deal with emotional needs or feelings of uselessness, and individuals report that their volunteer work is therapeutic (Musick & Wilson 2008). After the loss of a spouse, volunteering can help a person adjust to bereavement and protect against depressive symptoms (Li & Ferraro 2007). Brown and associates (2008) studied the effects of helping behavior on recovery from spousal loss and found that bereaved individual who engaged in helping others experienced a more rapid improvement in depression than those who did not, even after controlling for social support and health.

Given the potential of volunteering to increase the health and resiliency of our aging population, policymakers and program leaders increasingly are interested in strategies to maximize the involvement of older adults in volunteer activities.

Federal and State Government Programs

The federal government currently supports a variety of volunteer programs targeting older adults. Most prominent are the three national Senior Corps programs: the Foster Grandparent Program, the Senior Companion Program, and the Retired and Senior Volunteer Program (RSVP). Together these programs deploy over half a million older Americans in service to their communities each year (Eisner, Grimm, Maynard, & Washburn 2009).

The Foster Grandparent Program is Senior Corps' oldest program, dating back the 1960s (Freedman 1999). The Senior Companion Program pays a small stipend to low-income adults age 60 and over who serve as mentors, tutors, and caregivers for disadvantaged or disabled youth. RSVP is the newest program for promoting the engagement of seniors; it offers adults age 55 and older a diverse range of service activities, including organizing neighborhood watch programs, tutoring children, building homes, and assisting victims of natural disasters (Morrow-Howell et al. 2011).

The Senior Environmental Employment Program administered by the Environmental Protection Agency (EPA) provides an opportunity for retired and unemployed Americans age 55 and over to remain active, using their skills in meaningful tasks that support a wide variety of EPA's environmental goals. The Experience Corps Program, which began as a national demonstration project under the auspices of the Corporation for National and Community Service (CNCS) in 1995, supports adults age 55 and older who work in teams for at least 15 hours per week to tutor and mentor elementary school students, help teachers in the classroom, and lead after-school enrichment activities. Today the program operates in 23 cities with varied funding: from AmeriCorps (the national service program administered by CNCS); from state and local public and private funds; and from private foundations and in-kind donations.

Nonprofit organizations have spearheaded innovative efforts to create opportunities for volunteering, employment, life-long learning, advocacy, and public service in later life (e.g., "civic enterprise" at http://civicengagement .org). Other service networks include:

- Networks of retired healthcare professionals working in free clinics (e.g., Volunteers in Medicine);
- Networks of pro bono business consultants for nonprofits, schools, and government agencies (e.g., the Taproot Foundation);
- Faith-based initiatives to engage older adults in civic work (e.g., Shepherd's Centers, Faith in Action);
- National campaigns to advance federal and social innovation awards for individuals age 60 and older who have demonstrated vision and entrepreneurialism in addressing community and national problems (e.g., Civic Ventures Purpose Prize);

- Awards for employers and organizations creating pathways to social-impact work in the second half of life (Encore Opportunity Award);
- Clearinghouse-type organizations that facilitate the link between older adults and volunteering opportunities (e.g., Volunteer Match); and
- Initiatives to help working or retired adults transition into new careers in the public sector (Partnership for Public Service), non-profit sector (e.g., ReServe, the Transition Network, Bridgestar, Executive Service Corps), or international service (e.g., Encore!, Service Corps International, International Senior Lawyers Project).

In addition, three major nonprofit national professional associations in the aging field—the American Society on Aging (ASA), the Gerontological Society of America (GSA), and the National Council on Aging (NCOA)—recently have made civic engagement a focus of their programmatic research and policy efforts.

Policy, Politics, and the Changing Demographics of Baby Boomers

A doubling of the population of seniors in the coming decades and prolonged life spans will dictate necessary changes to governmental policies concerning retirement, Medicare eligibility age, continuous employment, and tax laws. The aging population of baby boomers in general is not interested in passive retirement; correspondingly, interest in civic engagement, part-time employment, and playing active roles in society is growing rapidly. In 2005, civic engagement was a focus of the fifth White House Conference on Aging. Among the 50 policy recommendations that delegates voted to bring forward, two were related to civic engagement. The first called for a national strategy to promote meaningful volunteer activities for older Americans; the second was a resolution calling for renewal of the laws that authorize national service programs (O'Neill 2007). One of the delegates' major policy goals was achieved in late 2006, when President Bush signed into law a five-year reauthorization of the Older Americans Act (H.R. 6197). This law (1) defined "civic engagement"; (2) required that the Assistant Secretary for Aging develop a comprehensive strategic plan for engaging older adults in meeting critical community needs; and (3) authorized a new program of demonstration, support, and research grants for projects that engage older adults in multigenerational and civic-engagement activities.

At the state level, new efforts to engage older adults in volunteer work have emerged as well. In 2007, California governor Arnold Schwarzenegger launched the EnCorps Teachers program, an initiative that recruits skilled, soon-to-be-retired employees to serve as math and science teachers in secondary schools. In 2008, California and New York were the first two states to create cabinet-level positions for service and volunteering, giving volunteers a more powerful voice. Facing tight budgets, states are experimenting with various other incentives to promote community volunteer opportunities. In several states, local districts offer residents over age 60 the opportunity to volunteer in schools and earn a modest tax credit against their property taxes (the Senior Tax Exchange Program, e.g., www.sunprairie.k12.wi.us/district/step_program.cfm).

In 2008, the 110th Congress also introduced and approved new bills: GIVE (Generations Invigorating Volunteerism and Education Act, H.R. 5366), the Encore Service Act (S. 3480), and the Serve America Act (S. 3487). Members of the U.S. House and Senate laid out their visions for service by Americans of all ages. In 2009, President Obama signed into law the Edward M. Kennedy Serve America Act of 2009—the largest expansion of national service programs since the depression-era Civilian Conservation Corps (Public Law 111-13 [H.R. 1388]). The act has several provisions that specifically benefit midlife and older adults. The law, in effect as of October 2009, establishes an Encore Fellowship program for individuals 55 years or older to serve in leadership or management positions in public or private nonprofit organizations for one year; it targets 10% of AmeriCorps funds for organizations that enroll adults age 55 and older; and it creates Silver Scholarships that provide a $1,000 higher-education award—transferable to children, foster children, and grandchildren—to older volunteers who contribute at least 350 hours of service per year. The law also requires the nation's 50 State Commissions on National and Community Service to complete detailed plans to recruit and leverage the resources of the baby boom generation. In addition, it expands service options for older Americans by lowering the age requirement for the Foster Grandparent and Senior Companion programs from 60 to 55 and increasing the hourly stipend eligibility requirement from 125% of the federal poverty level to 200%.

Evaluation of a program's accomplishments, as done by Senior Corps, is becoming ever-more important for continuous functioning (see www.nationalservice.gov/programs/senior-corps for a list of past research on program impacts).

Incentivized Resilience-Building Programs for Older Adults

The federal government can encourage more volunteering by helping to remove barriers such as transportation costs, competing caregiving demands, and limitations from chronic conditions. For instance, volunteers provide critical driving services to those who cannot otherwise conduct personal errands or get to and from medical appointments or other activities, yet individuals and nonprofit organizations must carry the cost of liability insurance. Driving services could be expanded if the Good Samaritan Laws were broadened to include volunteer drivers (Morrow-Howell et al. 2011).

Policymakers also can make use of rewards and incentives to encourage activities that benefit the public. Research suggests that small incentives such as education credits, access to group health insurance, or a modest monthly stipend might reap large benefits by attracting more participants into community service (Bridgeland, Putnam, & Wofford 2008). Going forward, policy experts have recommended that the president charge a national commission to develop a "blueprint" for tapping the time, energy, and talents of millions of older adults to strengthen America's communities. The commission might explore how tax, pension, education, retraining, and healthcare policies could be reformed to maximize the involvement of older adults and baby boomers (Gomperts 2007). The commission also might highlight existing individual and organizational role models and develop strategies for translating the most promising ideas into wider practice.

The corporate sector, too, can play an important role. Almost 70% of America's volunteers are part of the labor force (U.S. Bureau of Labor Statistics 2009). Volunteering peaks in midlife, not retirement. Therefore, the workplace is an ideal location to connect with potential volunteers, including future retirees. For example, IBM trains some of its most experienced employees to become fully accredited teachers in their local communities upon leaving the company. Moreover, policymakers might offer subsidies, tax credits, and other incentives to encourage businesses to create volunteer-time policies, such as paid and unpaid leave for volunteering (Gerontological Society of America 2005).

Conclusion

Research suggests that volunteering and civic engagement offer benefits for increasing resilience in older adults by providing purposeful living and community involvement. Efforts are under way to expand the availability and diversity of volunteering roles for older adults while policymakers are figuring out new infrastructure supports and more effective outreach programs, on both local and federal levels. The resilience process builds individual strengths and competencies. Through personal connections, older adults learn from others about their potentials and gifts; this awareness increases their self-efficacy and perseverance in the face of adversity. The meaningful relationships they have with friends and family provide them with resources to adapt to adversity, and their engagement in meaningful activities gives them a sense of purpose and the motivation to persevere and continue to learn. As a result, resilient older adults have a positive attitude and a forward-looking outlook that we should promote in all populations.

Baby boomers hold vast potential to leverage their skills, education, and experience to solve society's most challenging problems; policies and programs must continue to evolve in order to capitalize on this singular opportunity. For a first step, spreading the word about existing programs will help our older patients search for opportunities to contribute to their communities and maintain purposeful living. Clearinghouses and helpful Web sites can inform patients and caregivers about such existing opportunities. This area requires more research to accurately inform program and policy development in civic engagement.

Although we have accumulated evidence that civic engagement is good for older adults, we lack research to determine what programs and policy initiatives will maximize their engagement. We still need research that seeks to identify (1) the volunteer behaviors and motivations of the baby boom generation; (2) effective strategies to mobilize baby boomers and other older adults; (3) "best practices" for volunteer program structures and designs that will attract and support older volunteers; and (4) the extent of inclusion of diverse older adults by ethnicity and ranges of education, income, and functional abilities.

At the same time, outcomes research that tracks the economic impact of civic engagement will be critical in building support among legislators. To attract and retain older adult volunteers, we also need to develop strategies to support capacity-building by nonprofit groups. Researchers have observed that most nonprofit groups are not prepared for the challenge of engaging large numbers of older adults in meaningful volunteer roles (Casner-Lotto 2007; Eisner et al. 2009). Older volunteers generally are seen in low-skill service positions rather than in professional or leadership roles (National Council on Aging 2006). Nonprofit groups should be encouraged to invest more resources in senior-volunteer management and recognition—and to create more opportunities for highly skilled older volunteers to play a role in their operations.

References

AARP. (2003). *A synthesis of member volunteer experience.* Washington, DC: AARP.

Affleck, G., & Tennen, H. (1996). Construing benefits from adversity: Adaptational significance and dispositional underpinnings. *J Pers, 64*(4), 899–922.

Alvarez, J., & Hunt, M. (2005). Risk and resilience in canine search and rescue handlers after 9/11. *J Trauma Stress, 18*(5), 497–505.

Arnstein, P., Vidal, M., Wells-Federman, C., Morgan, B., & Caudill, M. (2002). From chronic pain patient to peer: Benefits and risks of volunteering. *Pain Manag Nurs, 3*(3), 94–103.

Beaton, R., Murphy, S., Johnson, C., Pike, K., & Corneil, W. (1999). Coping responses and posttraumatic stress symptomatology in urban fire service personnel. *J Trauma Stress, 12*(2), 293–308.

Bleuler, M. (1984). Different forms of childhood stress and patterns of adult psychiatric outcome. In N. F. Watt et al. (Eds.), *Children at risk for schizophrenia: A longitudinal perspective* (pp. 537–42). Cambridge: Cambridge University Press.

Bridgeland, J. M., Putnam, R. D., & Wofford, H. L. (2008). *More to give: Tapping the talents of the baby boomer, silent, and greatest generations.* Washington, DC: AARP. http://assets.aarp.org/rgcenter/general/moretogive.pdf.

Brown, S. L., Brown, R. M., House, J. S., & Smith, D. M. (2008). Coping with spousal loss: Potential buffering effects of self-reported helping behavior. *Pers Soc Psychol Bull, 34*(6), 849–61.

Carlson, M. C., Saczynski, J. S., Rebok, G. W., Seeman, T., Glass, T. A., McGill, S., . . . & Fried, L. P. (2008). Exploring the effects of an "everyday" activity program on executive function and memory in older adults: Experience Corps. *Gerontologist, 48*(6), 793–801.

Carver, C. S., Scheier, M. F., & Weintraub, J. K. (1989). Assessing coping strategies: A theoretically based approach. *J Pers Soc Psychol, 56*(2), 267–83.

Casner-Lotto, J. (2007). Boomers are ready for nonprofits, but are nonprofits ready for them? New York: Conference Board.

Cloitre, M., Koenen, K. C., Cohen, L. R., & Han, H. (2002). Skills training in affective and interpersonal regulation followed by exposure: A phase-based treatment for PTSD related to childhood abuse. *J Consult Clin Psychol, 70*(5), 1067–74.

Corporation for National and Community Service. (2009). *Volunteering and Civic Engagement in the United States.* Retrieved from www.volunteeringin america.gov/national.

Eisner, D., Grimm Jr., R. T., Maynard, S., & Washburn, S. (2009). The new volunteer workforce. *Stanford Social Innovation Review* (Winter), 32–37.

Florian, V., Mikulincer, M., & Taubman, O. (1995). Does hardiness contribute to mental health during a stressful real-life situation? The roles of appraisal and coping. *J Pers Soc Psychol, 68*(4), 687–95.

Folkman, S., & Moskowitz, J. T. (2000). Positive affect and the other side of coping. *Am Psychol, 55*(6), 647–54.

Fredrickson, B. L. (2001). The role of positive emotions in positive psychology. The broaden-and-build theory of positive emotions. *Am Psychol, 56*(3), 218–26.

Freedman, M. (1999). Prime time: How baby boomers will revolutionize retirement and transform America. New York: Public Affairs.

Fried, L. P., Carlson, M. C., Freedman, M. M., Frick, K. D., Glass, T. A., Hill, M. J., . . . & Zeger, S. (2004). A social model for health promotion for an aging population: Initial evidence on the Experience Corps model. *J Urban Health, 81*(1), 64–78.

Gerontological Society of America. (2005). *Civic engagement in an older America*. Retrieved from www.civicengagement.org/agingsociety/links/GSAfocus group_summary.pdf.

Gomperts, J. S. (2007). Toward a bold new policy agenda: Five ideas to advance civic engagement opportunities for older Americans. *Generations, 30*(4), 85–89.

Grimm, R., Spring, K., & Dietz, N. (2007). *The health benefits of volunteering: A review of recent research*. Corporation for National and Community Service.

Johnsen, B. H., Eid, J., Laberg, J. C., & Thayer, J. F. (2002). The effect of sensitization and coping style on post-traumatic stress symptoms and quality of life: Two longitudinal studies. *Scand J Psychol, 43*(2), 181–88.

Kent, M., & Davis, M. C. (2010). The emergence of capacity-building programs and models of resilience. In J. W. Reich, A. J. Zautra, & J. S. Hall (Eds.), *Handbook of adult resilience* (pp. 427–49). New York: Guilford Press.

King, L. A., King, D. W., Fairbank, J. A., Keane, T. M., & Adams, G. A. (1998). Resilience-recovery factors in post-traumatic stress disorder among female and male Vietnam veterans: Hardiness, postwar social support, and additional stressful life events. *J Pers Soc Psychol, 74*(2), 420–34.

Koenig, H. G., George, L. K., & Peterson, B. L. (1998). Religiosity and remission of depression in medically ill older patients. *Am J Psychiatry, 155*(4), 536–42.

Koenig, H. G., George, L. K., & Titus, P. (2004). Religion, spirituality, and health in medically ill hospitalized older patients. *J Am Geriatr Soc, 52*(4), 554–62.

Koppen, J. (2009). Volunteering perceptions and realities: A national survey of adults aged 18+. Washington, DC: AARP.

Li, Y., & Ferraro, K. F. (2007). Recovering from spousal bereavement in later life: Does volunteer participation play a role? *J Gerontol B Psychol Sci Soc Sci, 62*(4), S257–66.

Linehan, M. M. (1993a). Cognitive behavioral treatment for borderline personality disorder. New York: Guilford.

Linehan, M. M. (1993b). Skills training manual for treating borderline personality disorder. New York: Guilford.

Lum, T. Y., & Lightfoot, E. (2005). The effects of volunteering on the physical and mental health of older people. *Res Aging, 27*(1), 31–55.

Manne, S., Duhamel, K., Ostroff, J., Parsons, S., Martini, D. R., Williams, S. E., . . . & Redd, W. H. (2003). Coping and the course of mother's depressive symptoms during and after pediatric bone marrow transplantation. *J Am Acad Child Adolesc Psychiatry,* 42(9), 1055–68.

McCullough, M. E., Hoyt, W. T., Larson, D. B., Koenig, H. G., & Thoresen, C. (2000). Religious involvement and mortality: A meta-analytic review. *Health Psychol,* 19(3), 211–22.

Midlarsky, E. (1991). Helping as coping. In M. Clark (Ed.), *Prosocial behavior* (pp. 238–64). Newbury Park, CA: Sage.

Moen, P. (1995). A life course approach to post-retirement roles and well-being. In S. C. L. Bond, & A. Grams (Eds.), *Promoting successful and productive aging* (pp. 239–56). Thousand Oaks, CA: Sage.

Moen, P., Dempster-McClain, D., & Williams Jr., R. M. (1992). Successful aging: A life-course perspective on women's multiple roles and health. *Am J Sociol,* 97(6), 1612–38.

Morrow-Howell, N., Hinterlong, J., Rozario, P. A., & Tang, F. (2003). Effects of volunteering on the well-being of older adults. *J Gerontol B Psychol Sci Soc Sci,* 58(3), S137–45.

Morrow-Howell, N., Hong, S. I., & Tang, F. (2009). Who benefits from volunteering? Variations in perceived benefits. *Gerontologist,* 49(1), 91–102.

Morrow-Howell, N., O'Neill, G., & Greenfield, J. C. (2011). Civic engagement: Policies and programs to support a resilient aging society. In B. Resnick, L. P. Gwyther, & K. A. Roberto (Eds.), *Resilience in aging: Concepts, research, and outcomes* (pp. 147–62). New York: Springer.

Musick, M. A., Herzog, A. R., & House, J. S. (1999). Volunteering and mortality among older adults: Findings from a national sample. *J Gerontol B Psychol Sci Soc Sci,* 54(3), S173–80.

Musick, M. A., & Wilson, J. (2003). Volunteering and depression: The role of psychological and social resources in different age groups. *Soc Sci Med,* 56(2), 259–69.

Musick, M. A., & Wilson, J. (2008). *Volunteers.* Bloomington: Indiana University Press.

Najavits, L. M., Gastfriend, D. R., Barber, J. P., Reif, S., Muenz, L. R., Blaine, J., . . . & Weiss, R. D. (1998). Cocaine dependence with and without PTSD among subjects in the National Institute on Drug Abuse Collaborative Cocaine Treatment Study. *Am J Psychiatry,* 155(2), 214–19.

National Council on Aging. (2006). *Respectability in America: Promsing practices in civic engagement among adults 55+.* Retrieved from www.ncoa.org /Downloads/PromisingPracticesReport.pdf.

Omoto, A. M., Snyder, M., & Martino, S. C. (2000). Volunteerism and the life course: Investigating age-related agendas for action. *Basic Appl Soc Psych,* 22(3), 181–97.

O'Neill, G. (2007). Civic engagement on the agenda at the 2005 White Hour Conference on Aging. *Generations, 30*(4), 101–8.

Rachman, S. (1979). The concept of required helpfulness. *Behav Res Ther, 17*(1), 1–6.

Regehr, C., Hill, J., & Glancy, G. D. (2000). Individual predictors of traumatic reactions in firefighters. *J Nerv Ment Dis, 188*(6), 333–39.

Rozario, P. A. (2007). Volunteering among current cohorts of older adults and baby boomers. *Generations, 30*(4), 31–36.

Schaefer, J. A., & Moos, R. H. (1992). Life crisis and personal growth. In B. N. Carpenter (Eds.), *Personal coping: Theory, research, and application* (pp. 149–70). Westport, CT: Praeger.

Schaefer, J. A., & Moos, R. H. (1998). The context for posttraumatic growth: Life crises, individual and social resources, and coping. In I. B. Weinger (Eds.), *Posttraumatic growth: Positive changes in the aftermath of crisis* (pp. 99–125). Mahwah, NJ: Erlbaum.

Seligman, M. E. P. (2002). *Authentic happiness*. New York: Free Press.

Seligman, M. E. P., Castellon, C., Cacciola, J., Schulman, P., Luborsky, L., Ollove, M., & Downing, R. (1988). Explanatory style change during cognitive therapy for unipolar depression. *J Abnorm Psychol, 97*(1), 13–18.

Shmotkin, D., Blumstein, T., & Modan, B. (2003). Beyond keeping active: Concomitants of being a volunteer in old-old age. *Psychol Aging, 18*(3), 602–7.

Snyder, C. R., Rand, K. L., & Sigmon, D. R. (2002). Hope theory: A member of the positive psychology family. In C. R. Snyder & S. J. Lopez (Eds.), *Handbook of positive psychology* (pp. 257–76). New York: Oxford University Press.

Soet, J. E., Brack, G. A., & DiIorio, C. (2003). Prevalence and predictors of women's experience of psychological trauma during childbirth. *Birth, 30*(1), 36–46.

Southwick, S. M., & Charney, D. S. (2012). *Resilience: The science of mastering life's greatest challenges*. New York: Cambridge University Press.

Southwick, S. M., Vythilingam, M., & Charney, D. S. (2005). The psychobiology of depression and resilience to stress: Implications for prevention and treatment. *Annu Rev Clin Psychol, 1*, 255–91.

Stanton, A. L., Parsa, A., & Austenfeld, J. L. (2002). The adaptive potential of coping through emotional approach. In C. R. Snyder & S. J. Lopez (Eds.), *Handbook of positive psychology* (pp. 148–58). New York, Oxford University Press.

Tan, E. J., Xue, Q. L., Li, T., Carlson, M. C., & Fried, L. P. (2006). Volunteering: A physical activity intervention for older adults—The Experience Corps program in Baltimore. *J Urban Health, 83*(5), 954–69.

U.S. Bureau of Labor Statistics (2009). *Volunteering in the United States, 2008*. Washington, DC: U.S. Department of Labor.

Van Willigen, M. (2000). Differential benefits of volunteering across the life course. *J Gerontol B Psychol Sci Soc Sci, 55*(5), S308–18.

Wade, S. L., Borawski, E. A., Taylor, H. G., Drotar, D., Yeates, K. O., & Stancin, T. (2001). The relationship of caregiver coping to family outcomes during the initial year following pediatric traumatic injury. *J Consult Clin Psychol, 69*(3), 406–15.

Wuthnow, R. (1991). *Act of compassion.* Princeton, NJ: Princeton University Press.

Zedlewski, S. R., & Schaner, S. G. (2005). Older adults' engagement should be recognized and encouraged. In *The retirement project: Perspectives on productive aging.* Washington, DC: Urban Institute.

CHAPTER 9

Cultural and Ethnic Factors in Understanding and Building Resilience

CULTURAL CONTEXT INVOLVES shared systems of beliefs consisting of learned behaviors and meanings that are socially transferred in various life-activity settings for purposes of individual and collective adjustment and adaptation (Marsella, Johnson, Watson, & Gryczynski 2008b). The cultural context in which we are brought up shapes our realities by contributing to our worldviews, perceptions, and orientations with ideas, morals, and preferences (Marsella 2005). Culture is transmitted generation to generation; it is shaped by various inside and outside contexts and dynamics. This system of meaning comprises norms, beliefs, and values that both prescribe and proscribe behavior.

Effects of Cultural Context of Trauma and Individual Coping

Cultural context is immediately related to recovery from trauma. Since traumatic experience intimately involves reconstruction of meaning, consideration of resiliency must take into account a person's specific cultural norms, beliefs, and values, and cultural dynamics (e.g., the subject's culture of origin and the extent of the subject's acculturation or level of ethnic identification). Further, factors associated with ethnicity and culture strongly influence an individual's resilience, determining coping styles, cognitive responses to stress, experience of distress, and clusters of symptoms, as well as psychiatric outcomes (Charney et al. 2002). Hansen (2002) recommended consideration of multicultural competencies, such as the cultural context of the manifestation of mental illness and wellness, as dynamics of resilience or risk.

The specific type of cultural and societal context can shape the meaning of traumatic experiences. For example, American individualism correlates with high levels of stress, requiring increased awareness and coping (Lazarus & Folkman 1984), unlike in other more collectivism-oriented cultures (Bell 2011; Chun, Moos, & Cronkite 2006; Triandis 1995). Individualism and collective elements (Triandis 1995) are a set of values, attitudes, and behaviors that vary based on the value placed on the individual versus the group. Accordingly, individual freedoms, rights, and privileges are of utmost importance to many Americans. In collectivistic cultures, by contrast, the main emphasis is placed on the group's values, which can change the meaning of traumatic events and the locus of control (Chun et al. 2006). Cross-cultural studies show differences in the experience of locus of control in individuals from cultures like European Americans and New Zealanders, who tend to have a stronger sense of internal locus of control than individuals from collectivistic cultures, such as the Japanese (Bond & Tornatzky 1973; Mahler 1974), the Chinese (Hamid 1994), Asian Indians (Chandler, Shama, Wolf, & Planchard 1982), and individuals from Zambia and Zimbabwe (Munro 1979). Some authors have noted that cultural, racial, and ethnic minorities are more adversely affected by various traumas (Bell 2011; Bell et al. 2008; Norris & Alegria 2008). For example, Latinos and non-Hispanic blacks were more adversely affected by Hurricane Andrew than were non-Hispanic whites (Perilla, Norris, & Lavizzo 2002). Alternatively, Ryff, Keyes, and Hughes (2003) observed that blacks report higher levels of psychological well-being than whites, after controlling for education, income, perceived discrimination, and demographic variables. Keyes (2007) found also that African American women have the lowest suicide rates in the United States, which may have to do with their spiritual beliefs and upbringing counterbalancing the trauma of discrimination.

Hardiness is another concept that is close to resilience (Maddi & Harvey 2006). The notion of hardiness is present in all cultural, racial, and ethnic groups; it can be considered a generic aspect of human nature (Maddi & Harvey 2006). "Hardy attitudes" include commitment, control, and willingness to face challenges; "hardy skills" involve interacting with significant others in a fashion that enhances one's sense of social support. In other words, hardiness involves self-care aimed at maintaining "hardy coping" and social interactions. Self-efficacy, ego strength, optimism, resilience, post-traumatic growth, religiousness, endurance, patience, humility, and flexibility are all aspects of hardiness.

Both culture and spiritual beliefs shape individual coping and adaptation to trauma (Pargament 1997). Culture determines how people find meaning and gain control, comfort, and intimacy so that they can transform their traumatic experiences into growth experiences and perhaps gain a new sense of purpose (Klaasen, McDonald, & James 2006). Culture shapes how people engage in active coping, seeking social and emotional support, practicing religion, accepting and adapting to trauma, focusing on venting emotions, seeking peace and calmness, using alcohol or drugs, and engaging in humor (Carver, Scheier, & Weintraub 1989).

In multiple studies, spirituality has been found to be protective in dealing with trauma. High levels of religious involvement also predict lower risk of substance abuse (Koenig, George, Meador, & Blazer 1994; Larson & Wilson 1980; Payne, Bergin, Bielema, & Jenkins, 1991). In a population-based twin sample, Kendler et al. (2003) found that religiosity was inversely related to nicotine and alcohol dependence, drug misuse, and adult antisocial behavior. In the Netherlands Twin Register adult twin study, Koopmans and colleagues (1999) examined gene–environment interaction in the influence of religiosity on initiation of drinking, with results showing 0% between high religiosity and drinking and 40% between low religiosity and drinking.

Cultural Considerations for Cultivating Resiliency

The following is a brief outline of the cultural similarities and differences among some ethnic minority groups in the United States that could be helpful in providing individualized interventions for understanding and promoting resilience.

AFRICAN AMERICANS

African Americans have several characteristics that cultivate resiliency: historical experiences, cultural traits such as family characteristics, cultural values, ethnic orientation, strong kinship bonds, communal orientation, strong religious orientation, importance of tradition, strong work ethic (especially among women), individual and academic achievement, respect for elders, harmony with nature, holistic thinking, adherence to mainstream American cultural norms and values, religion, communication styles, food, holidays, and health considerations (Bell 2011; Billingsley 1992; Carswell & Carswell 2008; Jagers & Mock 1995; Sue & Sue 2003). Racial socialization is protective for African American families (Corneille & Belgrave 2007; Nasim,

Belgrave, Jagers, Wilson, & Owens 2007). Resiliency in African American families is strongly associated with facilitation of self-efficacy, parental supervision that is protective (Donenberg, Wilson, Emerson, & Bryant 2002), and orientation toward the future and spirituality (McCreary, Cunningham, Ingram, & Fife 2006). Racial socialization messages that promote a sense of affiliation and community have protective effects (Fischer & Shaw 1999; Stevenson, Reed, Bodison, & Bishop 1997). Miller and McIntosh (1999) stated that racial identity can create resilience by enhancing collective self-esteem (Bell 2011).

LATIN AMERICANS

Like other cultural and ethnic groups, Latin Americans display great diversity. Most Latinos have strong family-value and kinship systems, suggesting high regard for collectivism and interdependence. Catholic influence is still very strong, although it is becoming less true with assimilation and with each succeeding generation of U.S. Latinos (Bell 2011). Values that cultivate resilience include family ties and friendships, as well as respect, trust, caring, hope, and faith (Arredondo, Bordes, & Paniagua 2008; Padilla & Borrero 2006). Working with such cultures requires awareness of the roles of family and the recognition of religion and ethnic values.

NATIVE AMERICANS

Similar to African Americans, Native Americans face many challenges that cultivate their resiliency in the face of adversity (Johnson et al. 2008). The rates of death, disease, and substance abuse are greater among American Indians compared to Caucasians, with suicide rates being a close second to European American rates (Goldsmith, Pellmar, Kleinman, & Bunney 2002). Native American key values that foster resilience involve an emphasis on spirituality, sacredness of all living things, and respect (Lafromboise, Trimble, & Mohatt 1990). A major strength of Native American, Inuits, and Alaska Natives is that their medicine is oriented toward healing through restoring balance and harmony with the body, using strategies such as spiritual purification in sweat lodges.

ASIAN AMERICANS

"Asian American" is a very diverse group with different approaches to suffering, adaptation, and the environment, resulting in different coping strategies (Tweed & Conway 2006). There is a vast array of cultural subgroups within the general Asian culture, and these subgroups are influenced to varying degrees by three major religions and philosophies of Asian culture:

Taoism, Confucianism, and Buddhism. Taoism teaches a philosophy of living life serenely with equipoise (Bell 2011). Taoism also encourages mind-body practices, such as breathing exercises, that cultivate physical and mental well-being. Lao-tzu taught that entwined yin and yang qualities rule the nature of all things, as is shown in the saying, "Fortune owes its existence to misfortune and misfortune is hidden in fortune" (Chen 2006). This belief could be very adaptive, teaching flexibility in thought and action (Bell 2011).

Confucian tradition teaches the value of perseverance in response to difficulty; hence people from Asian cultures tend to believe in the utility of effort. Confucianism also emphasizes family piety, a moral duty to respect and serve elders, ancestor worship, dignified expression, reserved manner of speaking, and industriousness (Kaplan & Huynh 2008). Consequently, the tendency to catastrophize is minimized, which could decrease risk for disorders like post-traumatic stress disorder (PTSD) (Bryant & Guthrie 2005; Bell 2011).

Buddhism has been a very influential cultural force in Asia for more than 2,500 years (Chen 2006). Conservative Buddhism—prevalent in Sri Lanka, Burma, and Laos—adheres to the early scriptures believed to embody the authentic teachings of the Buddha. This form of Buddhism is called Hinayana ("lesser vehicle") because it is mainly focused on the enlightenment of its practitioners. Another form of Buddhism, Mahayana ("great vehicle")—dominant in China, Taiwan, Japan, Korea, and Vietnam—stresses the ideal of Bodhisattvas: compassionate enlightened beings whose goal is to save all humans from suffering. Zen developed out of Mahayana Buddhism and practices enlightenment through direct seeing of the true nature of the mind. Buddhist practices provide more than stress reduction; they provide a pathway that is free from life's troubles (Bell 2011).

Like Christianity, effective coping in Buddhism requires a personal spiritual transformation, which is cultivated by mental and physical discipline leading to enlightenment that provides inner serenity and compassion. Buddhism is based on *catvari aryasatyeni* ("four noble truths") (Byrom 1976; Chen 2006): (1) *Dukkha*, the truth of suffering, cravings, or greed, aversion or hatred, ignorance or delusions; (2) *Tnaha*, the truth of the arising of suffering; (3) *Nirvana*, the truth of liberation from suffering: freedom from suffering is possible through transforming cravings or greed, aversion, hatred, and ignorance or delusion by following the right path; and (4) *Magga*, the truth of the eightfold path: right speech, right action, right living, right effort, right mindfulness, right meditation, right thought, and right understanding. These eight aspects can be classified as morality, meditation, and wisdom (Chen 2006), leading to freedom from excessive pursuit, extravagance, and arrogance (Ajaya 1997; Bell 2011).

Indian community practices rooted in Hinduism are also very diverse, although they share the common features of transcendence, holistic values, collectivism, self-realization, and transformation of self (Prashantham 2008). Developing a sense of *Atman*, as soul or true self, is one way in which many Asian Indians cultivate their resiliency (Bell 2001). Other Asian Indian cultural values that cultivate resilience include humility, respect, responsibility, politeness, morality, tolerance, spirituality, holistic perception, hospitality, and nonviolence (Prashantham 2008). Hinduism and other folk religions that emphasize karma (the belief that the consequences of our actions and choices inevitably follows us through multiple reincarnations) are a large factor in encouraging people to be gracious and live in harmony with their "higher self" or soul. As in other cultures, Asian Indians have their own healing strategies, such as yoga, Ayurveda, naturopathy, homeopathy, tantra, shamans, reiki, pranic healing, kalari, and marma (Prashantham 2008). Family is important and resilience-cultivating practices that nurture a mind-body-spirit balance fit into their cosmology. Finally, belief in karma may lead to quicker acceptance of the inevitable, resulting in decreased risk for developing PTSD or mood disorders (Bryant & Guthrie 2005; Bell 2011).

Research on Resilience across Cultures

Culturally sensitive understandings are likely to require a research paradigm that is more tolerant of the individual's perspective, as well as multiple changes to Western-centered psychotherapy. Sanchez, Spector, and Cooper (2006) note that a serious limitation in cross-cultural, cross-national stress research is reliance on measures that are developed in a single country but then used in other cultures. Even if the items are successfully translated linguistically, there exists the possibility that the individual items do not reflect universal constructs. Culture is a more confounding variable when we appreciate that, for individual populations, the specificity of coping requires us to look for unique characteristics. Even among minority groups within a single country (e.g., Hispanic subpopulations in the United States), there may be great variability within groups when individuals claim different geographic and historical traditions. Mixed-method approaches and more focused quantitative research may provide results with greater construct validity (Luthar & Brown 2007; Ungar & Liebenberg 2005).

There are only a few examples of comprehensive resilience research in adults and older adults that take into account cultural diversity. One is

Weiss and Berger's (2006) study following the World Trade Center attacks in New York in 2001. They reported that the highest rates of PTSD among people living in New York were found among Hispanic women. Weiss and Berger speculated that these women's social isolation, lack of education, and low incomes made them more vulnerable to the effects of trauma. Nurturing resilience in these women would involve addressing each aspect of their vulnerabilities while emphasizing their strength and resiliency factors.

Immigrant Health and Cultural Resilience

Immigration is intrinsic to U.S. and worldwide cultural dynamics, influencing processes involved in cultural adaptation to new environments that could contain elements of trauma and evoke resilience mechanisms. Cultural adaptation is a complex process of adjustment in which daily experiences and individual, familial, and community factors influence the quality of life of diverse immigrants. In particular, discrimination based on race, gender, religion, physical appearance, or other factors constitutes a major stressor encountered by many immigrants—particularly within national environments in which economic downturns foment conditions of prejudice and discrimination against "foreigners" and "illegal aliens," who are perceived as "threats to society" that must be detained or deported.

Resilience theory provides a useful framework for understanding these experiences of migration. Resilience has been used widely and variably throughout the literature to describe life experiences within diverse populations (Rutter 1999). Castro and Murray (2010) defined resilience as positive adaptation to the stressors and challenges of migration and as coping with multiple and chronic stressors inherent in dealing with a new environment.

The strongest motivation for immigration is usually the search for a better life (Portes & Rumbaut 1996). However, distinct groups bring in distinctly different issues for coping mechanisms: manual laborers who migrate to conduct business and to enhance their standard of living, and refugees and asylum seekers who flee from war or persecution (Portes & Rumbaut 1996). The various stressors that typically influence this adaptation include language barriers, navigation of new cultural landscapes, changes in social networks and supports, and the logistical details of securing lodging, food, and other basic necessities (Padilla, Cervantes, Maldonado, & Garcia 1988). Resilience research examines how people respond to such challenges. The likelihood of positive adaptation is increased by (1) cultural competencies; (2) learning new occupational and linguistic skills;

and (3) establishing new networks of neighbors, friends, and others who can offer social support.

Acculturation occurs throughout the world in individuals who migrate to a new culture. *Assimilation* has been used to refer to the final outcome of the loss of ethnic identity leading to blending into the new culture. Among the most-cited models of acculturation, Berry's two-factor model defines four possible outcomes: (1) marginalization (low affiliation with the new culture, high affiliation with the native culture); (2) separation (high native country affiliation); (3) assimilation (high new culture affiliation, low native culture affiliation); and (4) integration (high affiliation with both cultures) (Berry 1997).

Acculturation research finds that immigrants do better if they participate in the larger community while maintaining their native heritage ("bicultural integration") (Berry 2005). However, experiences of minority groups in developed countries can be very different from those in developing countries. The definition of a resilient outcome may be influenced by the measures of positive adaptation (table 9.1). Ungar (2003) argues that researchers should use culturally appropriate outcomes. "Bottom-up" studies tend to use qualitative and mixed-method approaches (Hanson, Creswell, Clark, Petska, & Creswell 2005) that are essential for understanding the cultural meanings, nuances, and interpretations of the migration experience. "Top-down" approaches impose constraints on the definitions of successful adaptation. For example, an immigrant can achieve successful employment, have no physical or mental diseases, and enjoy good social support, yet mourn the loss of cultural identity from the native country, which will interfere with positive adaptation. Acculturation to either native or American culture can lead to different social outcomes but not differ in measures of social support (Birman, Trickett, & Vinokurov 2002). Resilience plays an important role in protecting from harm and promoting

TABLE 9.1   Risk and resilience factors in the acculturation process

Level of analysis	Risk	Resilience factors
Individual	Language barriers	Educational pursuits
	Social isolation	Social support
	Discrimination	Pursuit of happiness and locus of control
Family	Family conflict	Social support
	Parent-child acculturation gap	Cross-generational network and traditions

growth and goal attainment (Zautra, Hall, Murray, & the Resilience Solutions Group 2008). Ever-increasing intergenerational scenarios illustrate the diverse and intriguing patterns of cultural adaptation that should be examined in depth in future research.

Cross-Cultural Approaches to Resilience

Despite cultural differences, there are commonalities that can serve as bridges in operationalizing global positive mental health (Vaillant 2012). Several precautions are necessary. First, in defining mental health, cross-cultural differences and beliefs must be considered by practitioners in distinguishing mental disorders from health, and in recommending therapies. Next, mental health needs to be seen in the correct cultural context. Moreover, if mental health is "good," what is it good *for*? The self or the society? For "fitting in" or for creativity? Cultural anthropology teaches us that almost every form of behavior is considered healthy in some cultures, but that does not mean that the tolerated behavior is mentally healthy. The best way to enrich our understanding of what constitutes mental health is to study a variety of healthy populations from different perspectives, in different cultures, and for long periods of time.

At least seven promising perspectives should be considered for future research (Vaillant 2012). First, mental health can be conceptualized as above normal. Second, it can be regarded as the presence of multiple human strengths rather than the absence of weaknesses. Third, it can be conceptualized as maturity. Fourth, mental health can be seen as the dominance of positive emotions. Fifth, it can be conceptualized as high socioemotional intelligence. Sixth, it can be viewed as subjective well-being. Seventh, it can be conceptualized as resilience (Vaillant 2012).

The concept of mental health raises the issue of therapeutic interventions to achieve it. Which facets of mental health are fixed and which are susceptible to change? Drugs can alleviate symptoms of mental illness but do not necessarily restore brain function to optimal health. We can also enhance mental health through cognitive, behavioral, and psychodynamic education.

Research on mental health has to include culturally sensitive, inclusive definitions of health and resilience. Although mental health is one of humanity's important values, it should not be regarded as an ultimate good in itself. We must proceed in our efforts toward trying to achieve positive mental health while maintaining respect for individual autonomy in making their healthcare decisions and in choosing treatment and preventive approaches that are often rooted in their cultural origins.

General Issues

Essential issues in understanding the interface of trauma, culture, and resilience include the following: traditional mainstream *and* native cultures' healing practices; therapeutic context, such as cultural-based therapeutic practices (e.g., shamanic practices); beliefs about health and disease; perspective on the psychobiology of stress (mind-body-spiritual connections); and religious and spiritual involvement in healing and recovery (Wilson 2008). For example, Wilson (2004) describes the "abyss" experience as a confrontation with evil and death (soul death and nonbeing) combined with a sense of abandonment by humanity (loss of connectedness), ultimate aloneness, and a cosmic challenge of meaning (spirituality and the sense of mystical).

Marsella (2005) outlined the generic aspects of all cultural contexts as beliefs, catharsis, confession, cultural integration or separation, redefinition of problems of self, faith, forgiveness, hopes, identity, awareness, insight, locus of control, and so on. Historically, civilizations have experienced trauma and developed practices, techniques, wisdom, and other skills to ensure effective coping. Marsella (2005) also noted that all healing subcultures have the following assumptions and expectations: (1) a set of assumptions about the nature of the problems that matches their worldview and reality constructs; (2) a set of assumptions about context and requirements for healing to occur; (3) a set of assumptions and procedures to elicit expectations, emotions, and behaviors; (4) a set of expectations for the therapist. Unfortunately, there has been very little attention paid to mental health issues for different cultural and ethnic minority groups, and especially to the development of resilience-oriented interventions in these groups (Bell & Williamson 2002). Clinically, it would be important to have a basic understanding of these groups' cultural and spiritual beliefs, as well as strengths and weaknesses, in order to provide expert interventions that promote resilience and growth.

Conclusion

In the West, overcoming our monocultural ethnocentrism can lead to more culture-bound resilience-boosting interventions. To achieve this goal, we clinicians and researchers must develop a higher tolerance for what we don't understand and become more comfortable with a wide diversity of practices and beliefs. We must seek to study and research different cultural strategies to create protective factors, strength, and resilience within the many cultural and ethnic groups residing in the United States.

The first step toward this goal would be enhancing individual providers' understanding of the cultural roots of resiliency and helping them to be open to integrating those insights into treatment interventions. In addition, we need to be sure that care providers have the tools to perform a full assessment of cultural beliefs about health and disease and of expectations about treatment outcomes and end-of-life care. Frequently, asking patients to explain the cultural and religious context of their interpretation of trauma, their reaction and coping could be the first step to establishing a therapeutic alliance leading to recovery. Instead, if a different Western model of understanding of the disease, traumatic experiences, and coping is imposed on an individual, it could lead to broken communication and counter-therapeutic outcomes.

References

Ajaya, S. (1997). *Psychotherapy east and west: A unifying paradigm.* Honesdale, PA: Himalayan International Institute.

American Psychiatric Association. (1994). *Diagnostic and statistical manual of mental disorders: DSM-IV.* Washington, DC: APA.

Arredondo, P., Bordes, V., & Paniagua, F. A. (2008). Mexicans, Mexican Americans, Caribbean, and other Latin Americans. In Marsella, Johnson, Watson, & Gryczynski (2008a): 299–320.

Bell, C. C. (2001). Cultivating resiliency in youth. *J Adolesc Health,* 29(5), 375–81.

Bell C. C. (2011). Trauma, culture and resiliency. In S. M. Southwick, B. T. Litz, D. Charney, & M. J. Friedman (Eds.), *Resilience and mental health: Challenges across the lifespan* (pp. 176–87). Cambridge: Cambridge University Press.

Bell, C. C., Bhana, A., Petersen, I., McKay, M. M., Gibbons, R., Bannon, W., & Amatya, A. (2008). Building protective factors to offset sexually risky behaviors among black youths: A randomized control trial. *J Natl Med Assoc,* 100(8), 936–44.

Bell, C. C., Williamson, J. (2002). Articles on special populations published in Psychiatric Services between 1950 and 1999. *Psychiatr Serv,* 53(4), 419–24.

Berry, J. W. (1997). Immigration, acculturation, and adaptation. *Appl Psychol,* 46(1), 5–68.

Berry, J. W. (2005). Acculturation: Living successfully in two cultures. *Int J Intercult Relat,* 29(6), 697–712.

Billingsley, A. (1992). Climbing Jacob's ladder: The enduring legacy of African-American families. New York: Simon & Schuster.

Birman, D., Trickett, E. J., & Vinokurov, A. (2002). Acculturation and adaptation of Soviet Jewish refugee adolescents: Predictors of adjustment across life domains. *Am J Community Psychol,* 30(5), 585–607.

Bond, M. H., & Tornatzky, L. G. (1973). Locus of control in students in Japan and the United States: Dimensions and levels of response. *Psychologica: An International Jounal of Psychology in the Orient, 16,* 209–213.

Bryant, R., & Guthrie, R. M. (2005). Maladaptive appraisals as a risk factor for posttraumatic stress: A study of trainee firefighters. *Psychol Sci, 16*(10), 450–56.

Byrom, T. (1976). *The Dhammapada: The sayings of the Buddha.* New York: Vintage.

Carswell, S. B., & Carswell, M. A. (2008). Meeting the physical, psychological, and social needs of African Americans following disaster. In Marsella et al. (2008a), 39–71.

Carver, C. S., Scheier, M. F., & Weintraub, J. K. (1989). Assessing coping strategies: A theoretically based approach. *J Pers Soc Psychol, 56*(2), 267–83.

Castro, F. G., & Murray, K. E. (2010). Cultural adaptation and resilience: Controversies, issues, and emerging models. In J. W. Reich, A. J. Zautra, & J. S. Hall (Eds.), *Handbook of Adult Resilience* (375–403). New York: Guilford.

Chandler, T. A., Shama, D. D., Wolf, F. M., & Planchard, S. K. (1982). Multiattributional causality: A five cross-national samples study. *J Cross Cult Psychol, 12*(2), 207–21.

Charney, D. S., Barlow, D. H., Botteron, K. N., Cohen, J. D., Goldman, D., Gur, R. E., . . . & Zalcman, S. J. (2002). Neuroscience research agenda to guide development of a pathophysiologically based classification system. In D. J. Kupfer, M. B. First, & D. A. Regier (Eds.), *Research agenda for DSM V* (pp. 31–84). Washington, DC: APA.

Chen, Y. H. (2006). Coping with suffering: The Buddhist perspective. In Wong et al. (2006): 73–90.

Chun, C. A., Moos, R. H., & Cronkite, R. C. (2006). Culture: A fundamental concept for the stress and coping paradigm. In Wong et al. (2006): 29–53.

Corneille, M. A., & Belgrave, F. Z. (2007). Ethnic identity, neighborhood risk, and adolescent drug and sex attitudes and refusal efficacy: The urban African American girls' experience. *J Drug Educ, 37*(2), 177–90.

Donenberg, G. R., Wilson, H. W., Emerson, E., & Bryant, F. B. (2002). Holding the line with a watchful eye: the impact of perceived parental permissiveness and parental monitoring on risky sexual behavior among adolescents in psychiatric care. *AIDS Educ Prev, 14*(2), 138–57.

Fischer, A. R., & Shaw, C. M. (1999). African Americans' mental health and perception of racist discrimination: Moderating effects of racial socialization experiences and self-esteem. *J Couns Psychol, 46*(3), 395–407.

Goldsmith, S. K., Pellmar, T. C., Kleinman, A. M., & Bunney, W. E. (2002). *Reducing suicide: A national imperative.* Washington, DC: National Academies Press.

Hamid, P. N. (1994). Self-monitoring, locus of control, and social encounters of Chinese and New Zealnd students. *J Cross Cult Psychol, 25*(3), 353–68.

Hansen, N. D. (2002). Teaching cultural sensitivity in psychological assessment: A modular approach used in a distance education program. *J Pers Assess, 79*(2), 200–206.

Hanson, W. E., Creswell, J. W., Clark, V. L. P., Petska, K. S., & Creswell, J. D. (2005). Mixed methods research designs in counseling psychology. *J Couns Psychol, 52*(2), 224–35.

Jagers, R. J., & Mock, L. O. (1995). The Communalism Scale and collectivistic-individualistic tendencies: Some preliminary findings. *J Black Psychol, 21*(2), 153–67.

Johnson, J. L., Baldwin, J., Haring, R. C., Wiechelt, S. A., Roth, S., Gryczynski, J., & Lozano, H. (2008). Essential information for disaster management and trauma specialists working with American Indians. In Marsella et al. (2008a): 73–113.

Kaplan, A. S., & Huynh, U. K. (2008). Working with Vietnamese Americans in disasters. In Marsella et al. (2008a): 321–49.

Kendler, K. S., Aggen, S. H., Jacobson, K. C., & Neale, M. C. (2003). Does the level of family dysfunction moderate the impact of genetic factors on the personality trait of neuroticism? *Psychol Med, 33*(5), 817–25.

Keyes, C. L. (2007). Promoting and protecting mental health as flourishing: A complementary strategy for improving national mental health. *Am Psychol, 62*(2), 95–108.

Klaasen, D. W., McDonald, M. J. & James, S. (2006). Advance in the study of religious and spiritual coping. In Wong et al. (2006): 105–32.

Koenig, H. G., George, L. K., Meador, K. G., & Blazer, D. G. (1994). Religious practices and alcoholism in a southern adult population. *Hosp Community Psychiatry, 45*(3), 225–31.

Koopmans, J. R., Slutske, W. S., van Baal, G. C., & Boomsma, D. I. (1999). The influence of religion on alcohol use initiation: Evidence for genotype X environment interaction. *Behav Genet, 29*(6): 445–53.

Lafromboise, T. D., Trimble, J. E., & Mohatt, G. V. (1990). Counseling intervention and American-Indian tradition: An integrative approach. *Couns Psychol, 18*(4), 628–54.

Larson, D. B., & Wilson, W. P. (1980). Religious life of alcoholics. *South Med J, 73*(6), 723–27.

Lazarus, R. S., & Folkman, S. (1984). *Stress, appraisal, and coping.* New York: Springer.

Luthar, S. S., & Brown, P. J. (2007). Maximizing resilience through diverse levels of inquiry: Prevailing paradigms, possibilities, and priorities for the future. *Dev Psychopathol, 19*(3), 931–55.

Maddi, S. R., & Harvey, R. H. (2006). Hardiness considered across cultures. In Wong et al. (2006): 409–26.

Mahler, I. (1974). A comparative study of locus of control. *Psychologica: An International Journal of Psychology in the Orient, 17*, 135–39.

Marsella, A. J. (2005). Culture and conflict: Understanding and negotiating different cultural constructions of reality. *Int J Intercult Relat, 29*(6), 651–73.

Marsella, A. J., Johnson, J. L., Watson, P., & Gryczynski, J. (2008a). *Ethnocultural perspectives on disaster and trauma: Foundations, issues and applications.* New York: Springer.

Marsella, A. J., Johnson, J. L., Watson, P., & Gryczynski, J. (2008b). Essential concepts and foundations. In Marsella et al. (2008a): 3–14.

McCreary, M. L., Cunningham, J. N., Ingram, K. M., & Fife, J. E. (2006). Stress, culture, and racial socialization. In Wong et al. (2006): 487–513.

Miller, D. B., & MacIntosh, R. (1999). Promoting resilience in urban African American adolescents: Racial socialization and identity as protective factors. *Soc Work Res, 23*(3), 159–69.

Munro, D. (1979). Locus-of-control attribution: Factors among blacks and whites in Africa. *J Cross Cult Psychol, 10*: 157–72.

Nasim, A., Belgrave, F. Z., Jagers, R. J., Wilson, K. D., & Owens, K. (2007). The moderating effects of culture on peer deviance and alcohol use among high-risk African-American Adolescents. *J Drug Educ, 37*(3), 335–63.

Norris, F. H., & Alegria, M. (2008). Promoting disaster recovery in ethnic-minority individuals and communities. In Marsella et al. (2008a): 15–35.

Padilla, A. M., & Borrero, N. E. (2006). The effects of acculturative stress on the Hispanic family. In Wong et al. (2006): 299–317.

Padilla, A. M., Cervantes, R. C., Maldonado, M., & Garcia, R. E. (1988). Coping responses to psychosocial stressors among Mexican and Central American immigrants. *J Community Psychol, 16*(4), 418–27.

Pargament, K. I. (1997). *The psychology of religion and coping.* New York: Guilford.

Payne, I., Bergin, A. E., Bielema, K. A., & Jenkins, P. H. (1991). Review of religion and mental health: Prevention and enhancement of psychological functioning. *Prev Hum Serv, 9*(2), 11–40.

Perilla, J. L., F. H. Norris, & Lavizzo, E. A. (2002). Ethnicity, culture, and disaster response: Identifying and explaining ethnic differences in PTSD six months after Hurricane Andrew. *J Soc Clin Psychol, 21*(1), 20–45.

Portes, A., & Rumbaut, R. G. (1996). *Immigrant America: A portrait.* Berkeley: University of California Press.

Prashantham, B. J. (2008). Asian Indians: Cultural considerations for disaster workers. In Marsella et al. (2008a): 175–207.

Rutter, M. (1999). Resilience as the millennium Rorschach: Response to Smith and Gorrell Barnes. *J Fam Ther, 21*(2), 159–60.

Ryff, C. D., Keyes, C. L. & Hughes, D. L. (2003). Status inequalities, perceived discrimination, and eudaimonic well-being: Do the challenges of minority life hone purpose and growth? *J Health Soc Behav, 44*(3), 275–91.

Sanchez, J. I., Spector, P. E., & Cooper, C. L. (2006). Frequently ignored methodological issues in cross-cultural stress research. In Wong et al. (2006): 187–201.

Stevenson, H. C., Reed, J., Bodison, P., & Bishop, A. (1997). Racism stress management: Racial socialization beliefs and the experience of depression and anger in African American youth. *Youth Soc, 29*(2), 197–222.

Sue, D. W., & Sue, D. (2003). *Counseling the culturally diverse: Theory and practice.* New York: Wiley.

Triandis, H. C. (1995). *Individualism and collectivism.* Boulder, CO: Westview.

Tweed, R. G., & Conway, L. G. (2006). Coping strategies and culturally influenced beliefs about the world. In Wong et al. (2006): 133–53.

Ungar, M. (2003). Qualitative contributions to resilience research. *Qual Soc Work, 2*(1), 85–102.

Ungar, M., & Liebenberg, L. (2005). The International Resilience Project: A mixed methods approach to the study of resilience across cultures. In M. Ungar (Ed.), *Handbook for working with children and youth: Pathways to resilience across cultures and contexts* (pp. 211–26). Thousand Oaks, CA: Sage.

Vaillant, G. E. (2012). Positive mental health: Is there a cross-cultural definition? *World Psychiatry, 11*(2), 93–99.

Weiss, T., & Berger, R. (2006). Reliability and validity of a Spanish version of the Posttraumatic Growth Inventory. *Res Soc Work Pract, 16*(2), 191–99.

Wilson, J. P. (2004). The abyss experience and traumatic complex: A Jungian perspective on PTSD and dissociation. *J Trauma Dissociation, 5*(3), 43–68.

Wilson, J. P. (2008). Culture, trauma, and the treatment of post-traumatic syndromes: A global perspective. In Marsella et al. (2008a): 351–75.

Wong, P. T. P., Wong, L. C. J., & Lonner, W. J. (2006). *Handbook of multicultural perspectives on stress and coping.* New York: Springer.

Zautra, A. J., Hall A. J., Murray, K. E., & the Resilience Solutions Group (2008). Resilience: A new integrative approach to health and mental health research. *Health Psychol Rev, 2*(1), 41–64.

CHAPTER 10

Measuring Resilience in Older Adults

T HE ROOTS OF RESILIENCE concepts and measures typically emerge from two bodies of literature: the psychological aspects of coping and the physiological aspects of stress (Tusaie & Dyer 2004). Researchers argue that the concept of resilience may consist of a set of traits (Jacelon 1997), an outcome (Olsson, Bond, Burns, Vella-Brodrick, & Sawyer 2003; Vinson 2002), or a process (Olsson et al. 2003).

Assessment of resilience factors is typically based on theoretical models of successful coping and adaptation to stress (Hunter & Chandler 1999; Tusaie & Dyer 2004). Several key variables contribute to the resilience construct and, therefore, are frequently measured in research: coping style, personality style, cognitive flexibility, sense of purpose, positive emotional engagement, emotion regulation, and indicators of physiological biomarkers such as heart-rate variability, levels of cortisol, or inflammatory markers (Connor & Davidson 2003; Gerritsen et al. 2010; Heim et al. 2000; Lavretsky 2012; Lavretsky et al. 2011; Ryff & Singer 1998; Seligman & Csikszentmihalyi 2000). (Table 10.1 lists some questions used to assess resilience.) Research measures and interventions frequently take into account cultural values, beliefs, and norms, to increase understanding of resilience resources in individual experiences.

Aging-Specific Trauma and Resilience

Several theories address resilience and stress response to adversity in older adults. Most of these theories had been based on examining and measuring vulnerability, "stress inoculation," burden, and mortality effects (Yehuda, Golier, & Kaufman 2005), but more recently they have focused on measur-

TABLE 10.1 Questions for assessment of individual resilience

1. Why do you think you have lived such a long life?
2. What is your life philosophy?
3. How would you describe your relationships with your loved ones?
4. What do you do when you face difficulties in your life?
5. What does being healthy mean to you?
6. How do you handle change in your life?
7. Are you satisfied with your life?
8. Are you proud of your life?
9. Are there lessons to learn from life's difficulties?
10. Are there any benefits that come from stress?

ing psychological resilience. Older adults have a varied and extensive accumulation of traumas over a longer life span, affecting vulnerability to short- and long-term effects (L. Brown, Cohen, & Kohlmaier 2007; Phifer & Norris 1989). For example, in a sample of community-dwelling, predominantly Caucasian women over age 60 years, exploratory factor analysis using the Connor-Davidson Resilience Scale yielded four factors that contributed to resilience: (1) personal control and goal orientation; (2) adaptation and tolerance for negative effects; (3) leadership and trust in instincts; and (4) spiritual coping (Connor & Davidson 2003; Lamond et al. 2008). Consistent with this was the finding of Montross and colleagues (2006) that self-rated successful aging was positively associated with resiliency. Other predictors of resilience were higher emotional well-being, optimism, and social engagement, as well as fewer cognitive complaints. However, the authors found some differences in the coping styles of younger versus older adults. In younger adults resilience tends to be construed as "problem-focused active coping," while in older adults it could be described as "acceptance and tolerance of negative outcomes" (Montross et al. 2006).

At the level of the individual, resilience concepts have led researchers to develop indices of positive adaptation and effective coping. The majority tend to be self-reported measures of resilient outcomes or objective measures of pathological symptoms. In child development, this research has focused on competence and adaptation, identifying adaptation in this case as children successfully meeting developmental criteria (Luthar, Sawyer, & Brown 2006). For adults and older adults, preservation of health and well-being in the face of adversity provides key resilience outcomes. Resilient outcomes can focus on recovery from mental or physical illnesses and sustainability of an improved level of coping and functioning. The speed with which a person regains physiological homeostasis following inflammatory disease in an auto-immune flare-up is one example of the recovery aspects of resilience (Zautra, Hall, Murray, & the Resilience Solutions Group 2008). Recovery from a disease compared to improvement in mental health will require different measures for assessment, demonstrating improvement in health indices compared to the maintenance of a positive outcome (e.g., remission from depression).

In general, older adults experience stressful life events at a much greater frequency than younger adults (Hughes, Blazer, & George 1988). Dealing with chronic illnesses, cognitive or physical decline and disabilities, increasing dependence, widowhood, caregiver stress, and end-of-life issues is a daily struggle for older adults. Resilience is a key factor in maintaining their well-being, as well as a potentially important predictor of recovery from future illness and disability (Hardy, Concato, & Gill 2004). Other specific situations for the current cohort of older adults include existing cohorts of Holocaust survivors and World War II veterans now in their 80s and 90s, as well as aging Vietnam veterans just turning 60 to 70, all of whom have been extensively studied. More general measures exist to measure self-perceived stressors that are applicable across specific populations. Examples of more adversity-specific measures address caregiver stress and burden, as well as the severity of grief (Cummings et al. 1994; Graham, Christian, & Kiecolt-Glaser 2006; Zarit 2008). In clinical populations with depression or anxiety disorders, evidence of resilience would be an improvement on clinical rating scales that measure symptom severity (e.g., Beck Depression or Beck Anxiety scales) or maintenance of a remission state.

Trauma-Specific Coping and Measures

The severity and timing of trauma are important for measuring the actual traumatic experience. Earlier traumatic events that can later increase vulnerability of older adults include those that occurred during childhood (e.g., child abuse) and early in adulthood (e.g., military combat). Traumas during older adulthood bring yet another set of possible outcomes, which may be influenced by the developmental characteristics of this time-period. Individuals who experience trauma during older adulthood may respond more resiliently or recover relatively rapidly as a result of their prior successful coping with earlier adversity. Others may be less likely to ward off the negative effects of trauma because of decreases in physical or cognitive functioning, which may be compounded by fewer social and economic resources.

The response to different kinds of trauma (e.g., illness versus elder abuse) may be different. Empirical evidence specific to trauma in older adults reveals that most older adults recover more rapidly without intervention in the aftermath of trauma compared to younger adults (Boerner, Wortman, & Bonanno 2005; Bonanno, Wortman, & Nesse 2004; Norris 1992; Norris et al. 2002; Phifer & Norris 1989; Shalev 2002). Examples of emotional resilience in older adults include an age-associated reduction for negative emotional images (Charles, Mather, & Carstensen 2003). In large-scale disasters, such as hurricanes and earthquakes, older adults tend to downplay the extent of trauma or disruption they are experiencing (L. Brown et al. 2007). However, other studies emphasize reduction in resilience due to compromised cognition and health (Mancini, Bonanno, & Clark 2011). Regardless of the cause, minimizing losses can be problematic when such an appraisal means that needed services are not sought.

Resilient Personality

Personality styles and traits are relatively stable over the life span and contribute to both resilience and vulnerability to adversity. The five-factor model is a personality inventory that is widely used to describe such traits (John & Sirvastava 1999; Morey 2007). The inventory encompasses five dimensional measures of personality traits: openness, conscientiousness, extraversion, agreeableness, and neuroticism (OCEAN).

Neuroticism is closely associated with resilience across the life span (Ong, Bergeman, Bisconti, & Wallace 2006; van Os, Park, & Jones 2001). Neuroticism is the aspect of personality most relevant to adjustment, and those high on this dimension are likely to show evidence of maladjustment at all ages. Neuroticism reflects a person's stress tolerance, stability of emotions, and ability to adapt in response to change and evolving environmental demands (Costa & McCrae 1992). Current research indicates that people with poor stress tolerance and increased neuroticism are less resilient than those who are highly adaptive (van Os et al. 2001). Such personality dimensions as hardiness, self-enhancement, repressive coping, and positive emotions can play a role in a "resilient personality." Bonanno (2004) defined self-enhancement as an overly positive self-perception, while hardiness could be defined as being committed to finding meaningful purpose in life, the belief that one can influence one's surroundings and the outcome of events, and the belief that one can learn and grow from both positive and negative life experiences.

COPING STYLE

Coping style can influence the relationships between resilience and trauma. Coping has been defined as the cognitions and behaviors a person uses to reduce stress (Billings, Cronkite, & Moos 1983; Folkman 1984). Habitual coping strategies are believed to moderate the impact of stressful life events on functioning (Pearlin & Schooler 1978).

The starting point for much of this research is the conceptual analysis of stress and coping Lazarus first offered in 1966 (see also Carver, Scheier, & Weintraub 1989; Lazarus & Folkman 1984). Lazarus argued that stress consists of three processes: *Primary appraisal* is the process of perceiving a threat to oneself; *secondary appraisal* is the process of bringing to mind a potential response to the threat; and *coping* is the process of executing that response. The entire set of processes may cycle repeatedly in a stressful transaction. To study the coping process, Lazarus and his colleagues developed a measure called Ways of Coping (Folkman & Lazarus 1980), which has since been revised (Folkman & Lazarus 1985). This measure consists of a series of predicates, each of which portrays a coping thought or action that people sometimes engage in when under stress. Respondents indicate whether they used each of these responses in a given stressful transaction (or a given portion of such a transaction), either by giving a *yes* or *no* response or by making a rating on a multipoint scale. Embedded in the Ways of Coping Scale is a distinction between two general types of coping. The first, *problem-focused coping*, is aimed at problem solving or doing something to alter the source of the stress. The second, *emotion-focused coping*, is aimed at reducing or managing the emotional distress cued by the situation. Although most stressors elicit both types of coping, problem-focused coping tends to predominate when people feel they can do something constructive, whereas emotion-focused coping tends to predominate when people feel that the stressor is something they must endure (Folkman & Lazarus 1980).

Research typically finds that responses to the Ways of Coping Scale form several factors, rather than just two (Aldwin, Folkman, Schaefer, Coyne, & Lazarus 1980; Aldwin & Revenson 1987; Coyne, Aldwin et al. 1981; Folkman & Lazarus 1985). Many investigators have distinguished between problem-focused coping, emotion-focused coping, and avoidance coping (e.g., ignoring or denying) (Folkman & Lazarus 1980). Dysfunctional coping can lead to the development and maintenance of symptoms of posttraumatic stress disorder (PTSD). For example, neuroticism and emotion-focused coping can contribute to the development of PTSD symptoms in civilian flood survivors (Morgan, Matthews, & Winton 1995). Similar observations have also been made in other civilian samples (Amir et al. 1997) and in combat veterans (Blake, Cook, & Keane 1992; Nezu & Carnevale 1987). Therefore, individuals with negative emotionality or high neuroticism who engage in emotion-focused coping tend to have a higher dispo-

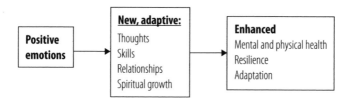

FIGURE 10.1 The relationship between positive emotions and enhanced resilience

sition toward developing PTSD and may require a corrective cognitive-affective processing approach to treatment—instead of the exposure method—for positive readjustment to trauma.

POSITIVE EMOTIONS

One of the most consistent findings associated with greater resilience to stress involves positive emotions (figure 10.1). It is widely acknowledged that positive emotions provide an array of adaptive benefits, both for everyday life and in response to stressful events (Bonanno, Galea, Bucciarelli, & Vlahov 2007; Fredrickson & Losada 2005; Keltner & Bonanno 1997; Lazarus, Kanner, & Folkman 1980; Tugade & Fredrickson 2004). Expression of positive emotions has consistently been shown to be a critical pathway toward healthy adaptation (Bonanno 2004). For example, individuals who exhibited genuine laughter and smiles when describing a recent loss were found to be better adjusted over the first several years of bereavement (Bonanno & Keltner 1997) and also evoked more favorable responses in observers (Keltner & Bonanno 1997). Resilient individuals tend to search for meaning to explain spousal death, whereas a ruminative practice leads to negative adjustment to loss (Nolen-Hoeksema, McBride, & Larson 1997).

The manner by which positive emotions facilitate coping with adversity suggest two independent mechanisms (Fredrickson 2001; Keltner & Bonanno 1997). One is that positive emotions quiet and "undo" negative emotions, which in turn helps to reduce levels of distress following trauma. A second is that positive emotions seem to facilitate coping by contagious influence on other people, thereby increasing social resources and support.

Positive emotions tend to attract close bonds in relationships. Studies have consistently shown that negative emotions do not lead to satisfactory and close relationships (Levenson & Gottman 1983; Schaap, Buunk, & Kerkstra 1988). It may be that negative emotions are enough to get people to talk to each other but not enough to build a firm relationship. If such affiliations do become relationships, it is most likely because the two

TABLE 10.2   Ten representative positive emotions

Ten positive emotions	Action equivalent	Resources	Description
Joy	Play, get involved	Skills gained via experiential learning	Joyful, glad, happy
Gratitude	Benefit	Showing care, loyalty, social bonds	Grateful, appreciative or thankful
Serenity, contentment	Savor and integrate	New priorities and new views of self	Serene, content, peaceful
Interest	Learn, discover	Knowledge, skills	Interested, alert, curious
Hope	Yearn for better, even if fearing the worst	Resilience, optimism	Hopeful, optimistic, encouraged
Pride	Achieve, share	Achievement, motivation	Proud, confident, self-assured,
Amusement	Joke, laugh	Social bonds	Amused, silly, fun
Inspiration	Appreciate human excellence	Motivation for personal growth	Inspired, uplifted, elevated
Awe	Absorb, adapt	New worldviews, shift in perception	Awed, wonder, amazed
Love	Feel, care	All of above, social bonds	Love, closeness, relatedness

SOURCE: Adapted from Fredrickson 2001

people were able to console each other, thus relieving the negative state; in other words, it may be the positive emotion of relief that is rewarding and begins to fuel relationship development.

Several measures of positive and negative emotions are available to researchers and clinicians. For example, a modified Differential Emotions Scale (see Izard 1977 for original; see Fredrickson, Tugade, Waugh, & Larkin 2003 for the modified version in table 10.2). The questionnaire asks participants to evaluate how often they experience 20 emotions over the course of a day, a week, or a month on a five-point scale (0 = never, 4 = most of the time). For daily measures of emotion, participants are instructed, "Looking back over the past 24 hours, please indicate the greatest amount that you have experienced of each of the following feelings." The positive emotion subscale consists of 11 items (amused, awed, contented, joyful, grateful, hopeful, interested, loving, proud, sympathetic, surprised). The negative emotion subscale consists of 8 items (angry, contemptuous, ashamed, disgusted, sad, scared, guilty, embarrassed).

Social Support

Social support is another factor that contributes to an individual's ability to cope. Examination of social support may be particularly important when considering the impact of trauma on older adults because diminishing social networks are part of the aging process. Death, relocation (e.g., moving to a nursing home or retirement community), and increased functional limitations (e.g., inability to drive or ambulate without assistance) may reduce contact with significant others and close friends.

Norris and Murrell (1990) found that social networks buffer the effects of bereavement in older adults. In a sample of community-residing older adults, formal volunteering was associated with more positive affect and moderated the negative effect of having role-identity absences in major life domains (e.g., partner, employment, and parental) on feelings of purpose in life (Greenfield & Marks 2004). Therefore, appropriately seeking social support, moving to an assisted-living facility, and volunteering may be ways to help older adults feel engaged and connected and thus more resilient.

Several measures of social support can be helpful. The Duke Social Support Index is a brief scale that has been extensively used with the chronically ill elderly (Koenig et al. 1993).

Measuring Psychological Resilience in Psychiatric Disorders and Treatment Outcomes

In order to study biological and psychosocial determinants of resilience, it is important to define and measure psychological resilience using standardized assessments. Ahern, Kiehl, Lou Sole, and Byers (2006) compared six instruments used to measure resilience and determined that two were particularly useful to assess resilience in adults: the Connor-Davidson Resilience Scale (CD-RISC) and the Resilience Scale for Adults (RSA). (See table 10.3 for the differences between four instruments in measuring adult resilience.) The CD-RISC consists of 25 self-rated items, with each item rated from zero to four and a scoring range from zero to 100 (Connor & Davidson 2003). Higher scores correspond to higher resilience. The scale builds upon the work of previous research on hardiness, action orientation, self-efficacy, confidence, adaptability, patience, and endurance in the face of adversity (Lyons 1991). The general-population mean is 80, whereas lower mean scores are observed in various treatment-seeking populations: primary care, 72; major depression, 58; PTSD, 50; and anxiety disorder, 62. Clinical

TABLE 10.3   Examples of research scales measuring resilience

Description	Research applications
Connor-Davidson Resilience Scale *(CD-RISC)* *(Connor & Davidson, 2003)*	
25 items, each rated on a five-point (0–4) scale, with higher scores reflecting more resilience. The rating scale assessing resilience was evaluated for reliability, validity, and factor structure. Data analyses indicate that the CD-RISC has sound psychometric properties and distinguishes between those with lesser and greater resilience.	A growing number of studies of mental illness use the CD-RISC.
Resilience Scale for Adults *(RSA)* *(Friborg, Hjemdal, Rosenvinge, & Martinussen, 2003)*	
37-item, five-point semantic differential scale. The scale is intended to measure the protective resources that promote adult resilience. The RSA contains five factors: *personal competence, social competence, family coherence, social support,* and *personal structure.*	The RSA is a valid and reliable measure in health and clinical psychology to assess the presence of protective factors important to regaining and maintaining mental health.
Baruth Protective Factors Inventory *(BPFI)* *(Baruth & Carroll 2002)*	
16-item, five-point (1–5) Likert Scale. The BPFI measures the construct of resilience by assessing four primary protective factors: *adaptable personality, supportive environments, fewer stressors,* and *compensating experiences.* The authors state that the reliability and validity of the BPFI will need further testing as the scale is refined.	There are no applications of the BPFI in the literature. The BPFI has been tested in the general population and in clinical settings, suggesting that there are many potential applications for its use.
Brief-Resilient Coping Scale *(BRCS)* *(Sinclair & Wallston 2004)*	
Four-item scale on a five-point rating (1–5), which is designed to measure tendencies to cope with stress in a highly adaptive manner. Due to the scale's brevity, it meets only minimal standards for reliability and validity. The authors indicate a need for further testing but suggest that the scale may be useful for identifying individuals in need of interventions designed to enhance resilient coping skills, especially in longitudinal studies.	There are no applications of the BRCS in the literature.

TABLE 10.3 (continued)

Description	Research applications
	Resilience Scale *(Wagnild & Young, 1993)*
25-item scale using a seven-point rating (1–7). The scale has two factors: *personal competence* and *acceptance of self and life*.	Although originally tested with adult subjects, several studies have validated that the scale has worked well with samples of all ages and ethnic groups.

improvement is accompanied by an up to 25% increase in resilience in proportion to global improvement. Sheehan's Stress Vulnerability Scale may also be considered a measure of resilience (Sheehan 1983). It is important to use standardized and validated assessments across clinical and neurobiological studies of resilience.

Culturally Based Assessment of Resilience

Cultural norms and values shape family belief systems, organizations, and communications. McCubbin and colleagues identified pathways of resilience in ethnic minority, native, and immigrant families (McCubbin, Thompson, Thompson, & Fromer 1998; McCubbin, Thompson, Thompson, & Futrell 1998). As societies become more culturally diverse, families are becoming increasingly multiethnic, multiracial, and multifaith, requiring mutual understanding and acceptance of differences (Walsh 2009). Socioeconomic conditions strongly impact family risk and resilience. Conditions of economic decline, unemployment, discrimination, neighborhood decay, crime and violence, and inadequate healthcare all have direct impact on resilience.

The assessment of family functioning is difficult because views of normality are imposed into every evaluation. A family-resilience framework offers several strengths under stress and adversity (Walsh 2003). Therefore, individual and family symptoms are best assessed in sociocultural and developmental contexts. A family genogram and timeline are essential tools for clinical assessment to schematize patterns of relationship-information track-systems over time and guide intervention planning (McGoldrick, Gerson, & Petry 2008). Particular attention should be paid to the timing of symptoms of distress, especially their co-occurrence with recent or threatening disruptive events in the family (Walsh & McGoldrick 2004).

Neurobiological Correlates of Resilience

Individual differences in the physiological aging process can be conceptualized as an accumulation of wear and tear caused by daily experiences and major life stressors that interact with genetic constitution and predisposing early life experiences. The adaptive physiological response to acute stress involves a process, initially referred to by Sterling and Eyer as *allostasis*—"maintaining stability through change" (Lavretsky & Irwin 2007)—in which the internal milieu varies to meet perceived and anticipated demand. McEwen (2003) extended this definition to include the concept of a setpoint that changes because of the process of maintaining homeostasis. The neuroendocrine system, autonomic nervous system, and immune system are mediators of this allostatic adaptation to the challenges of daily life. The aging process can undermine the maintenance of homeostasis by invoking changes in the endocrine, autonomic, and immune systems. The identified components of allostatic load are easily measured and monitored in clinical practice (see table 4.1).

NEUROENDOCRINE SYSTEM

Hypothalamic-pituitary-adrenal (HPA) dysregulation has been implicated in several late-life disorders—including anxiety, major depression, and cognitive impairment and decline (O'Hara et al. 2007). McEwen (2003) suggested that circulating catecholeamines are a key component of allostasis and can have synergistic and oppositional effects on the actions of glucocorticoids and arousal. Impaired hippocampal and medial temporal lobe function are implicated in stress-related disorders such as late-life depression and anxiety (O'Hara et al. 2007). Measures of cortisol, dehydroepiandrosterone (DHEA), or catecholamine levels are available clinically but need to be used in appropriate cases when failure of the HPA system is considered. Measures of hippocampal volumes are not provided routinely on clinical magnetic resonance imaging (MRI) or computerized tomography (CT) scans and are used in research only.

INFLAMMATORY MARKERS

Stress-related inflammation has also been implicated in late-life depression, anxiety, cognitive decline, and Alzheimer's disease, and many other chronic diseases of aging (e.g. cancer, arthritis, heart disease). The aging process alone is accompanied by a two- to four-fold increase in plasma or serum levels of inflammatory mediators, such as cytokines and acute-phase proteins. In addition, chronic inflammatory processes are implicated in diverse health outcomes associated with aging, such as atherosclerosis, insulin resistance, diabetes, and metabolic syndrome. Furthermore, there is some evidence that aging is associated with a dysregulated cytokine response following stimulation. Consistent with this research, inflammatory mediators are strong predictors of mortality independent of other known risk factors and of comorbidity in elderly cohorts. For example, interleukin-6 (IL-6)—a proinflammatory factor whose concentration generally increases in the blood with age—has been linked with Alzheimer's, osteoporosis, rheumatoid arthritis, cardiovascular disease, and some forms of cancer. It is also prospectively associated with general disability and mortality in large population-based studies (Harris et al. 1999; Kiecolt-Glaser et al. 2003).

The anti-inflammatory cytokines interleukin-4 (IL-4) and interleukin-10 (IL-10) may actually confer resilience to stress and serve a protective role for the immune system, involving phagocytosis of dying neurons and processing of beta-amyloid and microglia that have been implicated in late-life neuropsychiatric disorders. C-reactive protein has been used as a screening test for cardiovascular disease risk factors and is available for clinical use. These cytokines may be particularly important in conferring increased resilience to the inflammatory stress-response. Measures of metabolic syndrome are relatively easy to obtain. Obesity-related measures of hip-waist ratio or body-mass index (BMI) are easy-to-use measures and correlate with higher levels of proinflammatory cytokines. Measures of the cholesterol/HDL level can be helpful in establishing hypercholesterolemia. Hemoglobin A1c is an easy screen for hyperglycemia (Lavretsky 2012). All of these are components of metabolic syndrome and allostatic load (see table 4.1).

Methodological Issues and Future Directions

Several improvements can be made with regard to the assessment of resilience and related factors and the way they interact with genetic and personal risk/protective factors and various psychiatric disorders. First, it is important for clinicians to assess adversity history comprehensively so that they more precisely can delineate a history of the relationships *among* adversities and their contributions to psychiatric disorders late in life. Second, reporting bias continues to present a challenge, particularly in studies with older samples (O'Hara et al. 2007). It is possible that retrospective self-report measures misrepresent the levels of life stress, early adversity, and trauma experienced by older adults. Older individuals often have recall difficulties, and evidence suggests that they are more likely to pay attention to, and remember, positively valenced stimuli than negatively valenced stimuli (Reed & Carstensen 2012). Psychological resilience in those who are able to survive early life adversity may also potentially attenuate the effect of adversity exposure on risk for psychiatric disorders. In addition, distant traumatic events may be less relevant to older adults than the chronic, ongoing daily stress they experience. While recall of lifetime events has been found to be fairly reliable in research on depression (Brewin, Andrews, & Gotlib 1993), reliability is vastly improved by the use of interview measures (G. Brown & Harris 1998) that are designed to enhance recall and minimize reporting bias. Interview measures, however, present challenges in cost, manpower, and participant burden. Ideally, prospective studies, following participants from childhood into late adulthood with frequent assessments of adversity and symptoms, would be able to delineate longitudinal trajectories of risk, but these may take four to five decades to complete, which may be prohibitive in cost.

The few studies that have been able to look at predictors, moderators, and mediators of psychiatric disorders in a longitudinal design indicate that some of the risk associations between childhood adversity and psychiatric disorders in older adults may be mediated by psychopathology developed in early adulthood (Clark, Caldwell, Power, & Stansfeld 2010). Given that a broad range of experiences are subsumed under the term *adversity*, assessment needs to be comprehensive and to include measures of key dimensions of the experience, such as severity, chronicity, and onset. The use of biomarkers of resilience can help us understand the neurobiology of risk-versus-resilience factors for late-life neuropsychiatric disorders.

Efforts to identify moderators and mediators of the relationship between adversity and psychopathology have been largely focused on HPA functioning, which is just one marker of stress. Although emergent evidence points to the immune function as a potential mediator, relatively few studies have been conducted in this domain (Baram et al. 2012; Bauer, Wieck, Lopes, Teixeira, & Grassi-Oliveira 2010; Wilkin, Waters, McCormick, & Menard 2012). Nevertheless, several groups are pursuing translational and clinical research studies to determine whether therapies targeting immunological and inflammatory pathways can indeed modulate psychological symptoms linked to depression, leading to significant benefit for patients (reviewed in Haroon, Raison, & Miller 2012).

Evidence for genetic moderators similarly suggests that we need greater focus on gene–environment interactions on psychopathology (O'Hara et al.

2007), along with improved characterization and measurement of early adversity, before we can elucidate the mechanisms by which genetic susceptibility interacts with adversity, leading to increased risk for psychopathology in later life. Potential interventions targeting resilience should be based on precise measures of biological, individual, and interpersonal or community risk and resilience factors to shift the balance from maladjustment to positive coping (table 10.4). These measures can provide information about risk factors, moderators, and mediators (genetic, HPA axis, inflammatory markers, allostatic load, and metabolic syndrome), but they can also serve as outcomes of interventions (e.g., reduction in inflammation and symptom improvement).

TABLE 10.4   Examples of risk factors and resilience building interventions

Risk factors	Resilience-building interventions and outcomes
Biological (allostatic load)	
Blood pressure diastolic >90; systolic >140	Regular exercise
	Meditation, yoga
Decreased heart-rate variability	Spirituality
Cholesterol >240; resting glucose >124; body-mass index >25	Stress reduction
	Biofeedback
High C-reactive protein and other inflammatory markers	Improved immune response and regulation
Genetic factors	Reduced cortisol and increased DHEA levels
Chronic disease	
Individual vulnerability	
History of mental illness	Enhanced positive emotional resources
Depressed/hopeless/suicidal	Hope, optimism, mastery, antidepressant drugs
Traumatic brain injury	Increased cognitive functioning, executive functioning, cognitive training, rehabilitation
Interpersonal vulnerability	
Family history of mental illness	Secure family and social relationships
History of childhood trauma/adult abuse	Family or couples therapy
Chronic social stress	Therapy for trauma/abuse
	Positive reframing
	Stress-reduction, biofeedback, mind-body training, spirituality, adaptogens

Conclusion

This chapter reviewed the various key concepts and measures relevant to resilience that can be used in research and clinical practice when evaluating personality and trauma-specific coping abilities of an individual. It also provides an overview of measures that can be used to track clinical improvement with various disease—specific interventions, as well as neurobiological correlates that could be obtained to support clinical findings and to provide understanding of the neurobiological mechanisms of resilience-related treatment response. Comprehensive evaluation of individual strengths and weaknesses, social support, and cultural context can help develop more personalized treatment approaches by enhancing individual coping and resilience to stress.

References

Ahern, N. R., Kiehl, E. M., Lou Sole, M., & Byers, J. (2006). A review of instruments measuring resilience. *Issues Compr Pediatr Nurs, 29*(2), 103–25.

Aldwin, C., Folkman, S., Schaefer, C., Coyne, J. C., & Lazarus, R. S. (1980). Ways of coping: A process measure. Presented at the 88th annual meeting of the American Psychological Association, Montreal (September).

Aldwin, C. M., & Revenson, T. A. (1987). Does coping help? A reexamination of the relation between coping and mental health. *J Pers Soc Psychol, 53*(2), 337–48.

Amir, M., Kaplan, Z., Efroni, R., Levine, Y., Benjamin, J., & Kotler, M. (1997). Coping styles in post-traumatic stress disorder (PTSD) patients. *Pers Individ Dif, 23*(3), 399–405.

Baram, T. Z., Davis, E. P., Obenaus, A., Sandman, C. A., Small, S. L., Solodkin, A., & Stern, H. (2012). Fragmentation and unpredictability of early-life experience in mental disorders. *Am J Psychiatry, 169*(9), 907–15.

Baruth, K. E., & Caroll, J. J. (2002). A formal assessment of resilience: The Baruth Protective Factors. *J Individ Psychol, 58*, 235–44.

Bauer, M. E., Wieck, A., Lopes, R. P., Teixeira, A. L., & Grassi-Oliveira, R. (2010). Interplay between neuroimmunoendocrine systems during post-traumatic stress disorder: A minireview. *Neuroimmunomodulation, 17*(3), 192–95.

Billings, A. G., Cronkite, R. C., & Moos, R. H. (1983). Social-environmental factors in unipolar depression: Comparisons of depressed patients and nondepressed controls. *J Abnorm Psychol, 92*(2), 119–33.

Blake, D. D., Cook, J. D., & Keane, T. M. (1992). Post-traumatic stress disorder and coping in veterans who are seeking medical treatment. *J Clin Psychol, 48*(6), 695–704.

Boerner, K., Wortman, C. B., & Bonanno, G. A. (2005). Resilient or at risk? A 4-year study of older adults who initially showed high or low distress following conjugal loss. *J Gerontol B Psychol Sci Soc Sci, 60*(2), P67–73.

Bonanno, G. A. (2004). Loss, trauma, and human resilience: Have we underestimated the human capacity to thrive after extremely aversive events? *Am Psychol, 59*(1), 20–28.

Bonanno, G. A., Galea, S., Bucciarelli, A., & Vlahov, D. (2007). What predicts psychological resilience after disaster? The role of demographics, resources, and life stress. *J Consult Clin Psychol, 75*(5), 671–82.

Bonanno, G. A., & Keltner, D. (1997). Facial expressions of emotion and the course of conjugal bereavement. *J Abnorm Psychol, 106*(1), 126–37.

Bonanno, G. A., Wortman, C. B., & Nesse, R. M. (2004). Prospective patterns of resilience and maladjustment during widowhood. *Psychol Aging, 19*(2), 260–71.

Brewin, C. R., Andrews, B., & Gotlib, I. H. (1993). Psychopathology and early experience: A reappraisal of retrospective reports. *Psychol Bull, 113*(1), 82–98.

Brown, G. W., & Harris, T. O. (1998). *Social origins of depression: A study of psychiatric disorder in women.* New York: Free Press.

Brown, L. M., Cohen, D., & Kohlmaier, J. (2007). Older adults and terrorism. In B. Bongar, L. M. Brown, L. Beutler, P. Zimbardo, & J. Breckenridge, *Psychology of Terrorism* (pp. 288–310). New York: Oxford University Press.

Carver, C. S., Scheier, M. F., & Weintraub, J. K. (1989). Assessing coping strategies: A theoretically based approach. *J Pers Soc Psychol, 56*(2), 267–83.

Charles, S. T., Mather, M., & Carstensen, L. L. (2003). Aging and emotional memory: The forgettable nature of negative images for older adults. *J Exp Psychol Gen, 132*(2), 310–24.

Clark, C., Caldwell, T., Power, C., & Stansfeld, S. A. (2010). Does the influence of childhood adversity on psychopathology persist across the lifecourse? A 45-year prospective epidemiologic study. *Ann Epidemiol, 20*(5), 385–94.

Connor, K. M., & Davidson, J. R. (2003). Development of a new resilience scale: The Connor-Davidson Resilience Scale (CD-RISC). *Depress Anxiety, 18*(2), 76–82.

Costa, P. T., & McCrae, R. R. (1992). *Revised NEO Personality Inventory (NEO-PI-R) and NEO Five-Factor Inventory (NEO-FFI) professional manual.* Odessa, FL: Psychological Assessment Resources.

Coyne, J. C., Aldwin, C., & Lazarus, R. S. (1981). Depression and coping in stressful episodes. *J Abnorm Psychol, 90*(5), 439–47.

Cummings, J. L., Mega, M., Gray, K., Rosenberg-Thompson, S., Carusi, D. A., & Gornbein, J. (1994). The Neuropsychiatric Inventory comprehensive assessment of psychopathology in dementia. *Neurology, 44*(12), 2308–14.

Folkman, S. (1984). Personal control and stress and coping processes: A theoretical analysis. *J Pers Soc Psychol, 46*(4), 839–52.

Folkman, S., & Lazarus, R. S. (1980). An analysis of coping in a middle-aged community sample. *J Health Soc Behav*, 21(3), 219–39.

Folkman, S., & Lazarus, R. S. (1985). If it changes it must be a process: Study of emotion and coping during three stages of a college examination. *J Pers Soc Psychol*, 48(1), 150–70.

Fredrickson, B. L. (2001). The role of positive emotions in positive psychology. The broaden-and-build theory of positive emotions. *Am Psychol*, 56(3), 218–26.

Fredrickson, B. L., & Losada, M. F. (2005). Positive affect and the complex dynamics of human flourishing. *Am Psychol*, 60(7), 678–86.

Fredrickson, B. L., Tugade, M. M., Waugh, C. E., & Larkin, G. R. (2003). What good are positive emotions in crises? A prospective study of resilience and emotions following the terrorist attacks on the United States on September 11th, 2001. *J Pers Soc Psychol*, 84(2), 365–76.

Friborg, O., Hjemdal, O., Rosenvinge, J. H., & Martinussen, M. (2003). A new rating scale for adult resilience: What are the central protective resources behind healthy adjustment? *Int J Methods Psychiatr Res*, 12(2), 65–76.

Gerritsen, L., Geerlings, M. I., Beekman, A. T. F., Deeg, D. J. H., Penninx, B. W. J. H., & Comijs, H. C. (2010). Early and late life events and salivary cortisol in older persons. *Psychol Med*, 40(9), 1569–78.

Graham, J. E., Christian, L. M., & Kiecolt-Glaser, J. K. (2006). Stress, age, and immune function: Toward a lifespan approach. *J Behav Med*, 29(4), 389–400.

Greenfield, E. A., & Marks, N. F. (2004). Formal volunteering as a protective factor for older adults' psychological well-being. *J Gerontol B Psychol Sci Soc Sci*, 59(5), S258–64.

Hardy, S. E., Concato, J., & Gill, T. M. (2004). Resilience of community-dwelling older persons. *J Am Geriatr Soc*, 52(2), 257–62.

Haroon, E., Raison, C. L., & Miller, A. H. (2012). Psychoneuroimmunology meets neuropsychopharmacology: Translational implications of the impact of inflammation on behavior. *Neuropsychopharmacology*, 37(1), 137–62.

Harris, T. B., Ferrucci, L., Tracy, R. P., Corti, M. C., Wacholder, S., Ettinger Jr., W. H., . . . & Wallace, R. (1999). Associations of elevated interleukin-6 and C-reactive protein levels with mortality in the elderly. *Am J Med*, 106(5), 506–12.

Heim, C., Newport, D. J., Heit, S., Graham, Y. P., Wilcox, M., Bonsall, R., . . . & Nemeroff, C. B. (2000). Pituitary-adrenal and autonomic responses to stress in women after sexual and physical abuse in childhood. *JAMA*, 284(5), 592–97.

Hughes, D. C., Blazer, D. G., & George, L. K. (1988). Age differences in life events: A multivariate controlled analysis. *Int J Aging Hum Dev*, 27(3), 207–20.

Hunter, A. J., & Chandler, G. E. (1999). Adolescent resilience. *Image J Nurs Sch*, 31(3), 243–47.

Izard, C. E. (1977). *Human emotions.* New York: Plenum.

Jacelon, C. S. (1997). The trait and process of resilience. *J Adv Nurs, 25*(1), 123–29.

John, O. P., & Sirvastava, S. (1999). The big-five trait taxonomy: History, measurement, and theoretical perspectives. In L. A. Pervin & O. P. John (Eds.), *Handbook of personality: Theory and research* (Vol. 2, pp. 102–38). New York: Guilford.

Keltner, D., & Bonanno, G. A. (1997). A study of laughter and dissociation: Distinct correlates of laughter and smiling during bereavement. *J Pers Soc Psychol, 73*(4), 687–702.

Kiecolt-Glaser, J. K., Preacher, K. J., MacCallum, R. C., Atkinson, C., Malarkey, W. B., & Glaser, R. (2003). Chronic stress and age-related increases in the proinflammatory cytokine IL-6. *Proc Natl Acad Sci U S A, 100*(15), 9090–95.

Koenig, H. G., Westlund, R. E., George, L. K., Hughes, D. C., Blazer, D. G., & Hybels, C. (1993). Abbreviating the Duke Social Support Index for use in chronically ill elderly individuals. *Psychosomatics, 34*(1), 61–69.

Lamond, A. J., Depp, C. A., Allison, M., Langer, R., Reichstadt, J., Moore, D. J., . . . & Jeste, D. V. (2008). Measurement and predictors of resilience among community-dwelling older women. *J Psychiatr Res, 43*(2), 148–54.

Lavretsky, H. (2012). Resilience, stress, and late-life mood disorders. *Annu Rev Gerontol Geriatr, 32,* 49–72.

Lavretsky, H., Altstein, L., Olmstead, R. E., Ercoli, L., Riparetti-Brown, M., Cyr, N. S., & Irwin, M. R. (2011). Complementary use of tai chi chih augments escitalopram treatment of geriatric depression: A randomized controlled trial. *Am J Geriatr Psychiatry, 19*(10), 839.

Lavretsky, H., & Irwin, M. R. (2007). Resilience and aging. *Aging Health, 3*(3), 309–23.

Lazarus, R. S., & Folkman, S. (1984). *Stress, appraisal, and coping.* New York: Springer.

Lazarus, R. S., Kanner, A. D., & Folkman, S. (1980). Emotions: A cognitive-phenomenological analysis. In R. Plutchik & H. Kellerman (Eds.), *Emotions: Theory, research, and experience* (Vol. 1, pp. 189–217). New York: Academic.

Levenson, R. W., & Gottman, J. M. (1983). Marital interaction: Physiological linkage and affective exchange. *J Pers Soc Psychol, 45*(3), 587–97.

Luthar, S. S., Sawyer, J. A., & Brown, P. J. (2006). Conceptual issues in studies of resilience: Past, present, and future research. *Ann N Y Acad Sci, 1094,* 105–15.

Lyons, J. (1991). Strategies for assessing the potential for positive adjustment following trauma. *J Trauma Stress, 4*(1), 93–111.

Mancini, A. D., Bonanno, G. A., & Clark, A. E. (2011). Stepping off the hedonic treadmill: Individual differences in respose to major life events. *J Individ Dif, 32*(3), 144–52.

McCubbin, H. I., Thompson, E. A., Thompson, A. I., & Fromer, J. E. (1998). *Resiliency in Native American and immigrant families*. Resiliency in ethnic minority families, Vol. 1. Thousand Oaks, CA: Sage.

McCubbin, H. I., Thompson, E. A., Thompson, A. I., & Futrell, J. A. (1998). *Resiliency in African-American families*. Resiliency in ethnic minority families, Vol. 2. Thousand Oaks, CA: Sage.

McEwen, B. S. (2003). Interacting mediators of allostasis and allostatic load: Towards an understanding of resilience in aging. *Metabolism, 52*(10 Suppl 2), 10–16.

McGoldrick, M., Gerson, R., & Petry, S. S. (2008). *Genograms: Assessment and intervention*. New York: Norton.

Montross, L. P., Depp, C., Daly, J., Reichstadt, J., Golshan, S., Moore, D., ... & Jeste, D. V. (2006). Correlates of self-rated successful aging among community-dwelling older adults. *Am J Geriatr Psychiatry, 14*(1), 43–51.

Morey, L. C. (2007). *Personality Assessment Inventory, professional manual*. Odessa, FL: Psychological Assessment Resources.

Morgan, I. A., Matthews, G., & Winton, M. (1995). Coping and personality as predictors of posttraumatic intrusions, numbing, avoidance and general distress: A study of victims of the Perth flood. *Behav Cogn Psychother, 23*, 251–64.

Nezu, A. M., & Carnevale, G. J. (1987). Interpersonal problem solving and coping reactions of Vietnam veterans with posttraumatic stress disorder. *J Abnorm Psychol, 96*(2), 155–57.

Nolen-Hoeksema, S., McBride, A., & Larson, J. (1997). Rumination and psychological distress among bereaved partners. *J Pers Soc Psychol, 72*(4), 855–62.

Norris, F. H. (1992). Epidemiology of trauma: Frequency and impact of different potentially traumatic events on different demographic groups. *J Consult Clin Psychol, 60*(3), 409–18.

Norris, F. H., Friedman, M. J., Watson, P. J., Byrne, C. M., Diaz, E., & Kaniasty, K. (2002). 60,000 disaster victims speak: Part I. An empirical review of the empirical literature, 1981–2001. *Psychiatry, 65*(3), 207–39.

Norris, F. H., & Murrell, S. A. (1990). Social support, life events, and stress as modifiers of adjustment to bereavement by older adults. *Psychol Aging, 5*(3), 429–36.

O'Hara, R., C. M. Schroder, Schröder, C. M., Mahadevan, R., Schatzberg, A. F., Lindley, S., Fox, S., ... & Hallmayer, J. F. (2007). Serotonin transporter polymorphism, memory, and hippocampal volume in the elderly: Association and interaction with cortisol. *Mol Psychiatry, 12*(6), 544–55.

Olsson, C. A., Bond, L., Burns, J. M., Vella-Brodrick, D. A., & Sawyer, S. M. (2003). Adolescent resilience: A concept analysis. *J Adolesc, 26*(1), 1–11.

Ong, A. D., Bergeman, C. S., Bisconti, T. L., & Wallace, K. A. (2006). Psychological resilience, positive emotions, and successful adaptation to stress in later life. *J Pers Soc Psychol, 91*(4), 730–49.

Pearlin, L. I., & Schooler, C. (1978). The structure of coping. *J Health Soc Behav,* *19*(1), 2–21.

Phifer, J. F., & Norris, F. H. (1989). Psychological symptoms in older adults following natural disaster: Nature, timing, duration, and course. *J Gerontol,* *44*(6), S207–17.

Reed, A. E., & Carstensen, L. L. (2012). The theory behind the age-related positivity effect. *Front Psychol, 3,* 339.

Ryff, C. D., & Singer, B. H. (1998). The contours of positive human health. *Psychol Inq, 9*(1), 1–28.

Schaap, C., Buunk, B., & Kerkstra, A. (1988). Marital conflict resolution. In P. Noller & M. A. Fitzpatrick (Eds.), *Perspectives on marital interaction* (pp. 203–44). Clevedon, UK: Multilingual Matters.

Seligman, M. E., & Csikszentmihalyi, M. (2000). Positive psychology. An introduction. *Am Psychol, 55*(1), 5–14.

Shalev, A. Y. (2002). Acute stress reactions in adults. *Biol Psychiatry, 51*(7), 532–43.

Sheehan, D. V. (1983). *The anxiety disease.* New York: Scribner.

Sinclair, V. G., & Wallston, K. A. (2004). The development and psychometric evaluation of the Brief Resilient Coping Scale. *Assessment, 11*(1), 94–101.

Tugade, M. M., & Fredrickson, B. L. (2004). Resilient individuals use positive emotions to bounce back from negative emotional experiences. *J Pers Soc Psychol, 86*(2), 320–33.

Tusaie, K., & Dyer, J. (2004). Resilience: A historical review of the construct. *Holist Nurs Pract, 18*(1), 3–8; quiz 9–10.

van Os, J., Park, S. B. G., & Jones, P. B. (2001). Neuroticism, life events, and mental health: Evidence for person-environment correlation. *Br J Psychiatry Suppl, 40,* S72–77.

Vinson, J. A. (2002). Children with asthma: Initial development of the child resilience model. *Pediatr Nurs, 28*(2), 149–58.

Wagnild, G. M. & Young, H. M. (1993). Development and psychometric evaluation of the Resilience Scale. *J Nurs Meas, 1*(2), 165–78.

Walsh, F. (2003). Family resilience: A framework for clinical practice. *Fam Process, 42*(1), 1–18.

Walsh, F. (2009). Family transitions: Challenges and transitions. In M. Dulcan (Ed.), *Texbook of child and adolescent psychiatry.* Washington, DC: American Psychiatric Press.

Walsh, F., & McGoldrick, M. (2004). Loss and the family: A systemic perspective. In F. Walsh and M. McGoldrick (Eds.), *Living beyond loss: Death in the family* (pp. 3–26). New York, Norton.

Wilkin, M. M., Waters, P., McCormick, C. M., & Menard, J. L. (2012). Intermittent physical stress during early- and mid-adolescence differentially alters rats' anxiety- and depression-like behaviors in adulthood. *Behav Neurosci, 126*(2), 344–60.

Yehuda, R., Golier, J. A., & Kaufman, S. (2005). Circadian rhythm of salivary cortisol in Holocaust survivors with and without PTSD. *Am J Psychiatry*, *162*(5), 998–1000.

Zarit, S. H. (2008). Diagnosis and management of caregiver burden in dementia. *Handb Clin Neurol*, *89*, 101–6.

Zautra, A. J., Hall, J. S., Murray, K. E., & the Resilience Solutions Group. (2008). Resilience: A new integrative approach to health and mental health research. *Health Psychol Rev*, *2*, 41–64.

CHAPTER 11

Resilience-Promoting Interventions

RESILIENCE-PROMOTING INTERVENTIONS can be designed to enhance resilience or any other constructs associated with resilience (e.g., hardiness, well-being, etc.) and can be applied at the level of the individual, family, organization, or community. Interventions can target different time points: prior to, during, or after exposure to stress or trauma. Training administered prior to exposure is generally designed to enhance performance during stressful life events or traumas, with the intent to lessen or even prevent the development of stress-related morbidities; training at the time of or after exposure tends to provide treatment for developing conditions.

Developing approaches for enhancing psychological resilience as a way of preventing or treating late-life mood disorders may help to overcome health problems and resulting disability and mortality in older adults. The experience of frequent positive emotions such as feelings of joy and pride is the hallmark of happiness (Diener, Sandvik, & Pavot 1991; Urry et al. 2004). As discussed in chapter 10, positive emotions are advantageous during the process of recovery from negative experiences (Fredrickson 2001). Frequent positive emotions, high life satisfaction, feelings of happiness, and infrequent negative affect all make up subjective well-being (Diener & Lucas 1999).

The pursuit and attainment of happiness is part of the great American dream. Millions turn to self-help shelves in hopes of obtaining happier lives (although most of these "happiness claims" are not backed by scientific data). The implication from this self-help industry is that happiness lies outside the individual's grasp; it is something that needs to be learned from "experts." For example, a meta-analysis examined 225 cross-sectional longitudinal and experimental studies that relate happiness to success in multiple life domains (Lyubomirsky, King, & Diener 2005). This review found happiness to be associated with relatively stronger social relationships (Berry & Hansen 1996; Harker & Keltner 2001); superior work outcomes (Estrada, Isen, & Young 1994); and more energy, activity, and flow (Watson, Clark, McIntyre, & Hamaker 1992). In addition, the happiest of us have fewer psychopathological symptoms (Diener & Seligman 2002), show better coping abilities, enjoy stronger immune systems, and tend to live longer (Danner, Snowdon, & Friesen 2001). Therefore, developing interventions that increase happiness and resilience are important for improving successful outcomes in life.

Can Happiness Be Taught?

Despite some evidence for a genetically determined set-point of happiness from twin and adoption studies (Lykken & Tellegen 1996), the heritability of well-being is estimated to be about 50% (Braungart, Plomin, DeFries, & Fulker 1992; Suh, Diener, & Fujita 1996). In a longitudinal study, stable individual differences were found to be more accurate predictors of well-being than life circumstances (Costa, McCrae, & Zonderman 1987). Hedonic adaptation refers to human emotional "restlessness," wanting more than one already has, or adapting to negative stimuli over time (Frederick & Loewenstein 1999; Lyubomirsky 2009). Expressing gratitude, "counting blessings," and practicing acts of kindness have been shown to improve the level of happiness (Lyubomirsky et al. 2005). Happiness-enhancing strategies, by enhancing the ability to cope with stress and encouraging proactive control of one's emotional appraisals and reactions to events, can be important for boosting individual resilience (Folkman & Lazarus 1985). Positive emotions can reverse the harmful effects of negative emotions (Folkman & Moskowitz 2000). Thus, happiness interventions can help build resilience in the face of adversity through their enhancement of positive emotions, thoughts, and events. Positive emotions such as joy, satisfaction, and feelings of happiness can provide individuals with a psychological "time-out" in the face of stress and help them maintain hope for a better future. Other tested techniques include cognitive-behavioral therapy (CBT) (Beck, Rush, Shaw, & Emery 1979); mindfulness-based stress reduction (Kabat-Zinn 1990); and, when appropriate, psychopharmacological treatment (Klein, Gittelman-Klein, Quitkin, & Rifkin 1980).

Several psychotherapeutic approaches have already demonstrated promise in building resilience, such as positive affect skill-building (in cognitive behavioral or well-being therapy) in individuals with depression (Fava,

Rafanelli, Cazzaro, Conti, & Grandi 1998; Seligman, Rashid, & Parks 2006). Other approaches with documented success in building a positive attitude include gratitude, positive reappraisal, focusing on personal strengths and attainable goals, and altruism and volunteerism—all of which use cognitive reframing of the given individual circumstances.

Learning to enhance psychological resilience may help overcome disability, which will in turn increase happiness and quality of life. Successful stress-reduction and management in the vulnerable elderly can help prevent serious mental and physical illness. Integrated modalities to improve resilience and reduce stress in combination with pharmacotherapy and lifestyle changes are likely to improve the overall functioning and well-being of older adults.

The broaden-and-build theory states that positive emotions can broaden individuals' thought-action repertoires and assist them in building physical and social resources that boost their emotional well-being (Fredrickson & Branigan 2005; Fredrickson & Joiner 2002). This relationship was tested in U.S. college students (18 men and 28 women) who were first assessed in early 2001 and again in the weeks following the September 11 terrorist attacks (Fredrickson, Tugade, Waugh, & Larkin 2003). Mediational analyses showed that positive emotions experienced in the wake of the attacks—such as gratitude, interest, love—fully accounted for the relationship between (a) pre-crisis resilience and later development of depressive symptoms and (b) pre-crisis resilience and post-crisis growth in psychological resources. Findings suggest that in the aftermath of crises, positive emotions buffer resilient people against depression and fuel thriving, consistent with the broaden-and-build theory. On the grounds of the broaden-and-build theory, Tarrier and Gregg (2004) proposed that positive emotions (e.g., joy, hope, satisfaction) might represent a useful tool to incorporate into existing clinical interventions (such as CBT) because they may facilitate attentional processes that are a prerequisite for some clinical techniques (e.g., evaluation of evidence).

THE BROAD-MINDED AFFECTIVE COPING (BMAC) PROCEDURE

The broad-minded affective coping (BMAC) procedure is a recently developed clinical technique that aims to elicit positive emotions and reduce the experience of negative affective states through the recall of past positive events, such as positive autobiographical memories and mental imagery to elicit positive affect. Participants with a lifetime prevalence of post-traumatic stress disorder (PTSD) demonstrated greater increases in self-reported levels of positive emotions and greater reductions in self-reported levels of negative emotions following the BMAC technique, compared to those in the control condition (Panagioti, Gooding, & Tarrier 2012). These results suggest that BMAC is a useful clinical technique that can be incorporated into other clinical interventions (e.g., CBT) to elicit positive affect and promote resilience.

WELL-BEING THERAPY

Well-being therapy is a short-term, structured psychotherapeutic intervention designed to enhance well-being (Southwick, Pietrzak, & White 2011). While it shares many therapeutic features found in CBT, its primary goal is to engender positive outcomes (i.e. well-being, resilience) rather than to alleviate psychological distress. Well-being therapy is based on Ryff's multidimensional model, in which well-being is viewed as more than the absence of psychological distress (Ryff 1989). In this model, well-being incorporates six dimensions: autonomy, personal growth, environmental mastery, purpose in life, positive relations, and self-acceptance (Fava 1999; Fava & Ruini 2003; Ryff 1989). Well-being therapy has been described as structured, directive, and problem oriented (Fava 1999; Fava & Ruini 2003). It is conducted over six to eight sessions of 30–50 minutes, once a week. The initial sessions focus on learning to recognize personal episodes of well-being and rate the duration and intensity of well-being in a diary. Later, participants learn to recognize beliefs and thoughts that trigger premature interruption of a well-being episode. As in traditional CBT, the individual learns to challenge irrational negative beliefs, but this time related to well-being rather than to episodes of distress. The therapist also assigns the individual to engage in pleasurable activities and tasks and to self-monitor these experiences (Southwick et al. 2011). In the final phase, the therapist teaches the individual about the six dimensions in Ryff's model and provides guidelines for enhancing these dimensions (Fava 1999; Fava & Ruini 2003; Ryff 1989). Individuals learn to take greater control of their environment; recognize self-improvement (personal growth); search for a sense of meaning and develop life goals (purpose in life); become more assertive and resistant to social pressures (autonomy); develop greater self-acceptance; and build positive relationships with others. Throughout this phase of treatment, correction of irrational and automatic thoughts, as well as errors in thinking, is emphasized along with alternative interpretations.

Well-being therapy has been used in a number of small studies for treating the residual phase of affective disorders (Fava et al. 1998); preventing recurrent depression; and addressing residual symptoms in remitted patients suffering from panic disorder with agoraphobia (Fava et al. 2001).

Well-being therapy has also been found to increase psychological well-being, decrease distress, and improve long-term outcomes in individuals with generalized anxiety disorder (Fava et al. 2005) and PTSD (Belaise, Fava, & Marks 2005), lending preliminary evidence that it may possible to enhance psychological well-being and possibly resilience.

LEARNED OPTIMISM TRAINING

The teaching of optimistic thinking has been operationalized in a 12-week program called "Learned Optimism" (Seligman 1991). This program is based largely on Beck and colleagues' cognitive models of treatment for depression (Beck et al. 1979). In Learned Optimism, an individual learns to recognize the connections between adversity, beliefs, and consequences in everyday life. In an intervention study designed to prevent anxiety and depression, Seligman et al. (1999) reported improvements in hopelessness, dysfunctional attitudes, and cognitive style, as well as reduction in doctor visits and fewer physical symptoms at 6- to 30-month follow-ups.

HARDINESS TRAINING

Psychological hardiness is a construct that was developed to describe an inner resource (Florian, Mikulincer, & Taubman 1995) or constellation of personality characteristics (Westphal, Bonanno, & Bartone 2008) associated with good health and optimal performance under conditions of high stress (Eid & Morgan 2006). As defined by Kobasa, Maddi, and Kahn (1982), hardiness represents a pattern of behavior and beliefs that provides strategies of using adversity as growth opportunities (Maddi & Khoshaba 2005). Khoshaba and Maddi (2001) have developed a training program to increase hardiness. Small groups are taught techniques to handle stress and practice exercises designed to enhance attitudes of commitment, control, and challenge (Maddi 2008). In addition, they learn problem-solving skills. In what is termed *transformational coping*, trainees learn to broaden their perspective and deepen their understanding of the stressful experiences they face, and then develop and carry out a decisive course of action. Finally, they learn how to build and receive encouragement and assistance from others (Maddi & Khoshaba 2005).

Social Support Interventions

Interventions designed to increase social support have been shown to enhance physical and mental health and may be useful in promoting resilience to stress (Kaniasty & Norris 2008; King, King, Fairbank, Keane, & Adams

1998). While no studies have examined the effect of social support interventions on enhancing resilience, several have examined the impact of social support interventions on a variety of physical and mental health outcomes.

Lifestyle Interventions

Lifestyle changes can potentially improve resilience by providing better health and enhancing the sense of well-being.

NUTRITION

Large-scale epidemiological studies demonstrate a strong relationship between diet and inflammation and disorders such as depression or heart disease. Diets high in refined grains, processed meat, sugar, and saturated- and trans-fatty acids and low in fruits, vegetables, and whole grains promote inflammation (Kiecolt-Glaser et al. 2010). High-fat meals can increase glucose levels and triglycerides, which stimulate production of interleukin-6 and c-reactive protein (CRP) (Kiecolt-Glaser et al. 2010). In contrast, higher fruit and vegetable intake is associated with lower inflammation, which may counteract proinflammatory responses to high-saturated-fat meals (Kiecolt-Glaser et al. 2010).

In a recent study, Payne, Steck, George, and Steffens (2012) examined cross-sectional associations between clinically diagnosed depression and dietary intakes of anti-inflammatants in a cohort of older adults. Antioxidant, fruit, and vegetable intakes were assessed in 278 elderly participants (144 with depression, 134 without depression) using a food-frequency questionnaire administered between 1999 and 2007. Vitamin C, lutein, and beta cryptoxanthin intakes were significantly lower among individuals with depression than among comparison participants ($p < 0.05$). In addition, fruit and vegetable consumption, counted as antioxidant intake, was lower in individuals with depression. In multivariable models controlling for age, sex, education, vascular comorbidity score, body-mass index, total dietary fat, and alcohol use, findings showed that vitamin C, beta cryptoxanthin, fruits, and vegetables remained significant. Antioxidant, fruit, and vegetable intakes were lower in individuals with late-life depression than in comparison participants. These associations may partially explain the elevated risk of cardiovascular disease among older individuals with depression. In addition, these findings point to the importance of antioxidant food sources rather than dietary supplements. Because diet and stress both affect the immune system, the interaction of these two factors should be addressed in future studies.

CALORIC RESTRICTION

It has been well known for decades in gerontological research that restriction of caloric intake by between roughly one- and two-thirds, while maintaining nutritional balance ("under-nutrition without malnutrition," maintaining necessary vitamins, minerals, protein, etc.), can extend the mean and maximum life spans of model organisms and delay or prevent degenerative physiological changes and age-related disease (Weindruch & Walford 1982). It is less well known that the "classic" monastic or ascetic diet is actually similar or identical to the standard caloric restriction (CR) diet, being focused on nutrient-dense staples—including beans and legumes (such as lentils); nuts and seeds; milk, yogurt, and other nutrient-dense dairy products; and fruits and vegetables—often taken in one or two meals per day (which roughly amounts to caloric restriction of one- to two-thirds (see Bushell 1995; Thurman 1995). While most research has been conducted on model organisms (yeast, nematodes, Drosophila, rodents), nonhuman primate and human studies also have been undertaken. These studies are not of sufficient duration yet to determine whether CR will extend the mean or maximum life spans of nonhuman primates or humans, but data already generated have demonstrated apparent aging-slowing changes consistent with the results in model organisms (reductions in blood glucose, insulin resistance or its analogs, blood pressure in higher organisms, etc.) in which maximum life span has been extended (Fontana, Meyer, Klein, & Holloszy 2004; Roth et al. 2004; Walford, Mock, Verdery, & MacCallum 2002). More recent studies have determined that modifications of the CR paradigm—including decreased restriction of caloric intake (i.e., more food permitted than the typical CR regimen); increased time between meals rather than meal-skipping (independently of total calories); and "intermittent fasting" (an alternating daily eating schedule)—can also produce many of the salutary effects of the standard CR diet (Mattson 2005; Willcox et al. 2007). Whether or not this approach can improve resilience to stress is yet to be determined.

EXERCISE

Exercise also has been shown to be important in maintaining well-being. Exercise intensity, duration, frequency, and other factors appear to play important roles in anti-aging outcomes, as does the role of physical training (Salmon 2001; Tremblay, Mireault, Dessureault, Manning, & Sveistrup 2004). These effects appear to be most likely due to stress-reducing (Gotto & Brinton 2004), anti-inflammatory (Pedersen & Bruunsgaard 2003), and antioxidant effects (Ji 2002). Such effects may in turn be mediated by increases in the activity of melatonin (Buxton, L'Hermite-Baleriaux, Hirschfeld, & Van Cauter 1997), dehydroepiandrosterone (DHEA) (Lee, Hsieh, & Paffenbarger 1995), and interleukin-10 (Cadet et al. 2003) and interleukin-4 (Smith, Dykes, Douglas, Krishnaswamy, & Berk 1999), among others. While the exercise-induced enhancement of the latter three substances appears to be robust and replicated, the data with respect to exercise and melatonin appear to be more equivocal.

Human and other animal studies demonstrate that exercise targets many aspects of brain function, providing broad effects on overall brain health. The benefits of exercise have been best defined for learning and memory, protection from neurodegeneration, and alleviation of depression, particularly in elderly populations. Exercise increases synaptic plasticity by directly affecting synaptic structure and potentiating synaptic strength, as well as by strengthening the underlying systems that support plasticity, including neurogenesis, metabolism, and vascular function. Such exercise-induced structural and functional change has been documented in various brain regions but has been best studied in the hippocampus (Cotman, Berchtold, & Christie 2007).

Emerging evidence suggests that exercise has therapeutic and preventative effects on depression (Cotman et al. 2007). Depression is linked to cognitive decline and is considered to cause a worldwide health burden greater than that of ischemic heart disease, cerebrovascular disease, or tuberculosis. The therapeutic effects of exercise on depression have been most clearly established in human studies. Randomized and crossover clinical trials demonstrate the efficacy of aerobic or resistance-training exercise (two to four months) as a treatment for depression in both young and older individuals (Blumenthal et al. 1999; Singh et al. 2005). The benefits are similar to those achieved with antidepressants (Blumenthal et al. 1999). They are also dose dependent: greater improvements are seen with higher levels of exercise (Singh et al. 2005).

Although exercise seems to have both preventative and therapeutic effects on the course of depression, the underlying mechanisms are poorly understood. Studies of the protective effects of exercise on stress have focused on the hippocampus, where exercise-induced neurogenesis and growth-factor expression have been proposed as potential mediators, although not without controversy. Other proposed mechanisms include exercise-driven changes in the hypothalamic-pituitary-adrenal axis that regulates the stress response and altered activity of dorsal raphe serotonin neurons implicated in mediating learned-helplessness behaviors.

Complementary and Alternative Medicine

The use of complementary and alternative medicine (CAM) in the United States is increasing rapidly, exceeding a prevalence of 60% in a nationally representative survey conducted by the National Center for Health Statistics in 2002 (Ernst 2003; Meeks, Wetherell, Irwin, Redwine, & Jeste 2007). CAM therapies are defined as a group of diverse medical and health systems, practices, and products that are not currently considered to be part of conventional medicine (National Center for Complementary and Alternative Medicine [NCCAM] 2002). An alternative approach to mental healthcare is one that emphasizes the interrelationship between mind, body, and spirit. A national U.S. survey noted a 47% increase in total visits to CAM practitioners, from 427 million in 1990 to 629 million in 1997 (NCCAM 2002). Expenditures for CAM professional services were conservatively estimated at $21.2 billion in 1997, with at least $12.2 billion of out-of-pocket expenditures, exceeding out-of-pocket expenditures for all U.S. hospitalizations (NCCAM 2002). According to another nationwide survey, 36% of U.S. adults aged 18 years and over use some form of CAM, and aging baby boomers are expected to accelerate the use of CAM in the coming years (Barnes, Powell-Griner, McFann, & Nahin 2004).

Despite individuals' increasing use of CAM, scientific support for its efficacy is limited. The treatments with the best evidence of effectiveness are St. John's wort, exercise, and light therapy for seasonal depression. There is only some degree of evidence to support the effectiveness of acupuncture, light therapy for nonseasonal depression, massage therapy, negative air ionization (for winter depression), relaxation therapy, S-adenosyl-L-methionine, folate supplementations, and yoga breathing exercises (Jorm, Christensen, Griffiths, & Rodgers 2002). Use of CAM therapies is typically associated with higher levels of education, poorer health status, environmentalism, feminism, and interest in spirituality and personal-growth psychology (Astin 1998). Barnes and colleagues (2004) noted that nearly 33% of older adults had used CAM in the preceding year. In a survey, 42% of the patients in a managed-care organization reported using at least one CAM therapy, most commonly relaxation techniques (18%), massage (12%), herbal medicine (10%), or megavitamin therapy (9%). This review is devoted to the description of evidence-based CAM treatments applied to the care of older adults with late-life mood disorders (table 11.1).

Table 11.1   Complementary and alternative medicine interventions for treatment and prevention of late-life mood disorders

Mode of intervention	Postulated mechanism of action	Mood, depression	Main adverse effects and drug interactions
St. John's wort	MAOI and reduced monoamine reuptake and decreased amyloid production in rodent models of Alzheimer's disease	Close to 40 RCTs	Mania, serotonergic syndrome, photosensitivity, multiple drug interactions with HIV protease inhibitors, warfarin, digoxin, oral contraceptives, anticonvulsants
Omega-3 fatty acids (fish oil)	Mood stabilization, memory enhancement, neuroprotection, reduction in amyloid production	Several RCTs are mixed or negative in the effect on mood and well-being	Fishy aftertaste, gastrointestinal distress, increased effect of warfarin and NSAIDs
SAMe	Cofactor in neurotransmitter synthesis; methylation homocysteine to methionine	Several RCTs; parenteral SAMe is superior to placebo	Mania, gastrointestinal distress, headache, interaction with SSRIs
Folate and B12	Cofactor in neurotransmitter synthesis; methylation homocysteine to methionine; precursor to SAMe	Folic acid is an effective adjunct	Mania induction, interaction with SSRIs
Gingko biloba	Scavenging free radical; lowered oxidative stress; reduced neural damage; increased blood flow to the brain	Several RCTs in postmenopausal women, and for sexual side effects of antidepressants—mixed results	Increased bleeding time, allergic reactions
Adaptogens	New class of metabolic regulators of a natural origin (including ginsengs, maca, and rhodiola rosea) that protect against stress-related factors	Few animal and human studies identifying positive effects on mood, cognition libido	May increase bleeding (ginseng, rhodiola), anxiety, overstimulation

			Consistent with above side-effects of herbals
Ayurveda	Indian treatment system using herbs, diet, and lifestyle to achieve balance in cognition and well-being	Few studies suggestive of positive effect	
Acupuncture	Balancing energy flow through meridians in the body	Small RCTs with poor controls, randomization, and blinding, and with inconclusive results	Needle phobia, bleeding
Yoga	Postures, breath, meditation, rebalancing mind-body connections	Reduces depression and enhances well-being in a few studies	None
Spirituality	Lowers stress and enhances cognition via church attendance and prayer	Improves depression in practitioners	None
Exercise	Improved cardiovascular function, release of endorphins, increased energy, mental stimulation	Improved mood and well-being, especially in minor depression	Possible injury
Expressive therapies (art, music, dance)	Allows expression of emotional and cognitive facets of self	Improves mood, reduces stress	Possible injury

SOURCE: Adapted from Lavretsky 2009.
Notes: SAMe: S-adenosyl-L-methionine; RCT: randomized controlled trial

OMEGA-3 FATTY ACIDS

Fish oil and omega-3 fatty acids are commonly used as dietary supplements. Reductions in cardiovascular risk, depression, and rheumatoid arthritis symptoms have been correlated with omega-3 fatty acid intake, and there is increased interest in the use of omega-3 fatty acid supplementation for other psychiatric illnesses and prevention of Alzheimer's disease. Omega-3 fatty acids are found principally in fish and seafood, although some can be derived from green vegetables. By contrast, omega-6 fatty acids are found in soft margarine, most vegetable oils, and animal fat. Omega-6 is plentiful in most modern Western diets, while omega-3 is often relatively lacking. A high dietary ratio of omega-6 to omega-3 has been linked to vulnerability to many physical and mental disorders. Reported health benefits of increasing omega-3 intake include improvements in mood in unipolar and bipolar disorders, as well as in dementia (Andreescu, Mulsant, & Emanuel 2008; Fugh-Berman & Cott 1999; Jorm et al. 2002; Tanskanen et al. 2001).

Following the well-publicized promising results from a placebo-controlled study, there has been a broad interest in the use of omega-3 fatty acids for the treatment of bipolar disorder and depression. There is indeed mounting evidence that dietary supplementation with omega-3 fatty acids may be beneficial in treating a variety of conditions, including several psychiatric disorders (Tanskanen et al. 2001), although not all studies are in agreement. Most studies recommend omega-3 essential fatty acids with an EPA-DHA ratio of 7:1. In a recent trial, supplementation with omega-3 in patients with mild to moderate Alzheimer's did not result in marked effects on neuropsychiatric symptoms, except for possible positive effects on depressive and agitative symptoms (Freund-Levi et al. 2008). In summary, omega-3 fatty acids may have a role in the treatment of late-life neuropsychiatric disorders; however, additional studies are needed before their use can be recommended confidently to patients.

S-ADENOSYL-L-METHIONINE

S-adenosyl-L-methionine (SAMe) is one of the CAM products that has been studied under rigorous, controlled conditions. SAMe is derived from the amino acid L-methionine through the one-carbon cycle; it is a methyl donor involved in the synthesis of monoaminergic neurotransmitters. SAMe has been investigated for its antidepressant properties in both open (Andreescu et al. 2008) and randomized controlled (Mischoulon & Fava 2002) trials. SAMe dosages of 200-1,600 mg/day (orally or parenterally) have been shown to be superior to placebos and as effective as tricyclic antidepressants in alleviating depression, although some individuals may require higher doses (Mischoulon & Fava 2002). SAMe may have a faster onset of action than conventional antidepressants and may potentiate the effect of tricyclic antidepressants (Mischoulon & Fava 2002) or of serotonin reuptake inhibitors. At this time, the recommended dose range most commonly used is 200 mg twice daily up to 800 mg twice daily. Oral dosages of SAMe up to 1,600 mg/day appear to be significantly bioavailable and safe. SAMe has been associated with minor adverse effects, such as gastrointestinal symptoms and headaches. However, as with any antidepressant compound, some cases of mania have been reported in bipolar patients taking SAMe (Mischoulon & Fava 2002).

Overall, SAMe appears to be safe and efficacious in the treatment of depression, but further controlled studies are indicated, as current evidence comes mostly from open trials or small controlled studies. It may have a role in the management of patients with bipolar disorder, but more research is needed, in particular to determine its effective dose and to better assess the risk of a switch to mania or hypomania (Mischoulon & Fava 2002).

Additional research should be conducted on the role of omega-6 supplements, SAMe, and other natural products in the prevention and treatment of psychiatric symptoms.

ADAPTOGENS

Herbal adaptogens represent a new class of metabolic regulators of a natural origin, which increase the ability of an organism to adapt to environmental factors that are used to improve energy, mental focus, cognitive enhancement, and sexual function (Gerbarg & Brown 2013). Generally, adaptogens may be taken before and during a stressful period or continuously long-term for chronic conditions. Herbal adaptogens contain hundreds of bioactive compounds, including metabolic regulators, and have demonstrated abilities to protect from damage caused by oxidative stress, toxic chemicals, infection, neoplasm, heat, cold, radiation, hypoxia, physical exertion, and psychological stress in human and animal studies (Gerbarg & Brown 2013). Here I give examples of ginsengs, maca, and rhodiola rosea, which are commonly used by older adults.

GINSENGS: KOREAN OR ASIAN GINSENG (*PANAX GINSENG*) AND AMERICAN GINSENG (*PANAX QUINQUEFOLIUS*)

In practice, ginsengs are used to improve alertness, mental focus, energy, and cognitive function. Ginsengs contain numerous bioactive compounds, particularly ginsenocides or ginseng saponins (Gerbarg & Brown 2013).

P. ginseng increases nitric oxide production in endothelial cells, which is essential for blood flow and oxygen delivery. In a double-blind placebo-controlled crossover study of 32 healthy younger adults, 100 mg of *P. ginseng* significantly improved reaction time, accuracy, calmness, and working memory (Reay, Scholey, & Kennedy 2010). Average doses range between 300 and 800 mg per day. Side effects may include anxiety, insomnia, tachycardia, gastrointestinal disturbance, headache, and reduced platelet aggregation. American ginseng can reduce the anticoagulant effects of warfarin; therefore, the use of anticoagulants is a contraindication. In treating cognitive dysfunction due to stroke, trauma, or vascular disease, Gerbarg & Brown (2013) observed better results by combining *P. ginseng*, *P. quinquefolius*, and *E. senticosus*.

MACA (*LEPIDIUM MYENII*)

Maca, a Peruvian herb that grows at high altitudes in the Andes, is used to enhance sexual function, energy, alertness, mood, and physical resilience (Gonzalez 2012). Research on maca consists primarily of animal studies and a small number of methodologically limited human trials (Ernst, Posadzki, & Lee 2011). A randomized placebo-controlled pilot study found that maca (3 g/day) significantly reduced selective serotonin-reuptake-inhibitor-induced sexual dysfunction (Dording et al. 2008). Toxic effects have not been reported in animal or human studies using herb that has been boiled before consumption. In recommended doses, maca causes minimal side effects; excess doses may cause overactivation. In clinical practice, Gerbarg and Brown (2013) found that maca can be a useful adjunctive treatment for neural fatigue and sexual dysfunction.

ARCTIC ROOT (*R. ROSEA*)

R. rosea can be beneficial in many conditions: fatigue from any cause; cognitive dysfunction; memory problems; depression; stress-related conditions; sexual dysfunction; weakness; infection; and cancer (Brown, Gerbarg & Ramazanov 2002). When given alone or in combination with other adaptogens, it can enhance physical and intellectual performance, attention, and memory. *R. rosea* absorbs best when taken on an empty stomach 20 minutes before breakfast and 20 minutes before lunch. Capsules may contain 100 to 180 mg dry root extract. The usual starting dose is one capsule before breakfast, increasing by one capsule every 3 to 7 days as needed. For patients who are sensitive to stimulants, prone to anxiety, elderly, or medically ill, starting with a fraction of a capsule reduces the risk of overstimulation. The average adult doses range is 150 to 600 mg/day, although some respond to 25 mg/day (Gerbarg & Brown 2013). In some cases, the beneficial effects may fade after a few weeks or months. If this occurs, the dose could be increased, if necessary, up to a maximum tolerable dose (600–900 mg/day). Otherwise, "herbal holidays"—discontinuation for 1 to 3 weeks at a time—may be indicated. Patients usually report improved energy during the first week on adequate doses.

R. rosea is considered to be safe; adverse effects are rare. In some cases of individual sensitivity, anxiety, irritability, insomnia, headache, and, rarely, palpitations may occur. Because the effects of bleeding time are not known, the herb should be discontinued one week before surgery. Although *R. rosea* showed in-vitro inhibitory effects on CYP isoenzymes, in-vivo rat studies found no significant effects on CYP450 metabolism of theophylline or warfarin or on anticoagulant activity of warfarin (Panossian, Hovhannisyan, Abrahamyan, Gabrielyan, & Wikman 2009). In aging adults, *R. rosea* can reduce menopause-related symptoms of fatigue, impaired cognitive function and memory, depression, and loss of libido (Gerbarg & Brown 2013).

ACUPUNCTURE

The Chinese practice of inserting needles into the body at specific points manipulates the body's flow of energy to balance the endocrine system. This manipulation regulates functions such as heart rate, body temperature, and respiration, as well as sleep patterns and emotional changes. Acupuncture has been used in clinics to assist people with substance-abuse disorders through detoxification; to relieve stress and anxiety; to treat attention-deficit and hyperactivity disorders in children; to reduce symptoms of depression; and to help people with physical ailments. Compared to other empirically validated treatments, acupuncture designed specifically to treat major depression produced results that are comparable in terms of rates of response and of relapse or recurrence. One small study of acupuncture found positive subjective and objective effect on mood and well-being (Williams & Graham 2006). Moreover, in the Cochrane database review (Smith & Hay 2005) of seven trials comprising 517 subjects who generally had mild to moderate depression, there was no evidence that medication was better than acupuncture in reducing the severity of depression or in achieving remission. These results warrant a larger trial of acupuncture in the acute- and maintenance-phase treatment of depression.

AYURVEDA

Ayurveda is a comprehensive, natural healthcare system that originated in India more than 5,000 years ago and has been used for anti-aging, memory-enhancement, nerve-tonic, anxiolytic, anti-inflammatory, and immunopotentive effects. It is still widely used in India as a system of primary healthcare, and interest is growing worldwide as well. Ayurveda means "the science of life" (*ayur* means "life" and *veda* means "knowledge or science"). Ayurvedic medicine is described as "knowledge of how to live." It incorporates an individualized regimen, of diet, meditation, herbal preparations, and other techniques, to treat a variety of conditions (including depression), to facilitate lifestyle changes, and to teach people how to release stress and tension through yoga or transcendental meditation. There are encouraging results for its effectiveness in treating ailments, including chronic disorders associated with the aging process. Pilot studies of the effect of Ayurvedic therapies on depression, anxiety, sleep disorders, hypertension, diabetes mellitus, Parkinson's disease, and Alzheimer's disease have yielded positive results (Sharma, Chandola, Singh, & Basisht 2007).

YOGA AND MEDITATION

Practitioners of yoga, another ancient Indian system of healthcare, use breathing exercises, posture, stretching, and meditation to balance the body's energy centers. Mindful physical exercise has recently emerged as a therapeutic intervention for improving the psychosocial well-being of individuals. According to the IDEA Mind-Body Fitness Committee (1997–2001), mindful physical exercise is characterized by "physical exercise executed with a profound inwardly directed contemplative focus." (Abbot & Lavretsky 2013). A physical exercise is considered mindful if it (a) has a meditative or contemplative component that is noncompetitive and nonjudgmental; (b) has proprioceptive awareness that involves a low-to-moderate level of muscular activity with mental focus on muscular movement; (c) is breath-centering; (d) focuses on anatomic alignment, such as spine, trunk, and pelvis, or proper physical form; and (e) concerns energy-centric awareness of an individual's flow of intrinsic energy, vital life force, qi, and so on.

Yoga and qigong are two major streams of mindful physical exercise based on corresponding literature. Yoga is used in combination with other treatments for depression, anxiety, and stress-related disorders. Mindful physical exercise has been shown to provide an immediate source of relaxation and mental quiescence. Scientific evidence shows that medical conditions such as hypertension, cardiovascular disease, insulin resistance, depression, and anxiety disorders respond favorably to mindful physical exercise (Khalsa 2004).

The effects of yoga and Ayurveda on geriatric depression were evaluated in 69 persons older than 60 who were living in a residential home

(Krishnamurthy & Telles 2007). Depression-symptom scores of the yoga group at both three and six months decreased significantly, from a group-average baseline of 10.6 to 8.1 and 6.7, respectively ($p < .001$, paired t-test). Other groups showed no change. Hence, an integrated approach of yoga, including mental and philosophical aspects in addition to physical practices, was useful for institutionalized older persons.

MEDITATION, SPIRITUALITY, AND PASTORAL CARE

Some people prefer to seek help for mental-health problems from their pastor, rabbi, or priest rather than from therapists who are not affiliated with a religious community. Counselors working within traditional faith communities increasingly are recognizing the need to incorporate psychotherapy or medication along with prayer and spirituality to effectively help some people with mental disorders. Both religiousness and social support have been shown to influence depression outcomes, yet some researchers have theorized that religiousness largely reflects social support. In a recent study, religious coping was related to social support but was independently related to depression outcomes. The authors concluded that clinicians caring for older patients with depression should consider inquiring about spirituality and religious coping as a way of improving depressive outcomes (Bosworth et al. 2003). The protective effects of religion against late-life depression may depend on the broader sociocultural environment. Religious practice, church attendance, or prayer, especially when embedded within a traditional value-orientation, may facilitate coping with adversity in later life and promote stress reduction (Norton et al. 2008).

Addressing spirituality in clinical encounters also may lead to improved detection of depression and to treatments that are more congruent with patients' beliefs and values, as related in a study of older African American participants who described depression as being due to a "loss of faith." Faith and spiritual or religious activities were thought to be empowering in the way they can work together with medical treatments to provide the strength for healing to occur (Wittink, Joo, Lewis, & Barg 2009). That faith-based intervention can improve the outcomes of treatment was shown by employing "Christian Steps to Freedom" model prayers, used by individual patients personally or with a counselor, which reduced their psychiatric symptoms compared to those who did not practice prayer (Hurst, Williams, King, & Viken 2008).

The clinical effects of meditation affect a broad spectrum of physical and psychological symptoms and syndromes, including reduced anxiety, pain, and depression; enhanced mood and self-esteem; and decreased stress.

Meditation has been studied in populations with fibromyalgia, cancer, hypertension, and psoriasis. Meditation practice can positively influence the experience of chronic illness and can serve as a primary, secondary, or tertiary prevention strategy. Health professionals demonstrate commitment to holistic practices by asking patients about their use of meditation and can encourage this self-care activity. Simple techniques for mindfulness can be taught in clinical settings. Living mindfully with chronic illness is a fruitful area for research, and we can predict that evidence will grow to support the role of consciousness in the human experience of disease.

EXPRESSIVE THERAPIES

Creativity interventions have been shown to positively affect mental and physiological health indicators in older adults. Developing creative coping strategies can enable older adults to adapt more effectively to physical, psychological, and psychosocial changes that occur during old age. The process of creativity in relation to one's attitude toward life may be more important than the actual creative product or tangible outcome. Late-life creativity reflects aspects of late-life thinking: synthesis, reflection, and wisdom. From a problem-solving perspective, creativity is an asset in older adulthood, given the number of health, functional, and financial limitations likely to occur (Flood & Phillips 2007). However, many older adults who might benefit may not describe themselves as creative and could be reluctant to engage in typical creative endeavors, such as painting or drawing or writing about their lives (life review, journaling).

DANCE AND MOVEMENT THERAPY

The underlying premise to dance and movement therapy is that it can help a person to integrate emotional, physical, and cognitive facets of "self." A recent study designed a multimodal program aimed at influencing a group of 75 older-adult participants' purpose in life, depression, and hypochondriasis by targeting physical, mental, and spiritual well-being. Interventions included rhythm and dance exercises; general physical exercises; recreational exercise outdoors; relaxation exercises; a creativity-enhancement seminar; a seminar on psychology and philosophy of life; and a seminar on contact with other people and communication. Group sessions were conducted two days per week over a period of four months. Purpose in life, depression, and hypochondria were three parameters of well-being that were measured pre- and post-intervention. The Purpose in Life Scale (PIL) measured feelings of purpose, the Geriatric Depression Scale (GDS) assessed depressive symptoms, and the Hypochondriasis Scale Institutional-

Geriatric version (HIP-G) determined the presence of hypochondria. The first day each week consisted of an hour of some form exercise and a two-hour seminar. The second day each week was comprised of one hour of relaxation, an hour of exercise, and two hours of a seminar about stimulating creativity.

Significant changes in test scores were observed over time. Mean PIL scores increased from preintervention to postintervention, suggesting greater purpose in life, and these scores remained elevated at six months after intervention. Scores for the GDS and the HIP-G decreased from preintervention to postintervention, indicating a decrease in depressive symptoms and hypochondriasis, and these scores continued to be significantly reduced six months after intervention. These outcomes suggested that interventions were successful in improving quality of life for participants.

Those who prefer more structure or who feel they have "two left feet" gain a similar sense of release and inner peace from Eastern martial arts, such as tai chi chuan. There is considerable evidence that tai chi has positive health benefits that are physical, psychosocial, and therapeutic (Yau 2008). Furthermore, tai chi includes both a physical component and sociocultural and meditative ones that are believed to contribute to overall well-being. Tai chi exercise is often chosen by the elderly for its gentle, soft movements. Besides the physical aspect, these movements also include benefits to lifestyle issues, as well as psychological and social benefits (Irwin, Pike, Cole, & Oxman 2003; Motivala, Sollers, Thayer, & Irwin 2006). Evidence indicates that the improvement in physical and mental health through the practice of tai chi among older adults is related to their perceived level of quality of life (Chen et al. 2008). Since findings from several studies support the belief that the practice of tai chi has multiple benefits to practitioners, it is recommended as a strategy to promote successful cognitive and emotional aging.

Technology-Based Interventions

Technologies related to healthcare—including telehealth, electronic medical records, and telehomecare—can support independence and psychological resilience and safety and provide behavioral monitoring. Medical applications of the technology embodied in cell phones, Internet-connected computers, Wii, Facebook, and Twitter have the potential to enhance and support social resilience. Self-help communities can be created online to promote resilience via virtual support groups. Clearly, the use of social media can help to reduce the sense of loneliness and depression in many isolated older adults and to alleviate stress-related diseases.

Conclusion

Based on our review, resilience to stress can be promoted by enhancing protective factors. Successful stress reduction and management, particularly in the most vulnerable populations, can prevent serious mental and physical illness. Therefore, it will be crucial to develop effective treatment and preventive strategies to ensure successful aging by enhancing individual resilience and minimizing the burden of stress, anxiety, and depression—thereby leading to improved quality of life among our elderly (Charney et al. 2003). Novel interventions may become possible with increased understanding of the psychological predictors of resilience and the associated underlying genetic, neural, and neurochemical influences that shape psychological strength.

Future interventions enhancing resilience and reducing stress must (a) consider cultural, gender, and ethnic differences; (b) identify subjects at greatest risk (e.g., caregivers; those in bereavement); and (c) develop targeted programs that combine aspects of different interventional strategies. Future research should test culturally appropriate interventions, tailored to the needs of different populations that combine methods demonstrated to be effective in reducing stress and improving well-being and quality of life. Such methods include integrated use of cognitive-behavioral therapies that enhance individual resilience; complementary and alternative approaches to stress-reduction; pharmacological treatment; diet and exercise; and lifestyle changes. All are likely to improve overall functioning and well-being in older adults.

Neuroimaging and other biomarker studies can examine whether treatment-related changes in neuroplasticity and neural functioning can also reduce the likelihood of developing psychopathology in response to future stressors. Progress in understanding the neurobiological underpinnings of resilience and vulnerability to stress-related illnesses will also broaden pharmacological treatment approaches. Drug trials can target responsiveness to rewards and to dysregulated physiology.

Future research also should concentrate on discerning the specific psychological and biological mechanisms that underlie age-related changes in emotion regulation. Longitudinal studies are needed to better understand the dynamics between trajectories of emotional resilience and emotional growth and mature coping styles that engage mature defense mechanisms (i.e., suppression, anticipation, sublimation, humor, and altruism) and their role in promoting successful, positive aging. Culturally sensitive interventions can be developed to reflect the needs of aging ethnic groups in their cultural contexts.

New preventive interventions can focus on individuals at risk or on their environments. At the center of many communities are the physical capacities of housing, transportation, energy sources, sustainable environment, and land use, which can help support resilient communities. Therefore, interventions on the community level may affect sustainability of quality of life and interconnectedness between environmental and individual resilience. Investment in the infrastructure—such as affordable housing; home Internet access; increased social support, access to healthcare, public parks, and senior centers; air quality; and social programs addressing acculturation and adaptation of immigrant groups—would definitely increase.

Clinical Case

Mrs. M. was an 80-year-old nursing home resident with advanced dementia. She was a "wanderer"; she paced the floors of the facility for hours at a time; she was frequently agitated and rarely verbal. She was a former dancer and responded to music of the 1940s and '50s by calming down and dancing and singing along. She also responded to essential oils and brief massage using oils—especially lavender oil—by calming down and attending more to her grooming, and clothes. She also liked it when the group was reciting the loving-kindness meditation, though she would utter the words with difficulty: "May I be happy, may I be well, may I find peace, may I be filled with loving kindness. May all beings be happy, may all beings be well, may all beings find peace, may all beings be filled with loving kindness." A rare smile would fill her face instead of fear and anxiety, and she looked peaceful for a period of time before getting back to her routine. Overall, periods of better behavior and quality of life have improved for this patient.

. . .

References

Abbott, R., & Lavretsky, H. (2013) Tai Chi and Qigong for the treatment and prevention of mental disorders. *Psychiatr Clin North Am, 36*(1), 109–19.

Andreescu, C., Mulsant, B. H., & Emanuel, J. E. (2008). Complementary and alternative medicine in the treatment of bipolar disorder—a review of the evidence. *J Affect Disord, 110*(1–2), 16–26.

Astin, J. A. (1998). Why patients use alternative medicine: Results of a national study. *JAMA, 279*(19), 1548–53.

Barnes, P. M., Powell-Griner, E., McFann, K., & Nahin, R. L. (2004). Complementary and alternative medicine use among adults: United States, 2002. *Adv Data, 343*, 1–19.

Beck, A. T., Rush, A. J., Shaw, B. F., & Emery, G. (1979). *Cognitive therapy of depression*. New York: Guilford.

Belaise, C., Fava, G. A., & Marks, I. M. (2005). Alternatives to debriefing and modifications to cognitive behavior therapy for posttraumatic stress disorder. *Psychother Psychosom, 74*(4), 212–17.

Berry, D. S., & Hansen, J. S. (1996). Positive affect, negative affect, and social interaction. *J Pers Soc Psychol, 71*(4), 796–809.

Blumenthal, J. A., Babyak, M. A., Moore, K. A., Craighead, W. E., Herman, S., Khatri, P., . . . & Krishnan, K. R. (1999). Effects of exercise training on older patients with major depression. *Arch Intern Med, 159*(19), 2349–56.

Bosworth, H. B., Park, K. S., McQuoid, D. R., Hays, J. C., & Steffens, D. C. (2003). The impact of religious practice and religious coping on geriatric depression. *Int J Geriatr Psychiatry, 18*(10), 905–14.

Braungart, J. M., Plomin, R., DeFries, J. C., & Fulker, D. W. (1992). Genetic influence on tester rated infant temperament as assessed by Bayley's Infant Behavior Record: Nonadoptive and adoptive siblings and twins. *Dev Psychol, 28*(1), 40–47.

Brown, R. P., Gerbarg, P. L., & Ramazanov, Z. (2002). A phythomedical review of Rhodiola rosea. *Herbalgram, 56*, 40–62.

Bushell, W. C. (1995). Psychophysiological and comparative analysis of asceticomeditational discipline: Toward a new theory of asceticism. In V. L. Wimbush & R. Valantasis (Eds.), *Asceticism*. New York: Oxford University Press.

Buxton, O. M., L'Hermite-Balériaux, M., Hirschfeld, U., & Van Cauter, E. (1997). Acute and delayed effects of exercise on human melatonin secretion. *J Biol Rhythms, 12*(6), 568–74.

Cadet, P., Zhu, W., Mantione, K., Rymer, M., Dardik, I., Reisman, S., . . . & Stefano, G. B. (2003). Cyclic exercise induces anti-inflammatory signal molecule increases in the plasma of Parkinson's patients. *Int J Mol Med, 12*(4), 485–92.

Charney, D. S., Reynolds III, C. F., Lewis, L., Lebowitz, B. D., Sunderland, T., Alexopoulos, G. S., . . . & Young, R. C. (2003). Depression and Bipolar Support Alliance consensus statement on the unmet needs in diagnosis and treatment of mood disorders in late life. *Arch Gen Psychiatry, 60*(7), 664–72.

Chen, K. M., Lin, J. N., Lin, H. S., Wu, H. C., Chen, W. T., Li, C. H., & Kai Lo, S. (2008). The effects of a Simplified Tai-Chi Exercise Program (STEP) on the physical health of older adults living in long-term care facilities: A single group design with multiple time points. *Int J Nurs Stud, 45*(4), 501–7.

Costa, P. T., McCrae, R. R., & Zonderman, A. B. (1987). Environmental and dispositional influences on well-being: Longitudinal follow-up of an American national sample. *Br J Psychol, 78*(3), 299–306.

Cotman, C. W., Berchtold, N. C., & Christie, L. A. (2007). Exercise builds brain health: Key roles of growth factor cascades and inflammation. *Trends Neurosci, 30*(9), 464–72.

Danner, D. D., Snowdon, D. A., & Friesen, W. V. (2001). Positive emotions in early life and longevity: Findings from the nun study. *J Pers Soc Psychol, 80*(5), 804–13.

Diener, E., & Lucas, R. E. (1999). Personality and subjective well-being. In D. Kahneman, E. Diener, & N. Schwartz (Eds.), *Well-being: The foundations of hedonic psychology* (pp. 213–29). New York: Russell Sage Foundation.

Diener, E., Sandvik, E., & Pavot, W. (1991). Happiness is the frequency, not the intensity, of positive versus negative affect. In F. Strack, M. Argyle, & N. Schwarz (Eds.), *Subjective well-being: An interdisciplinary perspective* (pp. 119–39). Elmsford, NY: Pergamon.

Diener, E., & Seligman, M. E. (2002). Very happy people. *Psychol Sci, 13*(1), 81–84.

Dording, C. M., Fisher, L., Papakostas, G., Farabaugh, A., Sonawalla, S., Fava, M., & Mischoulon, D. (2008). A double-blind, randomized, pilot dose-finding study of maca root (L. meyenii) for the management of SSRI-induced sexual dysfunction. *CNS Neurosci Ther, 14*(3), 182–91.

Eid, J., & Morgan III, C. A. (2006). Dissociation, hardiness, and performance in military cadets participating in survival training. *Mil Med, 171*(5), 436–42.

Ernst, E. (2003). Complementary medicine: Where is the evidence? *J Fam Pract, 52*(8), 630–34.

Ernst, E., Posadzki, P., & Lee, M. S. (2011) Complementary and alternative medicine (CAM) for sexual dysfunction and erectile dysfunction in older men and women: An overview of systematic reviews. *Maturitas, 70*(1), 37–41.

Estrada, C., Isen, A. M., & Young, M. J. (1994). Positive affect influences creative problem solving and reported source of practice satisfaction in physicians. *Motiv Emot, 18*(4), 285–99.

Fava, G. A. (1999). Well-being therapy: Conceptual and technical issues. *Psychother Psychosom, 68*(4), 171–79.

Fava, G. A., Rafanelli, C., Cazzaro, M., Conti, S., & Grandi, S. (1998). Well-being therapy. A novel psychotherapeutic approach for residual symptoms of affective disorders. *Psychol Med, 28*(2), 475–80.

Fava, G. A., Rafanelli, C., Ottolini, F., Ruini, C., Cazzaro, M., & Grandi, S. (2001). Psychological well-being and residual symptoms in remitted patients with panic disorder and agoraphobia. *J Affect Disord, 65*(2), 185–90.

Fava, G. A., & Ruini, C. (2003). Development and characteristics of a well-being enhancing psychotherapeutic strategy: Well-being therapy. *J Behav Ther Exp Psychiatry, 34*(1), 45–63.

Fava, G. A., Ruini, C., Rafanelli, C., Finos, L., Salmaso, L., Mangelli, L., & Sirigatti, S. (2005). Well-being therapy of generalized anxiety disorder. *Psychother Psychosom, 74*(1), 26–30.

Flood, M., & Phillips, K. D. (2007). Creativity in older adults: A plethora of possibilities. *Issues Ment Health Nurs, 28*(4), 389–411.

Florian, V., Mikulincer, M., & Taubman, O. (1995). Does hardiness contribute to mental health during a stressful real-life situation? The roles of appraisal and coping. *J Pers Soc Psychol, 68*(4), 687–95.

Folkman, S., & Lazarus, R. S. (1985). If it changes it must be a process: Study of emotion and coping during three stages of a college examination. *J Pers Soc Psychol, 48*(1), 150–70.

Folkman, S., & Moskowitz, J. T. (2000). Positive affect and the other side of coping. *Am Psychol, 55*(6), 647–54.

Fontana, L., Meyer, T. E., Klein, S., & Holloszy, J. O. (2004). Long-term calorie restriction is highly effective in reducing the risk for atherosclerosis in humans. *Proc Natl Acad Sci U S A, 101*(17), 6659–63.

Frederick, S., & Loewenstein, G. (1999). Hedonic adaptation. In In D. Kahneman, E. Diener, & N. Schwartz (Eds.), *Well-being: The foundations of hedonic psychology* (302–29). New York: Russell Sage Foundation.

Fredrickson, B. L. (2001). The role of positive emotions in positive psychology. The broaden-and-build theory of positive emotions. *Am Psychol, 56*(3), 218–26.

Fredrickson, B. L., & Branigan, C. (2005). Positive emotions broaden the scope of attention and thought-action repertoires. *Cogn Emot, 19*(3), 313–32.

Fredrickson, B. L., & Joiner, T. (2002). Positive emotions trigger upward spirals toward emotional well-being. *Psychol Sci, 13*(2), 172–75.

Fredrickson, B. L., & Levenson, R. W. (1998). Positive emotions speed recovery from the cardiovascular sequelae of negative emotions. *Cogn Emot, 12*(2), 191–220.

Fredrickson, B. L., Tugade, M. M., Waugh, C. E., & Larkin, G. R. (2003). What good are positive emotions in crises? A prospective study of resilience and emotions following the terrorist attacks on the United States on September 11th, 2001. *J Pers Soc Psychol, 84*(2), 365–76.

Freund-Levi, Y., Basun, H., Cederholm, T., Faxén-Irving, G., Garlind, A., Grut, M., . . . & Eriksdotter-Jönhagen, M. (2008). Omega-3 supplementation in mild to moderate Alzheimer's disease: effects on neuropsychiatric symptoms. *Int J Geriatr Psychiatry, 23*(2), 161–69.

Fugh-Berman, A., & Cott, J. M. (1999). Dietary supplements and natural products as psychotherapeutic agents. *Psychosom Med, 61*(5), 712–28.

Gerbarg, P. L., & Brown, R. P. (2013). Phytomedicines for prevention and treatment of mental health disorders. *Psychiatr Clin North Am, 36*(1), 37–47.

Gonzales, G. F. (2012). Ethnobiology and ethnopharmacology of *Lepidium meyenii* (maca), a plant from the Peruvian Highlands. *Evid Based Complement Alternat Med, 193496.*

Gotto Jr., A. M., & Brinton, E. A. (2004). Assessing low levels of high-density lipoprotein cholesterol as a risk factor in coronary heart disease: A working group report and update. *J Am Coll Cardiol, 43*(5), 717–24.

Harker, L., & Keltner, D. (2001). Expressions of positive emotion in women's college yearbook pictures and their relationship to personality and life outcomes across adulthood. *J Pers Soc Psychol, 80*(1), 112–24.

Hurst, G. A., Williams, M. G., King, J. E., & Viken, R. (2008). Faith-based intervention in depression, anxiety, and other mental disturbances. *South Med J, 101*(4), 388–92.

Irwin, M. R., Pike, J. L., Cole, J. C., & Oxman, M. N. (2003). Effects of a behavioral intervention, Tai Chi Chih, on varicella-zoster virus specific immunity and health functioning in older adults. *Psychosom Med, 65*(5), 824–30.

Ji, L. L. (2002). Exercise-induced modulation of antioxidant defense. *Ann N Y Acad Sci, 959*, 82–92.

Jorm, A. F., Christensen, H., Griffiths, K. M., & Rodgers, B. (2002). Effectiveness of complementary and self-help treatments for depression. *Med J Aust, 176*(10), S84–96.

Kabat-Zinn, J. (1990). Full catastrophe living: The program of the Stress Reduction Clinic at the University of Massachusetts Medical Center. New York: Delta.

Kaniasty, K., & Norris, F. H. (2008). Longitudinal linkages between perceived social support and posttraumatic stress symptoms: Sequential roles of social causation and social selection. *J Trauma Stress, 21*(3), 274–81.

Khalsa, S. B. (2004). Yoga as a therapeutic intervention: A bibliometric analysis of published research studies. *Indian J Physiol Pharmacol, 48*(3), 269–85.

Khoshaba, D. M., & Maddi, S. R. (2001). *HardiTraining*. Newport Beach, CA: Hardiness Institute.

Kiecolt-Glaser, J. K., Christian, L., Preston, H., Houts, C. R., Malarkey, W. B., Emery, C. F., & Glaser, R. (2010). Stress, inflammation, and yoga practice. *Psychosom Med, 72*(2), 113–21.

King, L. A., King, D. W., Fairbank, J. A., Keane, T. M., & Adams, G. A. (1998). Resilience-recovery factors in post-traumatic stress disorder among female and male Vietnam veterans: Hardiness, postwar social support, and additional stressful life events. *J Pers Soc Psychol, 74*(2), 420–34.

Klein, D. F., Gittelman-Klein, R., Quitkin, F., & Rifkin, A. (1980). *Diagnosis and drug treatment of psychiatric disorders*. Baltimore: Williams & Wilkins.

Kobasa, S. C., Maddi, S. R., & Kahn, S. (1982). Hardiness and health: A prospective study. *J Pers Soc Psychol, 42*(1), 168–77.

Krishnamurthy, M. N., & Telles, S. (2007). Assessing depression following two ancient Indian interventions: Effects of yoga and Ayurveda on older adults in a residential home. *J Gerontol Nurs, 33*(2), 17–23.

Lavretsky, H. (2009). Complementary and alternative medicine use for treatment and prevention of late-life mood and cognitive disorders. *Aging Health, 5*(1), 61–78.

Lee, I. M., Hsieh, C. C., & Paffenbarger Jr., R. S. (1995). Exercise intensity and longevity in men. The Harvard Alumni Health Study. *JAMA, 273*(15), 1179–84.

Lykken, D., & Tellegen, A. (1996). Happiness is a stochastic phenomenon. *Psychol Sci, 7*(3), 186–89.

Lyubomirsky, S. (2009). Hedonic adaptation to positive and negative experiences. In S. Folkman (Ed.), *The Oxford handbook of stress, health, and coping*. New York: Oxford University Press.

Lyubomirsky, S., King, L., & Diener, E. (2005). The benefits of frequent positive affect: Does happiness lead to success? *Psychol Bull, 131*(6), 803–55.

Maddi, S. R. (2008). The courage and strategies of hardiness as helpful in growing despite major, disruptive stresses. *Am Psychol, 63*(6), 563–64.

Maddi, S. R., & Khoshaba, D. M. (2005). *Resilience at work*. New York: AMACOM.

Mattson, M. P. (2005). Energy intake, meal frequency, and health: A neurobiological perspective. *Annu Rev Nutr, 25*, 237–60.

Meeks, T. W., Wetherell, J. L., Irwin, M. R., Redwine, L. S., & Jeste, D. V. (2007). Complementary and alternative treatments for late-life depression, anxiety, and sleep disturbance: A review of randomized controlled trials. *J Clin Psychiatry, 68*(10), 1461–71.

Mischoulon, D., & Fava, M. (2002). Role of S-adenosyl-L-methionine in the treatment of depression: A review of the evidence. *Am J Clin Nutr, 76*(5), 1158S–61S.

Motivala, S. J., Sollers, J., Thayer, J., & Irwin, M. R. (2006). Tai Chi Chih acutely decreases sympathetic nervous system activity in older adults. *J Gerontol A Biol Sci Med Sci, 61*(11), 1177–80.

National Center for Complementary and Alternative Medicine. (2002). *Complementary, alternative, or integrative health: What's in a name?* Retrieved from http://nccam.nih.gov/health/whatiscam.

Norton, M. C., Singh, A., Skoog, I., Corcoran, C., Tschanz, J. T., Zandi, P. P., . . . & Steffens, D. C. (2008). Church attendance and new episodes of major depression in a community study of older adults: The Cache County Study. *J Gerontol B Psychol Sci Soc Sci, 63*(3), P129–37.

Panagioti, M., Gooding, P. A., & Tarrier, N. (2012). An empirical investigation of the effectiveness of the broad-minded affective coping procedure (BMAC) to boost mood among individuals with posttraumatic stress disorder (PTSD). *Behav Res Ther, 50*(10), 589–95.

Panossian A., Hovhannisyan, A., Abrahamyan, H., Gabrielyan, E., & Wikman, G. (2009). Pharmacokinetic and pharmacodynamic study of interaction of Rhodiola rosea SHR-5 extract with warfarin and theophylline in rats. *Phytother Res, 23*(3), 351–57.

Payne, M. E., Steck, S. E., George, R. R., & Steffens, D. C. (2012). Fruit, vegetable, and antioxidant intakes are lower in older adults with depression. *J Acad Nutr Diet, 112*(12), 2022–27.

Pedersen, B. K., & Bruunsgaard, H. (2003). Possible beneficial role of exercise in modulating low-grade inflammation in the elderly. *Scand J Med Sci Sports, 13*(1), 56–62.

Reay, J. L., Scholey, A. B., & Kennedy, D. O. (2010). Panax ginseng (G115) improves aspects of working memory performance and subjective ratings of calmness in healthy young adults. *Hum Psychopharmacol, 25*(6), 462–71.

Roth, G. S., Mattison, J. A., Ottinger, M. A., Chachich, M. E., Lane, M. A., & Ingram, D. K. (2004). Aging in rhesus monkeys: Relevance to human health interventions. *Science, 305*(5689), 1423–26.

Ryff, C. D. (1989). Happiness is everything, or is it? Explorations on the meaning of psychological well-being. *J Pers Soc Psychol, 57*(6), 1069–81.

Salmon, P. (2001). Effects of physical exercise on anxiety, depression, and sensitivity to stress: A unifying theory. *Clin Psychol Rev, 21*(1), 33–61.

Seligman, M. E. (1991). *Learned optimism.* New York: Pocket.

Seligman, M. E., Rashid, T., & Parks, A. C. (2006). Positive psychotherapy. *Am Psychol, 61*(8), 774–88.

Seligman, M. E., Schulman, P., DeRubeis, R. J., & Hollon, S. D. (1999). The prevention of depression and anxiety. *Prevention & Treatment, 2*(1), 8a.

Sharma, H., Chandola, H. M., Singh, G., & Basisht, G. (2007). Utilization of Ayurveda in health care: An approach for prevention, health promotion, and treatment of disease. Part 1—Ayurveda, the science of life. *J Altern Complement Med, 13*(9), 1011–19.

Singh, N. A., Stavrinos, T. M., Scarbek, Y., Galambos, G., Liber, C., & Singh, M. A. F. (2005). A randomized controlled trial of high versus low intensity weight training versus general practitioner care for clinical depression in older adults. *J Gerontol A Biol Sci Med Sci, 60*(6), 768–76.

Smith, C. A., & Hay, P. P. (2005). Acupuncture for depression. *Cochrane Database Syst Rev, 2,* CD004046.

Smith, J. K., Dykes, R., Douglas, J. E., Krishnaswamy, G., & Berk, S. (1999). Long-term exercise and atherogenic activity of blood mononuclear cells in persons at risk of developing ischemic heart disease. *JAMA, 281*(18), 1722–27.

Southwick, S. M., Pietrzak, R. H., & White, G. (2011). Interventions to enhance resilience and resilience-related constructs in adults. In S. M. Southwick, B. T. Litz, D. Charney, & M. J. Friedman (Eds.). *Resilience and mental health: Challenges across the lifespan* (pp. 289–306). Cambridge: Cambridge University Press.

Suh, E., Diener, E., & Fujita, F. (1996). Events and subjective well-being: Only recent events matter. *J Pers Soc Psychol, 70*(5), 1091–102.

Tanskanen, A., Hibbeln, J. R., Hintikka, J., Haatainen, K., Honkalampi, K., Viinamaki, H., & Stoll, A. L. (2001). Fish consumption, depression, and suicidality in a general population. *Arch Gen Psychiatry, 58*(5), 512–13.

Tarrier, N., & Gregg, L. (2004). Suicide risk in civilian PTSD patients—predictors of suicidal ideation, planning, and attempts. *Soc Psychiatry Psychiatr Epidemiol, 39*(8), 655–61.

Thurman, R. A. F. (1995). Tibetan Buddhist perspectives on asceticism. In V. L. Wimbush & R. Valantasis (Eds.), *Asceticism.* New York: Oxford University Press.

Tremblay, F., Mireault, A. C., Dessureault, L., Manning, H., & Sveistrup, H. (2004). Postural stabilization from fingertip contact: I. Variations in sway attenuation, perceived stability and contact forces with aging. *Exp Brain Res, 157*(3), 275–85.

Urry, H. L., Nitschke, J. B., Dolski, I., Jackson, D. C., Dalton, K. M., Mueller, C. J., . . . & Davidson, R. J. (2004). Making a life worth living: Neural correlates of well-being. *Psychol Sci, 15*(6), 367–72.

Walford, R. L., Mock, D., Verdery, R., & MacCallum, T. (2002). Calorie restriction in biosphere 2: alterations in physiologic, hematologic, hormonal, and biochemical parameters in humans restricted for a 2-year period. *J Gerontol A Biol Sci Med Sci, 57*(6), B211–24.

Watson, D., Clark, L. A., McIntyre, C. W., & Hamaker, S. (1992). Affect, personality, and social activity. *J Pers Soc Psychol, 63*(6), 1011–25.

Weindruch, R., & Walford, R. L. (1982). Dietary restriction in mice beginning at 1 year of age: Effect on life-span and spontaneous cancer incidence. *Science, 215*(4538), 1415–18.

Westphal, M., Bonanno, G. A., & Bartone, P. T. (2008). Resilience and personality. In B. J. Lukey & V. Tepe (Eds.), *Biobehavioral resilience to stress* (pp. 219–44). Boca Raton, FL: CRC.

Willcox, B. J., Willcox, D. C., Todoriki, H., Fujiyoshi, A., Yano, K., He, Q., . . . & Suzuki, M. (2007). Caloric restriction, the traditional Okinawan diet, and healthy aging: The diet of the world's longest-lived people and its potential impact on morbidity and life span. *Ann N Y Acad Sci, 1114*, 434–55.

Williams, J., & Graham, C. (2006). Acupuncture for older adults with depression: A pilot study to assess acceptability and feasibility. *Int J Geriatr Psychiatry, 21*(6), 599–600.

Wittink, M. N., Joo, J. H., Lewis, L. M., & Barg, F. K. (2009). Losing faith and using faith: Older African Americans discuss spirituality, religious activities, and depression. *J Gen Intern Med, 24*(3), 402–7.

Yau, M. K. (2008). Tai Chi exercise and the improvement of health and well-being in older adults. *Med Sport Sci, 52*, 155–65.

CHAPTER 12

Building Resilient Communities
for Older Adults

GOVERNMENTS AROUND THE WORLD are recognizing the importance of measuring subjective well-being as an indicator of progress (Huppert & So 2013). Nonetheless, Western society continues to struggle with anti-aging attitudes that tend to ignore the talents and creative contributions of older adults. These attitudes are expressed in a lack of opportunities for either vocational retraining and employment or community service. An alternative strategy, such as focusing on increasing resilience in the aging population, can lead to improved well-being and positive mental health, which in turn lead to flourishing.

Huppert and So (2013) examined international diagnostic criteria for depression and anxiety in the *Diagnostic and Statistical Manual* (DSM) and the International Classification of Diseases (ICD) classifications and identified ten features of positive well-being: competence, emotional stability, engagement, meaning, optimism, positive emotion, positive relationships, resilience, self-esteem, and vitality. An operational definition of flourishing was developed based on psychometric analysis of indicators of these ten features, using data from a representative sample of 43,000 Europeans. Application of this definition to respondents from the 23 countries of the European Social Survey revealed a fourfold difference in flourishing rates, from 41% in Denmark to less than 10% in Slovakia, Russia, and Portugal. There are also striking differences in country profiles across the ten features. These profiles offer insight into cultural- and country-specific differences in well-being, and they indicate which features may provide the most promising targets for policies to improve well-being. These findings can be used in designing community programs for building resilience in older adults, given the economic challenges global aging presents for different countries.

Aging Workforce, Economic Challenges, and Vocational Rehabilitation

In the United States and abroad, older workers are vulnerable to negative perceptions, stereotyping, and discrimination (Hedge, Borman, & Lammlein 2006). One persistent notion is that they are hard to train and slow to learn new technologies and information. In addition, they are thought to be less productive, physically able, ambitious, and adaptable than younger workers (Hassell & Perrewe 1995; Ng & Feldman 2008). However, demographic trends are changing with the aging of baby boomers—including delays in the labor participation of younger workers, the aging of the large baby boom cohort, changes in retirement age requiring dramatic changes in policies on retirement, and Social Security programs—all requiring longer labor force participation among older adults. By 2010 the number of workers age 55 and older reached 26 million, a 46% increase since 2000; by 2025 this number will increase to approximately 33 million. The number of workers over age 65 will also increase accordingly (Fullerton & Toosi 2001).

However, in today's economy, seniority no longer means job security, as layoffs of older workers from their career jobs become more common and more stressful for the health and well-being of individuals and their families. Older dual-earner couples are in double jeopardy of job layoffs. Once laid off or facing early retirement, older workers find that they cannot get hired for comparable jobs and salaries. Most older workers have minimal savings or pension prospects, as their mortgages, children's tuition bills, and other costs require two incomes. Financial burdens and anxiety about the future become very toxic for their health and well-being.

Both internal and external factors can contribute to resilience and hardiness. Studies of resilience tend to focus on individuals as the unit of analysis and to deal with all types of stressors that come with job loss or retirement. Several possible strategies allow for a positive adaptation in case of job loss or retirement, thereby promoting resilient life courses, including changing the situation (e.g., changing jobs); reframing the situation and its severity (e.g., "retirement," not "layoff"); and managing strains and tensions. Three components seem to be crucial for positive adaptation: (1) taking control or mastery over one's life; (2) social connections and support (within the couple or social network); and (3) making a meaningful contribution through paid work, civic engagement, or family work. Future stress-management resources are developed from this positive adaptation—the sense of control, connectedness, and contribution—overall leading to increased resilience (Moen, Sweet, & Hill 2010).

Society can help older workers manage stress and ill-health consequences of job and income loss by providing professional retraining, part-time employment, volunteering opportunities, and counseling—all of which will allow older adults to adapt at an easier pace. Ultimately, the question for policymakers may be not how to promote resilience (though this would be important, too) but rather how to set standards for an acceptable threshold of the "toxicity" of layoffs (e.g., rights to advanced notification, reasonable work schedules, access to breaks, etc.) and the expanding of resources and options available to individuals vulnerable to displacement (e.g., retraining, unemployment compensation, family leave). If the global economy continues to sustain flexibility for employers (e.g., the ability to lay off employees regardless of prior agreements), it may be possible to create an infrastructure that will support flexibility for career transitions, providing retraining, bridge income, and alternative arrangements for part-time employment (Moen et al. 2010). For older workers, policies and practices that facilitate the creation of second, third, and fourth careers would facilitate their recovery and renewal in the face of an uncertain economy and an uncharted course in the second half of life (Moen et al. 2010). Such policies and practices will also help to revive the viability of the notion of the role of elders in society.

Boosting the Role of Elders in Society

Historically, the elders of a society functioned as transmitters of sacred knowledge and rituals. They established an awareness of the culture and its roots that is necessary for the health and growth of the community (Moberg 2006). With a growing population of older adults, the role of elders in society should be expanded, to enrich and give meaning to the lives of its aging citizens.

"Elder" is a role played in organized communities, most commonly in subsistence cultures, with *elderhood* being the condition or quality of being an elder. It is essentially the state of being in the latter portion of one's life and being looked to for leadership, of either a passive or an active nature, by one's peers or subordinates almost exclusively because of one's age (Jones 2006). Sometimes this role involves a definite chronological milestone that must be surpassed, while at other times the required age is simply relative to the ages of all the other members of the group. Once they have met the requirements of their individual group, however, all elders are generally expected to mentor, share their experience, create a sense of oneness for their followers, and, most especially, act as the spiritual embodiments of their communities.

An example of informal elderhood is the role of the matriarchal grandmother as it appears in many parts of the so-called global South (the nations of Africa, Central and Latin America, and most of Asia). Grandmothers in these areas tend to serve both as the heads of their groups of descendants and as the catalysts of their periodic reunions and meetings. By so doing, they provide their families with a cohesion that would probably be absent otherwise. Another example is that of the vocational mentor who guides her or his apprentices with sponsorship, advocacy, and skill training. Mentors facilitate creativity by caring and teaching traditions of various occupations.

How can different countries establish programs promoting successful and positive aging? This will become an ever more crucial question as we move into the future.

Capacity-Building Programs

Interventions to stimulate and build resilience are focused on three areas: (1) developing disposition attributes of the individual, such as vigor, optimism, and physical robustness; (2) improving socialization practices; and (3) strengthening self-efficacy, self-esteem, and motivation through interpersonal interactions and experiences. These three areas are not mutually exclusive but can be complementary. For example, participating in a dance class can improve physical strength, provide social support, and strengthen self-efficacy (Pargament & Cummings 2010).

In studies of resilience, researchers are increasingly aware of complexity, which extends beyond protective factors of traits and risk factors of context or environment (Curtis & Cicchetti 2003). An example would be multifaceted approaches to optimizing resilience while considering risk-oriented strategies. Environmental interventions—such as safe chairs, beds, and toilets—can facilitate successful transfers required for boosting resilience. Social-networking systems that help disseminate opportunities for activities and increase outreach to older adults are likewise important and useful interventions to consider when trying to strengthen resilience. The interventions of the Strength-Focused and Meaning-Oriented Approach to Resilience and Transformation (SMART) are another example of a multifaceted approach to strengthen resilience in response to trauma; SMART incorporated Eastern spiritual teachings, physical techniques such as yoga, and psychoeducation to promote the reconstruction of meaning (Chan, Chan, & Ng 2006).

Interventions to Strengthen Motivation

Low motivation, or apathy, interferes with successful coping (Marin 1991) and can unfortunately increase with age and accompany many aging-related diseases such as Parkinson's, stroke, or dementia. An intervention devoted to increasing motivation can help improve coping, quality of life, and recovery from illness.

Motivation refers to the need, drive, or desire to act in a goal-directed fashion. Resilience relies on the individual's experiencing a life challenge of some type of adversity. The challenge may be a developmental change, such as impaired vision or mobility, or a social or economic challenge (retirement, bereavement, movement to an assisted-living facility). Conversely, motivation may not be dependent on an adverse event but may be a necessary component of pursuing recovery and achieving balance. Resilient reintegration requires increased energy and motivation. An example of the interaction between resilience and motivation is exercise or medication adherence. Interventions are directed at increasing self-efficacy while taking into account interpersonal, intrapersonal, and environmental factors (table 12.1). Interventions addressing apathy in a variety of neuropsychiatric conditions require the use of stimulants or dopaminergic agents (e.g., methylphenidate, bupropion, amantadine, bromocriptine, and selegiline) (Marin, Fogel, Hawkins, Duffy, & Krupp et al. 1995). It may be necessary to encourage and require a behavioral activity or intervention in a person with apathy.

Wellness-Oriented Holistic Interventions

Western medicine tends to focus on illness and acute care rather than on prevention or wellness. Both patients and care providers lose sight of their strengths and abilities. Holistic, integrative, and complementary and alternative medicine (CAM) focuses on whole persons, with all their strength and weaknesses (McBee 2008). In addition, holistic medicine tends to be preventative and wellness oriented. We will see the burgeoning number of baby boomers increasingly use Western *and* Oriental holistic medicine approaches to the treatment and prevention of the most common diseases of aging. These therapies can be practiced mindfully to promote awareness in

TABLE 12.1   Interventions to increase resilience and motivation

Focus of intervention	Examples of intervention techniques
Beliefs	Verbally encourage capability to perform. Expose older adults to role models. Decrease unpleasant sensations associated with activities. Encourage actual practice of activities. Educate about the benefits of the behavior and reinforce and underline those benefits. Teach realistic beliefs. Relate behavior to outcomes (e.g., exercise reduces blood pressure and aids weight loss).
Relief of symptoms of pain or fear	Facilitate appropriate use of medications and therapy. Use alternative measures such as heat or ice to relieve pain associated with activities. Employ cognitive behavioral therapy to explore thoughts and feelings, and triggers related to sensations and help patients develop a more realistic attitude to pain and fear and prevent episodes. Teach relaxation and distraction techniques. Use graded exposure to overcome fear (e.g., of falling, heights).
Individualized care	Demonstrate kindness and caring to the patient. Use humor. Positively reinforce desired behaviors. Recognize individual needs and differences, such as setting a rest period. Clearly communicate recommendations, write them out.
Social support	Evaluate social support of patient. Teach communication skills. Use social support and activities as a goal for intervention.
Goal setting	Develop realistic goals with the older adult. Set goals that can be met in a short time as well as longer-range goals. Use meaningful rewards. Teach to adapt to the current level of functioning and adjust expectations.
Successful performance	Review goals, skills, and utilized techniques. Expose individuals to successful activities that they can accomplish. Take small steps toward achievement. Build challenges into activities so that new successes can be incorporated. Celebrate and note accomplishments.

SOURCE: Adapted from Resnick 2011

the practitioner and the patient. Studies already report increasing use of mind-body medicine—especially meditation, imagery, and yoga—among older adults in the United States (Lavretsky 2009). Moreover, mindfulness practice has a demonstrated acceptability with elders and their caregivers (McBee 2004). Mindfulness and mindfulness-based stress reduction can be taught to anybody who can understand instructions, and they impart stress-reducing techniques that can reduce suffering.

Humor and laughter therapy also promote healing and well-being. In 1964, Norman Cousins documented the role of humor as a source for his own healing in *Anatomy of an Illness* (Cousins 1979). In 1995 in Bombay, India, Madan Kataria founded Laughing Clubs International by simply inviting people to laugh in a park each morning before work. Today there are over 3,000 laughing clubs throughout the world, including in the United States. Physiologically, laughter can increase breath, aid circulation, release endorphins, protect the immune system, and tone muscles. And laughter can be easily shared with others.

Another technique, which can be used in cognitively impaired individuals or those open to aromatherapy, is the use of essential oils with different intended actions. For example, lavender oil is used for relaxation, balance, and insomnia (Ballard et al. 2002). A few drops can be put in bathwater or on a pillow to help with relaxation and sleep; this oil may also be used for headaches, premenstrual syndrome, flu, and asthma (McBee 2008). Other examples include the use of peppermint oil for lifting energy and fighting fatigue, lemongrass oil for reducing stress and depression or infections, cinnamon oil for low mood and appetite; and ylang ylang oil for depression and as an aphrodisiac (McBee 2008).

Yet another holistic technique is hand massage, which can be utilized to increase balance, energy, and the sense of well-being (McBee 2008). Simple touching alone or as a part of full massage can reduce the sense of isolation and loneliness in socially isolated persons (McBee 2008). In over 90 studies, massage has been shown to be effective in enhancing health and alleviating symptoms, including promoting sleep, reducing anxiety, and decreasing physical agitation in people with dementia (Kennedy & Chapman 2006; Rowe & Alfred 1999). Table 12.2 offers examples of other CAM approaches used in wellness- and balance-oriented holistic medicine.

Activity-Oriented Therapies

Expressive therapies, such as art, music, drama, and movement, traditionally have been intertwined with spirituality and healing. Drumming, cave

TABLE 12.2   Integrative and holistic interventions domains and examples

Domain	Examples of the interventions	Comments
Biologically based therapies	Herbal (botanical) medicines, vitamins, nonvitamin/ nonmineral natural products (e.g., omega-3 fatty acids; adaptogens)	Nonvitamin/nonmineral natural products are used by 18% of U.S. adults.
Mind-body medicine	Biofeedback, meditation techniques, yoga, tai chi, energy therapies (e.g., light therapy, qigong, healing touch), exercise	Focuses on interactions among brain, mind, body, and behavior to affect physical function and promote health.
Manipulative and body-based practices	Chiropractic spinal manipulation, massage therapies, movement therapies (e.g., Pilates)	Focuses on structural and functional systems of the body, including bones and joints, soft tissues, circulatory, and lymphatic systems.
Alternative medical systems	Acupuncture, Ayurveda, homeopathy/ naturopathy, traditional healers (e.g., Native American healers)	Focuses on achieving optimal health and well-being.
Other complementary and alternative medicine (CAM) practices	Spirituality, pastoral care, expressive therapies	Approaches not formally categorized, but easily accepted by individuals.

painting, sacred music, and ritual dances can serve as examples of creative healing tools. Religious settings and services integrate creative expression into worship. The use of creative therapies aligns with other CAM modalities, affecting and empowering the whole person. Physical exercise, both aerobic and mindful, works to benefit physical and mental health and cognitive function (Merrill, Payne, & Lavretsky 2013). These therapies tend to improve quality of life.

The use of creativity is especially helpful for persons in crisis—undergoing significant changes or challenges—when a search for meaning may arise. Art and music can be used with any patient, no matter how ill (Boso, Politi, Barale, & Emanuele 2006; Cohen 2006; Hannemann 2006). Elderly persons with dementia may particularly benefit from creative modalities for expression and communication (Bober, McClellan, McBee, & Westreich 2002; Roome 2005).

Intergenerational Communities

For centuries, in both traditional and modern cultures, intergenerational learning has been the informal vehicle within families for "systematic transfer of knowledge, skills, competencies, norms and values between generations—and is as old as mankind" (Hoff 2007; Newman & Hatton-Yeo 2008). Typically, the elders or grandparents of the family share their wisdom and are valued for their role in perpetuating the values, culture, and uniqueness of the family. Intergenerational exchange within the family is intended to keep new generations grounded in the history of their culture and to provide a link to the past (Newman & Hatton-Yeo 2008). Familial intergenerational learning is informal and involves multigenerational interaction.

In modern, more complex societies, however, intergenerational learning is no longer transmitted by the family alone and increasingly occurs outside the family. While traditional families still may value the elder as the transmitter of cultural lore, preparing younger individuals for life in the modern world has become a function of wider social groups that are nonfamilial. The new model is "extrafamilial" (Newman & Hatton-Yeo 2008).

Intergenerational programs contribute to achieving the objectives of lifelong and intergenerational learning in four ways. They (1) lay the foundation for a lifelong culture for young and old; (2) develop positive attitudes among generations; (3) integrate benefits for children, youth, and older adults, schools, and community; and (4) create shared learning activities for all age groups, thus contributing to social inclusion, social cohesion, and solidarity (Hatton-Yeo 2007).

Toward the end of the twentieth century, another social paradigm emerged that has further advanced the notion of cooperation between various generations within a community's social structure. It is derived from, and nurtured in, social contexts in which people are working toward a common goal, creating synergy, and providing cohesiveness, trust, and solidarity. Though the culture, values, and infrastructure of communities differ, there are several characteristics associated with intergenerational learning that can provide programmatic cohesiveness and enable global application. *Benefits* of intergenerational learning refer to immediate or long-term positive gains. They are accrued by both older and younger learners and may be complementary or shared. Benefits for older learners include appreciations of their personal contributions and as a generational cohort. For younger learners, benefits include increased self-esteem and self-confidence and a deeper understanding of older adults. Both generations benefit from (1) feeling valued, accepted, and respected; (2) enhanced knowledge and skills; and (3) the creation of a meaningful, trusting intergenerational relationship (Newman & Hatton-Yeo 2008). Representative of intergenerational learning are "Engaged University" programs that develop educational opportunities for older scholars who join young students in the university classroom.

Intergenerational learning is emerging as a means for older adults to make valuable contributions to children, youth, and young adults while enhancing their own learning and growth. It is a concept that includes cross-generational and cross-system partnerships. Intergenerational learning will become even more important in the context of demographic aging.

Since the beginning of the twenty-first century, there have been efforts in Spain, England, and Germany to promote intergenerational learning as part of the policy debate. In 2002, the Second World Assembly on Ageing convened in Madrid and developed the Madrid International Plan of Action on Ageing (MIPAA), which recognized the dramatic transformation that has taken place in the world and the profound consequences this has for every aspect of individual, community, national, and international life. The MIPAA went on to stress the importance of "strengthening of solidarity through equity and reciprocity between generations" and called for initiatives aimed at promoting mutual, productive exchange and learning between generations, focusing on older people as a societal resource in building "a society for all ages" (Newman & Hatton-Yeo 2008).

Conclusion

Building resilient communities and programs for older adults will enhance their health, functioning, and well-being, but it also will require multifaceted management. Recognition and revival of the role of society elders will be required to sustain older adults' resilience and provide them with opportunities to flourish. Such initiatives will involve wellness interventions, increased socialization and opportunities for learning, vocational retraining, and opportunities for volunteering, intergenerational learning, and contributing to society.

The urgency of this issue has been reinforced in several ways as the baby boomers age. First, there is now a global recognition of the need to see older people as learning resources and as assets to their communities. Capacity-building programs will become essential for maintaining the well-being of the society at large and for reducing the costs of retirement and chronic diseases. Therefore, policymakers need to provide frameworks that promote the active aging of their citizens. Second, there is increasing acknowledgement of the role of lifelong and intergenerational learning, not only for its personal benefits but also to take account of the needs for an aging workforce to remain engaged longer and to take an active part in supporting young people as we work together to develop a successful, sustainable economy. Third, as education grows more important for individual economic success and younger people grow more concerned over the failures of existing educational systems, older people can gain a developing role as mentors.

References

Ballard, C., Stephens, S., McLaren, A., Wesnes, K., Kenny, R. A., Burton, E., . . . & Kalaria, R. (2002). Neuropsychological deficits in older stroke patients. *Ann N Y Acad Sci, 977*, 179–82.

Bober, S., McLellan, E., McBee, L., & Westreich, L. (2002). The Feelings Art Group: A vehicle of personal expression in skilled nursing home residents with dementia. *Journal of Social Work in Long Term Care, 1*(4), 73–87.

Boso, M., Politi, P., Barale, F., & Emanuele, E. (2006). Neurophysiology and neurobiology of the musical experience. *Funct Neurol, 21*(4), 187–91.

Chan, C. L., Chan, T. H., & Ng, S. M. (2006). The Strength-Focused and Meaning-Oriented Approach to Resilience and Transformation (SMART): A body-mind-spirit approach to trauma management. *Soc Work Health Care, 43*(2–3), 9–36.

Cohen, G. (2006). *The creativity and aging study: The impact of professionally conducted cultural programs on older adults. Final report: April 2006*. Retrieved from http://cahh.gwu.edu/arts-aging-study.

Cousins, N. (1979). *Anatomy of an illness as perceived by the patient: Reflections on healing and regeneration*. New York: W. W. Norton.

Curtis, W. J., & Cicchetti, D. (2003). Moving research on resilience into the 21st century: Theoretical and methodological considerations in examining the biological contributors to resilience. *Dev Psychopathol, 15*(3), 773–810.

Fullerton, H. N., & Toosi, M. (2001). Labor force projections to 2010: Steady growth and changing composition. *Monthly Labor Review, 124*, 21–38.

Hannemann, B. T. (2006). Creativity with dementia patients. Can creativity and art stimulate dementia patients positively? *Gerontology, 52*(1), 59–65.

Hassell, B. L., & Perrewe, P. L. (1995). An examination of beliefs about older workers: Do stereotypes still exist? *J Organ Behav, 16*(5), 457–68.

Hatton-Yeo, A. (2007). *Intergenerational practice: Active participation across the generations.* Beth Johnson Foundation. Retrieved from www.centreforip.org .uk/res/documents/publication/intergenerational_practice_report.pdf.

Hedge, J. W., Borman, W. C., & Lammlein, S. E. (2006). *The aging workforce: Realities, myths, and implications for organizations.* Washington, DC: APA.

Hoff, A. (2007). Intergenerational learning as an adaptation strategy in aging knowledge societies. In European Commission (Ed.), *Education, Employment, Europe* (pp. 126–29). Warsaw: National Contact Point for Research Programmes of the European Union.

Huppert, F. A., & So, T. T. (2013). Flourishing across Europe: Application of a new conceptual framework for defining well-being. *Soc Indic Res, 110*(3), 837–61.

Jones, T. (2006). *Elder: A spiritual alternative to being elderly.* Portland, OR: Elderhood Institute.

Kennedy, E., & Chapman, C. (2006). *Massage therapy and older adults.* New York: Springer.

Lavretsky, H. (2009). Complementary and alternative medicine use for treatment and prevention of late-life mood and cognitive disorders. *Aging Health, 5*(1), 61–78.

Marin, R. S. (1991). Apathy: A neuropsychiatric syndrome. *J Neuropsychiatry Clin Neurosci, 3*(3), 243–54.

Marin, R. S., Fogel, B. S., Hawkins, J., Duffy, J., & Krupp, B. (1995). Apathy: A treatable syndrome. *J Neuropsychiatry Clin Neurosci, 7*(1), 23–30.

McBee, L. (2004). Mindfulness practice with the frail elderly and their caregivers: Changing the practitioner-patient relationship. *Top Geriatr Rehabil, 19*(4), 257–264.

McBee, L. (2008). *Mindfulness-Based Elder Care.* New York, Springer.

Merrill, D., Payne, M., & Lavretsky, H. (2013). Complementary and alternative medicine approaches for treatment and prevention in late-life mood disorders. In H. Lavretsky, M. Sajatovic, & C. F. Reynolds III (Eds.), *Late-life mood disorders* (pp. 432–47). Oxford: Oxford University Press.

Moberg, D. O. (2006). *Aging and spirituality: Spiritual dimensions of aging theory, research, practice, and policy.* Binghampton, NY: Haworth Pastoral Press.

Moen, P., Sweet, S., & Hill, R. (2010). Risk, resilience, and life-course fit: Older couples' encores following job loss. In P. S. Fry & C. L. M. Keyes (Eds.), *New frontiers in resilient aging: Life-strengths and well-being in late life* (pp. 283–309). New York: Cambridge University Press.

Newman, S., & Hatton-Yeo, A. (2008). Intergenerational learning and the contributions of older people. *Ageing Horizons, 8,* 31–39.

Ng, T. W., & Feldman, D. C. (2008). The relationship of age to ten dimensions of job performance. *J Appl Psychol, 93*(2), 392–423.

Pargament, K. I., & Cummings, J. (2010). Anchored by faith: Religion as a resilience factor. In J. W. Reich, A. J. Zautra, & J. S. Hall (Eds.), *Handbook of Adult Resilience* (pp. 193–210). New York: Guilford Press.

Resnick B. (2011). The relationship between resilience and motivation. In B. Resnick, L. P. Gwyther, & K. A. Roberto (Eds.), *Resilience in aging: Concepts, research, and outcomes* (pp. 199–216). New York: Springer.

Roome, D. R. (2005). Painting memories: Art is therapy for Alzheimer's patients. *Mountain View Voice.* Retrieved from www.mv-voice.com/morgue/2005/2005_03_11.alzheime.shtml.

Rowe, M., & Alfred, D. (1999). The effectiveness of slow-stroke massage in diffusing agitated behaviors in individuals with Alzheimer's disease. *J Gerontol Nurs, 25*(6), 22–34.

CHAPTER 13

Resilience-Building Interventions and Prevention of Chronic Diseases of Aging

THERE ARE SOME COMMONALITIES and differences in approaching resilience, depending on the life settings and circumstances of older adults. In this chapter, I review the most common health and living situations that may benefit from resilience-building interventions. Older Americans, in both rural and urban communities, tend to experience hardships due to a decline in physical health; moreover, losing a spouse or close friend can cause significant distress and impairment of mental health.

In developing interventions, mental health providers are turning toward resilience to increase the likelihood of maintaining good health, aging well, and contributing to the vitality of the community. According to the resiliency framework, if stressors disrupt individuals' lives, both internal protective factors, such as self-reliance, and external protective factors, such as social networks, can restore balance; this process is referred to as "resilient reintegration" (Richardson, Neiger, Jensen, & Kumpfer 1990). Based on the resiliency process, interventions to promote protective factors can be initiated to help individuals adjust to hardships in a positive, growth-oriented manner.

Focus on boosting protective factors can be helpful in preventing disorders of aging and improving quality of life. Social networks have been found to be associated with resilience in multiple studies (Adams, Sanders, & Auth 2004; Easley & Schaller 2003; Felten 2000; Hinck 2004; Kinsel 2005; Montross et al. 2006; Tusaie, Puskar, & Sereika 2007; Yoon & Lee 2007); however, some studies found no relationship (Hunter & Chandler 1999; Markstrom, Marshall, & Tryon 2000). Several studies found a relationship between physical health status and resilience (Adams et al. 2004; Felten 2000; Hardy, Concato, & Gill 2004; Heilemann, Lee, & Kury 2005;

Hinck 2004; Humphreys 2003; Montross et al. 2006; Nygren et al. 2005; Wagnild 2003). In general, better self-reported physical health status was associated with higher levels of resilience. Many studies found a relationship between positive emotions and resilience (Christopher 2000; Lothe & Heggen 2003; Markstrom et al. 2000; Tugade & Fredrickson 2004; Tusaie & Patterson 2006; Tusaie et al. 2007; Wagnild 2003). An inverse relationship between mental health disorders, such as depression, and resilience was also found in many studies (Aroian & Norris 2000; Hardy et al. 2004; Heilemann et al. 2005; Humphreys 2003; Miller & Chandler 2002; Tusaie et al. 2007).

Creative engagement, as an expression of resilience, may have a neuroprotective effect among older adults, contributing to retention of cognitive capacity (McFadden & Basting 2010). Recent research on creative activities shows that they strengthen social networks and give persons a sense of control; both outcomes have been associated with brain health. McFadden and Basting (2010) cite evidence suggesting that positive social interactions can nurture resilience and creative engagement among older persons, including those living with dementia. The motivational, attentional, affective, and social components of creative activities combine to offer older persons meaningful opportunities to express and strengthen their resilience, regardless of their cognitive status, despite the biopsychosocial challenges of aging.

Increasing evidence suggests that an active lifestyle with physical and mental activities has a protective effect on brain functioning in the elderly population. Preventive approaches to the disorders of aging, including cognitive decline and dementia, could then be the basis of recommendations to the community. Such a nonpharmacological therapeutic approach may be an appealing low-cost, low-risk alternative treatment of this major public health priority. Even a modest decrease in the incidence of the disease would have a significant effect on social and economic cost. It has been reported that a five-year delay in the onset of dementia would result in a 50% decrease in the number of dementia cases (Felten 2000).

In the absence of curative treatment, physical exercise seems a reasonable basis for prevention trials (Hinck 2004). Only a few large randomized controlled trials (RCTs) (Kinsel 2005; Montross et al. 2006) have been conducted to show the benefit of physical activity on brain health. They support the benefit of physical activity on cognitive decline, but none has shown that physical activity can prevent dementia. Trials involving physical activity in the prevention of cognitive decline and dementia have specific design challenges. Individuals who agree to engage in physical activity programs are likely to differ in many other lifestyle domains (Hardy et al.

2004). Further, it may be difficult for subjects to maintain compliance with a physical activity program for a long period.

The main challenge is how to change lifestyle habits and promote physical activity in the older population over the long term. In primary care, prevention of many diseases already relies on a healthy diet and lifestyle, control of cardiovascular risk factors, ongoing learning experiences, and regular physical activity. During the past two decades, it has been shown that increasing physical activity can reduce the risk of chronic diseases such as congestive heart disease (Sasaki 2008) or colon (Akishita et al. 2004) and breast (Akishita 2007) cancer. The benefits that exercise can provide to brain functioning have been less thoroughly studied. However, the occurrence of dementia can be attributed to an accumulation of risk and protective factors during the life span (Iguchi 2005), and physical activity may contribute to the maintenance of a healthy aging brain. Recently, arguments from epidemiologic and basic research have emphasized that inactivity, a modifiable lifestyle factor, may affect age-related cognitive decline and the development of Alzheimer's disease. Prevention of cognitive decline and dementia could be a decisive argument to convince patients to increase their physical activity, as well as to modify public health policy.

Promoting Resilience as a Tool for Primary Prevention of Chronic Diseases

Primary prevention could well be the most important component of healthcare. However, only 2–3% of total healthcare spending goes for prevention (Woolf 2009). Resilience offers a framework that recognizes the preponderance of positive outcomes in patients with chronic disease and examines their antecedents, such as personality traits, coping style, and social support. Intervention programs can test whether fostering these can build resilience in a population at risk for certain diseases.

Self-help resources are available to maintain resilience. The American Psychological Association's online help center (www.apahelpcenter.org) provides a comprehensive overview along with an assessment tool and self-help tips (table 13.1) to build and maintain resilience (American Psychological Association 2007). The Web site highlights key factors that can help sustain resilience, including self-efficacy, setting and meeting realistic goals, communication and problem-solving skills, and controlling impulsive responses. In addition, it focuses on resilience as an ongoing process of growth, providing guidelines for learning from previous life experiences and actively facing sources of distress.

TABLE 13.1 Top ten ways to build resilience

1. Make connections.
2. Avoid seeing crises as insurmountable problems.
3. Accept that change is a part of living.
4. Move toward your goals.
5. Take decisive action.
6. Look for opportunities for self-discovery.
7. Nurture a positive view of yourself.
8. Keep things in perspective.
9. Maintain a hopeful outlook.
10. Take care of yourself.

SOURCE: American Psychological Association Help Center, www.apa.org/help center/road-resilience.aspx

Researchers are also developing clinical interventions to improve emotional well-being in chronically ill patients. Perhaps the most widely studied are interventions designed using Jon Kabat-Zinn's Mindfulness-Based Stress Reduction Program (MBSR), based on Buddhist practices. As mentioned in chapter 7, mindfulness emphasizes consistent, dispassionate, and nonevaluative moment-to-moment awareness of mental activities (Grossman, Niemann, Schmidt, & Walach 2004). A recent meta-analysis evaluated both physical and mental well-being across a variety of studies and concluded that mindfulness may enhance coping and reduce distress and disability (Grossman et al. 2004).

A variety of lifestyle changes, which may be either common across diseases or disease specific, typically can be recommended to improve the quality of life. For example, patients with most chronic conditions—whether cardiovascular disease, diabetes, depression, or pain—are advised to increase physical activity (Blumenthal et al. 2000; Boule, Haddad, Kenny, Wells, & Sigal 2001). Dietary recommendations could be disease specific, such as the DASH (Dietary Approach to Stop Hypertension) diet for heart disease and a low-carbohydrate diet for diabetic patients (Knowler et al. 2002).

A practical tool for primary care providers and specialists is the "5A" construct of behavioral counseling, first developed for tobacco-cessation programs, which allows assessment and recommendations that boost resilience (Glasgow, Emont, & Miller 2006).

1. *Assess:* Evaluate patient's disease knowledge (e.g., exercise is important); attitudes (e.g., self-efficacy for doing exercise); and

preferences (e.g., the type of exercise). The provider should also address barriers to the desired behavior.

2. *Advise*: Give personalized advice for maintaining or changing behaviors, incorporating specific recommendations of behavior change based on personal health risk, with gradual increase in exercise intensity.

3. *Agree*: Collaborate in goal-setting to improve chronic illness self-management, discussing realistic goals.

4. *Assist*: Develop an action plan that responds to patient's needs and barriers (e.g., where to get a pedometer; where to walk).

5. *Arrange*: Help to arrange for specific steps needed for goal achievement and provide assistance.

In summary, resilience can be built and maintained through the proactive efforts of patients using self-help or wellness-community models and support groups. The importance of examining resilience in chronic diseases and developing interventions to enhance it is likely to grow with the increasing prevalence of chronic disease in our aging society.

Primary and Secondary Prevention of the Mental Disorders of Aging

Another approach to boosting resilience in older community-dwelling adults would include primary prevention of the mental disorders of aging, including depression, anxiety, and cognitive decline (Okereke, Lyness, Lotrich, & Reynolds 2013). The famous aphorism "An ounce of prevention is worth a pound of cure" recognizes the value of prevention. Yet it is only recently that scientific attention has been paid to preventing the mental disorders of later adulthood, mostly focusing on prevention of late-life depression and cognitive decline.

Most clinicians are familiar with classifying prevention efforts into the following three categories: *primary*, preventing newly incident disease; *secondary*, detecting disease early and preventing progression; and *tertiary*, preventing or limiting the impact of the disease (American Medical Association 2012). This scheme, while useful, is based on the status of the disease in question.

A more useful framework for preventive interventions can be built around the target population. Such a framework was summarized by the Institute of Medicine (IOM) and entails *universal*, *selective*, and *indicated* prevention. Universal prevention focuses on the general population of interest. Selective prevention focuses on persons at risk to develop a particular disease. Indicated prevention is directed at people who have some symptoms but are below the symptom threshold that would indicate disease. These types of prevention may be viewed as part of a larger continuum of health promotion, as described by the IOM (Mrazek & Haggerty 1994).

Prevention in Primary Care Settings

Since the incidence of depression is elevated with most chronic medical conditions (Lyness 2008), there is a clear advantage to conducting preventive trials in medically ill populations. Indeed, the prevalence of subsyndromal depressive symptoms (e.g., sadness, anhedonia) is relatively high among such persons. Focusing on primary care recognizes that most older adults with subsyndromal depressive symptoms do see their primary care providers (Gallo & Coyne 2000); in fact, most seniors who die by suicide have been seen in primary care within a month of their death (Conwell 2004). Accordingly, efforts to improve detection and treatment of late-life depression have focused on primary care settings (Katon et al. 2005).

Mental-health policies targeting the prevention of depression across the life span could also have global implications for other problems in aging. For example, in a recent study, Barnes and Yaffe (2011) estimated that prevalent cases of Alzheimer's disease attributable to depression range from 506,000 to 1,078,000 subjects in the United States. Accordingly, the prevention of 10% and 25% of lifetime cases of depression may reduce the prevalence of Alzheimer's by 68,000 and 173,000, respectively.

Selective Prevention

Research groups from the Netherlands and the United States have found that identifying persons at high risk for depression—based on risk markers such as medical comorbidity, low social support, or functional disability—can yield theoretical numbers needed to treat (NNTs) of approximately 5 to 7 in primary care settings (Lyness, Yu, Tang, Tu, & Conwell 2009; Smit, Beekman, Cuijpers, de Graaf, & Vollebergh 2004; Smit, Ederveen, Cuijpers, Deeg, & Beekman 2006; Smits et al. 2008). Furthermore, a few pioneering RCTs of selective prevention have been conducted in specialty settings by focusing on high-risk populations with medical comorbidity. In one study, short-term problem-solving therapy (PST) approximately halved the two-month incidence of depression as compared with usual care in patients with macular degeneration (Rovner et al. 2007); however, the two groups did not differ significantly at a six-month follow-up.

In another study among patients who had suffered stroke, selective prevention was tested using a three-group design: escitalopram, PST, or placebo control. Those receiving escitalopram had about one-quarter the incidence of major depression at one year compared to placebo-receiving controls; patients who received PST had an intermediate outcome not significantly different from placebo in intent-to-treat analyses (Robinson et al. 2008). However, by six months after discontinuation of preventive intervention, the group that had previously received escitalopram had greater levels of depressive symptoms than either of the other comparison groups (Mikami et al. 2011). Thus it is clear that future research needs to identify the optimal methods for achieving a more enduring benefit of preventive interventions.

Opportunities for Using Universal Prevention Strategies

A remaining important question is whether general health- and wellness-oriented strategies can be developed to allow selective *and* universal prevention of depression. VITAL-DEP (Depression Endpoint Prevention in the VITamin D and OmegA-3 TriaL, NCT01696435) using nutritional supplements is one example of an ongoing trial.

VITAL-DEP is a depression-prevention ancillary study of the VITamin D and OmegA-3 TriaL (VITAL, NCT01169259), which is an RCT of supplementation with vitamin D (in the form of vitamin D3 [cholecalciferol], 2,000 IU daily) and marine omega-3 fatty acid (eicosapentaenoic acid [EPA] + docosahexaenoic acid [DHA], 1 g daily), for the primary prevention of heart disease and cancer among 20,000 U.S. adults (10,000 men aged 50+ years, 10,000 women aged 55+ years); the randomized treatment period will be five years (Manson et al. 2012). Current evidence from laboratory studies, observational research, and limited clinical trials suggest that these particular nutritional supplements have strong plausibility as tools to reduce risk of depression or improve mood (Appleton et al. 2006; Berk et al. 2007; Freeman et al. 2006; Garcion, Wion-Barbot, Montero-Menei, Berger, & Wion 2002; Hoogendijk et al. 2008; Jorde, Sneve, Figenschau, Svartberg, & Waterloo 2008; Kuningas et al. 2009; Mischoulon & Fava 2000; Pan et al. 2009; Tanskanen et al. 2001; Tiemeier, van Tuijl, Hofman, Kiliaan, & Breteler 2003; Timonen et al. 2004; Vieth, Kimball, Hu, & Walfish 2004; Wilkins et al. 2006). The trial utilizes a 2 × 2 factorial design, such that both independent main effects and possible agent synergies may be explicitly tested. Participants are randomized to one of four groups ($n = 5,000$ per group): (1) daily vitamin D3 and omega-3; (2) daily vitamin D3 and omega-3 placebo; (3) daily vitamin D placebo and omega-3; or (4) daily vitamin D and omega-3 placebos. Primary aims are to test whether these agents reduce the risk of clinical depressive syndrome and yield better mood scores over time in the full cohort of 20,000 generally healthy late-midlife and older participants, which is a true test of *universal* prevention.

Depression Prevention in Home-Bound Elders

Another growing population at high risk for depression is homebound elders, who tend to have multiple medical problems and mobility issues and face social isolation as well. Of the almost 40 million people over the age of 65 in the United States, nearly a tenth (9.2%) are considered housebound and in need of home-based care (Qiu et al. 2010; U. S. Census Bureau 2012). Based on epidemiological studies of community-dwelling older adults, the burden of depression and other mood disorders in this population is exceptionally high (Bruce & Hoff 1994; Bruce et al. 2011; Charlson et al. 2008; Ganguli, Fox, Gilby, & Belle 1996). Untreated depression leads to higher rates of healthcare use, premature institutionalization, and mortality (Arean, Hegel, Vannoy, Fan, & Unuzter 2008; Cuijpers, van Straten, & Warmerdam 2007; Lyness, Chapman, McGriff, Drayer, & Duberstein 2009; Malouff, Thorsteinsson et al. 2007). A common goal of many researchers and interested institutions is to develop interventions that efficiently reach as many depressed, homebound older adults as possible. To that end, studies build upon existing home-based care in the health or aging services sector or take advantage of remote communication technologies.

While treatment using antidepressant medication can be considered in homebound older adults, evidence suggests that they have a limited response to antidepressants alone, in part because of poor patient adherence or inadequate monitoring by the treating clinicians. Poor response may also reflect lack of attention to the psychosocial and physical needs of this population, such as multiple chronic medical conditions, disability, social isolation, and limited financial resources (Arean & Reynolds 2005; Cohen et al. 2006; Miranda, Azocar, Organista, Dwyer, & Areane 2003). Different psychotherapies, such as problem-solving therapy, problem-adaptation therapy, and supportive-interpersonal therapy, have been adapted for in-home use with homebound seniors. A major challenge to in-person psychotherapy is the added financial burden on both homebound seniors and care agencies, given the need either to transport disabled individuals to outpatient settings or to reimburse therapists for travel to the home setting.

Internet-guided and telepsychiatry interventions may save costs and time for patients and therapists. They may also reach depressed older adults not reached by traditional therapies, solve transportation problems, stimulate empowerment of patients, and reduce the stigma associated with mental illness. Although a growing number of studies have looked at the effects of Internet-based and telephone-supported interventions, few have examined these in older adults. However, research shows that these interventions are promising, and there is no reason to assume that they are not effective in older adults.

For example, Sheeran and colleagues (2011) embedded depression clinical management (DCM) components (e.g., assessment of depressive symptoms, antidepressant treatment adherence, and side effects) into remote monitoring devices commonly used by home healthcare agencies to transmit temperature, blood pressure, and other health-related information to "telehealth" nurses based at the agency. They reported high levels of feasibility, acceptability by patients and nurses, and preliminary evidence of effectiveness. Kroenke developed a telecare-management intervention that includes nurse telephone-care management, automated symptom monitoring, and medication management (Kroenke et al. 2010). In a trial of 309 patients (mean age, 58 years), patients in the intervention group had significantly greater increase in depressive-symptom improvement than those in usual-care group (over 12 months). Although not designed specifically for homebound older adults, the trial demonstrated the feasibility of providing DCM across multiple geographically dispersed, community-based practices in both urban and rural areas by coupling human with technology-augmented patient interactions.

More research into resilience-building interventions in the homebound elderly is needed, especially since technology develops so quickly, and innovative types of interventions and new possibilities to reduce the disease burden in depressed older adults are emerging rapidly.

Resilience Interventions in Assisted-Living and Nursing-Home Elders

The population of older adults living in assisted-living facilities and nursing homes faces multiple challenges and is in great need of resilience-building interventions. Although the majority of people with dementia live at home, long-term institutional care can be inevitable as the disease progresses. Care for dementia sufferers has been based on a medical somatic model, emphasizing illness and treatment of underlying pathology. Physically and functionally, long-term care facilities resemble hospitals, with nursing stations and visiting physicians. Their rules and routines governing daily life permit little individualization. However, there is a shift toward strength-based and person-centered care for people with dementia living in care facilities, with care aimed at building on a patient's personal strengths and supporting the overall well-being of the individual (Verbeek, Kane, van Rossum, & Hamers 2011). Implementation of person-centered care requires changes in environmental design practices to promote greater autonomy, privacy, personal identity, personhood, and socialization (Calkins & Keane 2008; Cutler et al. 2006; Zeisel et al. 2003).

The process of cultural change promotes resident-directed care and quality of life, emphasizing the care-based relationship between residents and direct-care workers (White-Chu et al. 2009). This cultural change movement is reflected in architecture and physical design to promote home-like environments and in care that focuses on residents' autonomy and opportunity for choice, as well as on sustaining a sense of self and control. Everyday quality of life in nursing homes is thereby improved. Staff training focuses on increased flexibility and individualization of care.

Other trends include the creation of dementia special-care units designed for residents with few nursing needs but with behavioral problems that require specialized staff training and architectural designs to protect them from wondering off or harming themselves or others. Another trend is an increasing number of small residential facilities with a family setting, frequently referred to as board-and-care facilities, which try to "normalize" the lifestyle of the residents. Findings from a few studies that assessed the effects of small-scale living suggest resilience-promoting outcomes for the residents (de Rooij, Luijkx, Emmerink, Declerq, & Schols 2009). For example, residents of small-scale living communities are more socially engaged and have more things to do and enjoy compared to residents of large nursing homes. Caregivers also have more opportunities for involvement (Verbeek, van Rossum, Zwakhalen, Kempen, & Hamers 2008).

Additional resilience-promoting interventions can include psychotherapy, activities-oriented interventions (e.g., art, physical exercise, occupational and physical therapy, dance, music, pet therapies), and any number of complementary and alternative interventions that these facilities and residents are open to, which could be culture- or spirituality-based.

Resilience-Building Interventions in Palliative- and Hospice-Care Settings

From the earliest stages of the modern hospice movement, there has been an acknowledgment of the depth of psychological distress that many dying patients experience. The British physician Cicely Saunders is widely credited with establishing modern standards of hospice care in a 1963 address to the Royal Society of Medicine (Irwin 2013). Describing the management of pain in patients with terminal cancer, Saunders observed that "mental distress may be perhaps the most intractable pain of all" (Ferris et al. 2002). In her later writings, Saunders articulated the concept of "total pain," now embodied in the interdisciplinary approach to patient care that characterizes modern-day palliative medicine. Within total pain, Saunders placed emotional distress alongside physical pain and social and spiritual problems, arguing that effective care of dying patients required attention to the relief of suffering in each of these domains (Center to Advance Palliative Care 2011).

The most important elements of hospice care are (1) focus on preserving quality of life; (2) attention to suffering in both the patient and caregivers; (3) care that is provided by a team with interdisciplinary expertise; and (4) support that can complement disease-oriented treatments throughout the entire course of an illness for persons of any age. When a cure is no longer possible, or when disease-modifying treatment is no longer desired, palliative care may become the sole focus. When prognosis is short and the goals of therapy are to optimize quality of life and function in the final phase of life, hospice delivers enhanced palliative care wherever patients live. Uniquely, hospice services also include bereavement care for family members up to and after a patient's death (Byock, Twohig, Merriman, & Collins 2006). In the United States, hospice care is available to patients with a prognosis of six months or less, and the services provided are largely governed by the guidelines of the federal healthcare benefit.

Can Positive Outcomes Be Achieved in End-of-Life Healthcare Settings?

Some studies that have looked at clinical outcomes in different palliative-care settings show improvements in symptom relief, and most show improvements in quality of life. For example, in a retrospective study of more than 400 cancer patients, an outpatient palliative-care intervention was associated with significant reductions in pain, fatigue, dyspnea, insomnia, depression, and anxiety, as well as significant improvements in overall quality of life (Yennurajalingam et al. 2012). In addition, surveys have consistently reported high levels of satisfaction among family and caregivers. In a nationally representative sample of family members of deceased patients, for example, those who used home-based hospice services (as compared to home health, nursing home, or hospital) reported improved relief of pain, higher levels of emotional support for both patient and family, increased treatment with respect, and higher overall quality of care (Teno et al. 2004).

Several psychotherapies have been adapted to or developed for the setting of advanced life-threatening illness. Of these, two of the most prominent—meaning-centered psychotherapy and dignity therapy—have been recently tested in randomized controlled trials. Dignity therapy is a brief individual psychotherapy derived from an empirical model of dignity in terminally ill patients (Chochinov 2002), with promising data for effectiveness from a phase-one trial (Chochinov et al. 2005). In a multisite randomized controlled trial, dignity therapy (relative to client-centered care or standard palliative care) was associated with greater levels of perceived helpfulness, improved quality of life, greater sense of dignity, and a higher degree of helpfulness to the family. Of note, there were no significant differences in global distress levels, the primary outcome (Chochinov et al. 2011).

Meaning-centered psychotherapy is a short-term intervention grounded in the writings and logotherapy of Viktor Frankl. The treatment seeks to bolster meaning and spiritual well-being in terminally ill patients, through individual and group applications (Breitbart, Gibson, Poppito, & Berg 2004). In a small RCT in group format, participants received either the meaning-centered intervention or supportive group psychotherapy. Subjects in the meaning-centered psychotherapy arm reported significantly greater improvements in their sense of meaning and spiritual well-being, as well as reductions in both anxiety and desire for death (Breitbart et al. 2010). In a follow-up trial of similar design, the individual format of meaning-centered psychotherapy was also tested. Here the comparator was therapeutic massage. Again, participants who received the meaning-centered intervention reported significant improvements in spiritual well-being and quality of life relative to their counterparts in the massage arm. The effect was short lived, however, as differences in the treatment arms were absent by the two-month assessment (Breitbart et al. 2012).

Psychiatric conditions are often difficult to differentiate in the setting of serious illness, due to symptom overlap with medical conditions (Irwin & Ferris 2008). In hospice patients, for example, roughly 50% will experience symptoms of depression, approximately 70% will experience clinically significant anxiety, and nearly all patients will experience delirium as death nears. However, increasing evidence suggests that palliative care achieves better clinical outcomes than standard care alone. Patients feel better and report improved quality of life, and caregivers report higher levels of satisfaction. What's more, when matched by diagnosis and severity of illness, palliative care appears to be less costly than standard care alone. Finally, emerging data suggest that under some circumstances there may be improvements in length of survival as well.

Conclusion

This chapter has focused on different approaches and models of care to targeting resilience and prevention of chronic diseases of aging. Fortunately, in the last decade, efforts have demonstrated that universal, population-wide prevention and selective prevention can be successful in reducing morbidity and mortality, as occurred with the smoking cessation campaigns. The difficulties of addressing mental disorders of aging have to do with the stigma of mental illness and stigma of aging, but we are making strides in these areas by educating governments, communities, and general public, as well as clinicians, about simple lifestyle and more complex therapeutic approaches to improve resilience and quality of life in older adults.

References

Adams, K. B., Sanders, S., & Auth, E. A. (2004). Loneliness and depression in independent living retirement communities: Risk and resilience factors. *Aging Ment Health, 8*(6), 475–85.

Akishita M. (2007). [Guidelines for medical treatment and its safety in the elderly]. *Nihon Ronen Igakkai Zasshi, 44*(1), 31–34.

Akishita, M., Teramoto, S., Arai, H., Mizukami, K., Morimoto, S., & Toba, K. (2004). Incidence of adverse drug reactions in geriatric wards of university hospitals. *Nihon Ronen Igakkai Zasshi, 41*(3), 303–6.

American Medical Association. (2012). *Glossary term "Prevent."* Retrieved from http://jamaevidence.com/JAMAevidence_Glossary_Final.pdf.

American Psychological Association. (2007). *The road to resilience.* Retrieved from www.apa.org/helpcenter/road-resilience.aspx.

Appleton, K. M., Hayward, R. C., Gunnell, D., Peters, T. J., Rogers, P. J., Kessler, D., & Ness, A. R. (2006). Effects of n-3 long-chain polyunsaturated fatty acids on depressed mood: systematic review of published trials. *Am J Clin Nutr, 84*(6), 1308–16.

Arai, H., Ouchi, Y., Yokode, M., Ito, H., Uematsu, H., Eto, F., . . . & Kita, T. (2012). Toward the realization of a better aged society: Messages from gerontology and geriatrics. *Geriatr Gerontol Int, 12*(1), 16–22.

Arean, P., Hegel, M., Vannoy, S., Fan, M. Y., & Unuzter, J. (2008). Effectiveness of problem-solving therapy for older, primary care patients with depression: Results from the IMPACT project. *Gerontologist, 48*(3), 311–23.

Arean, P. A., Reynolds III, C. F. (2005). The impact of psychosocial factors on late-life depression. *Biol Psychiatry, 58*(4), 277–82.

Aroian, K. J., & Norris, A. E. (2000). Resilience, stress, and depression among Russian immigrants to Israel. *West J Nurs Res, 22*(1), 54–67.

Barnes, D. E., & Yaffe, K. (2011). The projected effect of risk factor reduction on Alzheimer's disease prevalence. *Lancet Neurol, 10*(9), 819–28.

Berk, M., Sanders, K. M., Pasco, J. A., Jacka, F. N., Williams, L. J., Hayles, A. L., & Dodd, S. (2007). Vitamin D deficiency may play a role in depression. *Med Hypotheses, 69*(6), 1316–19.

Blumenthal, J. A., Sherwood, A., Gullette, E. C., Babyak, M., Waugh, R., Georgiades, A., . . . & Hinderliter, A. (2000). Exercise and weight loss reduce blood pressure in men and women with mild hypertension: Effects on cardiovascular, metabolic, and hemodynamic functioning. *Arch Intern Med, 160*(13), 1947–58.

Boule, N. G., Haddad, E., Kenny, G. P., Wells, G. A., & Sigal, R. J. (2001). Effects of exercise on glycemic control and body mass in type 2 diabetes mellitus: A meta-analysis of controlled clinical trials. *JAMA, 286*(10), 1218–27.

Breitbart, W., Gibson, C., Poppito, S. R., & Berg, A. (2004). Psychotherapeutic interventions at the end of life: A focus on meaning and spirituality. *Can J Psychiatry, 49*(6), 366–72.

Breitbart, W., Poppito, S., Rosenfeld, B., Vickers, A. J., Li, Y., Abbey, J., . . . & Cassileth, B. R. (2012). Pilot randomized controlled trial of individual meaning-centered psychotherapy for patients with advanced cancer. *J Clin Oncol, 30*(12), 1304–9.

Breitbart, W., Rosenfeld, B., Gibson, C., Pessin, H., Poppito, S., Nelson, C., . . . & Olden, M. (2010). Meaning-centered group psychotherapy for patients with advanced cancer: A pilot randomized controlled trial. *Psychooncology, 19*(1), 21–28.

Bruce, M. L., & Hoff, R. A. (1994). Social and physical health risk factors for first-onset major depressive disorder in a community sample. *Soc Psychiatry Psychiatr Epidemiol, 29*(4), 165–71.

Bruce, M. L., Sheeran, T., Raue, P. J., Reilly, C. F., Greenberg, R. L., Pomerantz, J. C., . . . & Johnston, C. L. (2011). Depression Care for Patients at Home (Depression CAREPATH): Home care depression care management protocol, part 2. *Home Healthc Nurse, 29*(8), 480–89.

Byock, I., Twohig, J. S., Merriman, M., & Collins, K. (2006). Promoting excellence in end-of-life care: A report on innovative models of palliative care. *J Palliat Med, 9*(1), 137–51.

Calkins, M. P., & Keane, W. (2008). Tomorrow's assisted living and nursing homes: The converging worlds of residential long-term care. In S. M. Golant & J. Hyde (Eds.) *The Assisted living residence: a vision for the future* (pp. 86–118). Baltimore: Johns Hopkins University Press.

Center to Advance Palliative Care. (2011). *2011 Public Opinion Research on Palliative Care*. Retrieved from www.capc.org/tools-for-palliative-care-programs /marketing/public-opinion-research/2011-public-opinion-research-on-palliative -care.pdf. {AU: See note on p. 26.}

Charlson, M. E., Peterson, J. C., Syat, B. L., Briggs, W. M., Kline, R., Dodd, M., . . . & Dionne, W. (2008). Outcomes of community-based social service interventions in homebound elders. *Int J Geriatr Psychiatry, 23*(4), 427–32.

Chochinov, H. M. (2002). Dignity-conserving care—a new model for palliative care: Helping the patient feel valued. *JAMA, 287*(17), 2253–60.

Chochinov, H. M., Hack, T., Hassard, T., Kristjanson, L. J., McClement, S., & Harlos, M. (2005). Dignity therapy: A novel psychotherapeutic intervention for patients near the end of life. *J Clin Oncol 23*(24), 5520–25.

Chochinov, H. M., Kristjanson, L. J., Breitbart, W., McClement, S., Hack, T. F., Hassard, T., & Harlos, M. (2011). Effect of dignity therapy on distress and end-of-life experience in terminally ill patients: A randomised controlled trial. *Lancet Oncol, 12*(8), 753–62.

Christopher, K. A. (2000). Determinants of psychological well-being in Irish immigrants. *West J Nurs Res, 22*(2), 123–40; discussion 140–43.

Cohen, A., Houck, P. R., Szanto, K., Dew, M. A., Gilman, S. E., & Reynolds III, C. F. (2006). Social inequalities in response to antidepressant treatment in older adults. *Arch Gen Psychiatry, 63*(1), 50–56.

Conwell, Y. (2004). Suicide. In S. P. Roose & H. A. Sackeim (Eds.), *Late-life depression* (pp. 95–106). Oxford, Oxford University Press.

Cuijpers, P., van Straten, A., & Warmerdam, L. (2007). Problem solving therapies for depression: A meta-analysis. *Eur Psychiatry, 22*(1), 9–15.

Cutler, L. J., Kane, R. A., Degenholtz, H. B., Miller, M. J., & Grant, L. (2006). Assessing and comparing physical environments for nursing home residents: Using new tools for greater specificity. *Gerontologist, 46*(1), 42–51.

de Rooij, I., Luijkx, K. G., Emmerink, P. M. J., Declerq, A., & Schols, J. M. G. A. (2009). Does small-scale living increase quality of life for older people with dementia? In I. de Rooij & H. Stoop (Eds.), *Grote kwaliteit op kleine schaal. Is kleinschalig wonen voor mensen met dementie een succesvolle parel in de ouderenzorg?* (pp. 43–52). Tilburg, NL: Programmaraad Zorgvernieuwing Psychogeriatrie en De kievitshorst / De Wever.

Easley, C., & Schaller, J. (2003). The experience of being old-old: Life after 85. *Geriatr Nurs, 24*(5), 273–77.

Felten, B. S. (2000). Resilience in a multicultural sample of community-dwelling women older than age 85. *Clin Nurs Res, 9*(2), 102–23.

Ferris, F. D., Balfour, H. M., Bowen, K., Farley, J., Hardwick, M., Lamontagne, C., . . . & West, P. J. (2002). A model to guide patient and family care: Based on nationally accepted principles and norms of practice. *J Pain Symptom Manage, 24*(2), 106–23.

Freeman, M. P., Hibbeln, J. R., Wisner, K. L., Davis, J. M., Mischoulon, D., Peet, M., . . . & Stoll, A. L. (2006). Omega-3 fatty acids: Evidence basis for treatment and future research in psychiatry. *J Clin Psychiatry, 67*(12), 1954–67.

Gallo, J. J., & Coyne, J. C. (2000). The challenge of depression in late life: Bridging science and service in primary care. *JAMA, 284*(12), 1570–72.

Ganguli, M., Fox, A., Gilby, J., & Belle, S. (1996). Characteristics of rural homebound older adults: A community-based study. *J Am Geriatr Soc, 44*(4), 363–70.

Garcion, E., Wion-Barbot, N., Montero-Menei, C. N., Berger, F., & Wion, D. (2002). New clues about vitamin D functions in the nervous system. *Trends Endocrinol Metab, 13*(3), 100–105.

Glasgow, R. E., Emont, S., & Miller, D. C. (2006). Assessing delivery of the five "A"s for patient-centered counseling. *Health Promot Int, 21*(3), 245–55.

Grossman, P., Niemann, L., Schmidt, S., & Walach, H. (2004). Mindfulness-based stress reduction and health benefits. A meta-analysis. *J Psychosom Res, 57*(1), 35–43.

Hardy, S. E., Concato, J., & Gill, T. M. (2004). Resilience of community-dwelling older persons. *J Am Geriatr Soc, 52*(2), 257–62.

Heilemann, M. V., Lee, K. A., & Kury, F. S. (2005). Strength factors among women of Mexican descent. *West J Nurs Res, 27*(8), 949–65; discussion, 966–76.

Hinck, S. (2004). The lived experience of oldest-old rural adults. *Qual Health Res, 14*(6), 779–91.

Hoogendijk, W. J., Lips, P., Dik, M. G., Deeg, D. J., Beekman, A. T., & Penninx, B. W. (2008). Depression is associated with decreased 25-hydroxyvitamin D and increased parathyroid hormone levels in older adults. *Arch Gen Psychiatry, 65*(5), 508–12.

Humphreys, J. (2003). Resilience in sheltered battered women. *Issues Ment Health Nurs, 24*(2), 137–52.

Hunter, A. J., & Chandler, G. E. (1999). Adolescent resilience. *Image J Nurs Sch, 31*(3), 243–47.

Iguchi, A. (2005). [Terminal care of the elderly]. *Nihon Ronen Igakkai Zasshi, 42*(3), 285–87.

Irwin, S. A. (2013). Palliative Care. *FOCUS, 11*(1), 48–51.

Irwin, S. A., & Ferris, F. D. (2008). The opportunity for psychiatry in palliative care. *Can J Psychiatry, 53*(11), 713–24.

Jorde, R., Sneve, M., Figenschau, Y., Svartberg, J., & Waterloo, K. (2008). Effects of vitamin D supplementation on symptoms of depression in overweight and obese subjects: Randomized double blind trial. *J Intern Med,* 264(6), 599–609.

Katon, W. J., Schoenbaum, M., Fan, M. Y., Callahan, C. M., Williams Jr., J., Hunkeler, E., . . . & Unutzer, J. (2005). Cost-effectiveness of improving primary care treatment of late-life depression. *Arch Gen Psychiatry,* 62(12), 1313–20.

Kinsel, B. (2005). Resilience as adaptation in older women. *J Women Aging,* 17(3), 23–39.

Knowler, W. C., Barrett-Connor, E., Fowler, S. E., Hamman, R. F., Lachin, J. M., Walker, E. A., & Nathan, D. M. (2002). Reduction in the incidence of type 2 diabetes with lifestyle intervention or metformin. *N Engl J Med,* 346(6), 393–403.

Kroenke, K., Theobald, D., Wu, J., Norton, K., Morrison, G., Carpenter, J., & Tu, W. (2010). Effect of telecare management on pain and depression in patients with cancer: A randomized trial. *JAMA,* 304(2), 163–71.

Kuningas, M., Mooijaart, S. P., Jolles, J., Slagboom, P. E., Westendorp, R. G., & van Heemst, D. (2009). VDR gene variants associate with cognitive function and depressive symptoms in old age. *Neurobiol Aging,* 30(3), 466–73.

Lothe, E. A., & Heggen, K. (2003). A study of resilience in young Ethiopian famine survivors. *J Transcult Nurs,* 14(4), 313–20.

Lyness, J. M. (2008). Depression and comorbidity: Objects in the mirror are more complex than they appear. *Am J Geriatr Psychiatry,* 16(3), 181–85.

Lyness, J. M., Chapman, B. P., McGriff, J., Drayer, R., & Duberstein, P. R. (2009). One-year outcomes of minor and subsyndromal depression in older primary care patients. *Int Psychogeriatr,* 21(1), 60–68.

Lyness, J. M., Yu, Q., Tang, W., Tu, X., & Conwell, Y. (2009). Risks for depression onset in primary care elderly patients: potential targets for preventive interventions. *Am J Psychiatry,* 166(12), 1375–383.

Malouff, J. M., Thorsteinsson, E. B., & Schutte, N. S. (2007). The efficacy of problem solving therapy in reducing mental and physical health problems: A meta-analysis. *Clin Psychol Rev,* 27(1), 46–57.

Manson, J. E., Bassuk, S. S., Lee, I. M., Cook, N. R., Albert, M. A., Gordon, D., . . . & Buring, J. E. (2012). The VITamin D and OmegA-3 TriaL (VITAL): Rationale and design of a large randomized controlled trial of vitamin D and marine omega-3 fatty acid supplements for the primary prevention of cancer and cardiovascular disease. *Contemp Clin Trials,* 33(1), 159–71.

Markstrom, C. A., Marshall, S. K., & Tryon, R. J. (2000). Resiliency, social support, and coping in rural low-income Appalachian adolescents from two racial groups. *J Adolesc,* 23(6), 693–703.

McFadden, S. H., & Basting, A. D. (2010). Healthy aging persons and their brains: Promoting resilience through creative engagement. *Clin Geriatr Med,* 26(1), 149–61.

Mikami, K., Jorge, R. E., Moser, D. J., Arndt, S., Jang, M., Solodkin, A., . . . & Robinson, R. G. (2011). Increased frequency of first-episode poststroke depression after discontinuation of escitalopram. *Stroke,* 42(11), 3281–83.

Miller, A. M., & Chandler, P. J. (2002). Acculturation, resilience, and depression in midlife women from the former Soviet Union. *Nurs Res, 51*(1), 26–32.

Miranda, J., Azocar, F., Organista, K. C., Dwyer, E., & Areane, P. (2003). Treatment of depression among impoverished primary care patients from ethnic minority groups. *Psychiatr Serv, 54*(2), 219–25.

Mischoulon, D., & Fava, M. (2000). Docosahexanoic acid and omega-3 fatty acids in depression. *Psychiatr Clin North Am, 23*(4), 785–94.

Montross, L. P., Depp, C., Daly, J., Reichstadt, J., Golshan, S., Moore, D., . . . & Jeste, D. V. (2006). Correlates of self-rated successful aging among community-dwelling older adults. *Am J Geriatr Psychiatry, 14*(1), 43–51.

Mrazek, P. B., & Haggerty, R. J. (1994). *Reducing risks for mental disorders.* Washington, D.C, National Academy Press.

Nygren, B., Alex, L., Jonsen, E., Gustafson, Y., Norberg, A., & Lundman, B. (2005). Resilience, sense of coherence, purpose in life, and self-transcendence in relation to perceived physical and mental health among the oldest old. *Aging Ment Health, 9*(4), 354–62.

Okereke, O. I., Lyness, J. M., Lotrich, F. E., & Reynolds, C. F. (2013). Depression in late-life: A focus on prevention *FOCUS, 11*, 22–31.

Pan, A., Lu, L., Franco, O. H., Yu, Z., Li, H., & Lin, X. (2009). Association between depressive symptoms and 25-hydroxyvitamin D in middle-aged and elderly Chinese. *J Affect Disord, 118*(1–3), 240–43.

Qiu, W. Q., Dean, M., Liu, T., George, L., Gann, M., Cohen, J., & Bruce, M. L. (2010). Physical and mental health of homebound older adults: An overlooked population. *J Am Geriatr Soc, 58*(12), 2423–28.

Richardson, G. E., Neiger, B. L., Jensen, S., & Kumpfer, K. L. (1990). The resiliency model. *Health Education, 21*, 33–39.

Robinson, R. G., Jorge, R. E., Moser, D. J., Acion, L., Solodkin, A., Small, S. L., . . . & Arndt, S. (2008). Escitalopram and problem-solving therapy for prevention of poststroke depression: A randomized controlled trial. *JAMA, 299*(20), 2391–400.

Rovner, B. W., Casten, R. J., Hegel, M. T., Leiby, B. E., & Tasman, W. S. (2007). Preventing depression in age-related macular degeneration. *Arch Gen Psychiatry, 64*(8), 886–92.

Sasaki, H. (2008). [Medical economy]. In [Geriatrics textbook (Japanese)] (pp. 248–49).

Sheeran, T., Rabinowitz, T., Lotterman, J., Reilly, C. F., Brown, S., Donehower, P., . . . & Bruce, M. L. (2011). Feasibility and impact of telemonitor-based depression care management for geriatric homecare patients. *Telemed J E Health, 17*(8), 620–26.

Smit, F., Beekman, A., Cuijpers, P., de Graaf, R., & Vollebergh, W. (2004). Selecting key variables for depression prevention: Results from a population-based prospective epidemiological study. *J Affect Disord, 81*(3), 241–49.

Smit, F., Ederveen, A., Cuijpers, P., Deeg, D., & Beekman, A. (2006). Opportunities for cost-effective prevention of late-life depression: An epidemiological approach. *Arch Gen Psychiatry, 63*(3), 290–96.

Smits, F., Smits, N., Schoevers, R., Deeg, D., Beekman, A., & Cuijpers, P. (2008). An epidemiological approach to depression prevention in old age. *Am J Geriatr Psychiatry, 16*(6), 444–53.

Tanskanen, A., Hibbeln, J. R., Tuomilehto, J., Uutela, A., Haukkala, A., Viinamäki, H., . . . & Vartiainen, E. (2001). Fish consumption and depressive symptoms in the general population in Finland. *Psychiatr Serv, 52*(4), 529–31.

Teno, J. M., Clarridge, B. R., Casey, V., Welch, L. C., Wetle, T., Shield, R., & Mor, V. (2004). Family perspectives on end-of-life care at the last place of care. *JAMA, 291*(1), 88–93.

Tiemeier, H., van Tuijl, H. R., Hofman, A., Kiliaan, A. J., & Breteler, M. M. (2003). Plasma fatty acid composition and depression are associated in the elderly: the Rotterdam Study. *Am J Clin Nutr 78*(1), 40–46.

Timonen, M., Horrobin, D., Jokelainen, J., Laitinen, J., Herva, A., & Räsänen, P. (2004). Fish consumption and depression: the Northern Finland 1966 birth cohort study. *J Affect Disord, 82*(3), 447–52.

Tugade, M. M., & Fredrickson, B. L. (2004). Resilient individuals use positive emotions to bounce back from negative emotional experiences. *J Pers Soc Psychol, 86*(2), 320–33.

Tusaie, K. R., & Patterson, K. (2006). Relationships among trait, situational, and comparative optimism: Clarifying concepts for a theoretically consistent and evidence-based intervention to maximize resilience. *Arch Psychiatr Nurs, 20*(3), 144–50.

Tusaie, K., Puskar, K., & Sereika, S. M. (2007). A predictive and moderating model of psychosocial resilience in adolescents. *J Nurs Scholarsh, 39*(1), 54–60.

U.S. Census Bureau. (2012). *USA quick facts*. Retrieved from http://quickfacts .census.gov/qfd/states/00000.html.

Verbeek, H., Kane, R. A., van Rossum, E., & Hamers, J. P. (2011). Promoting resilience in small-scale, homelike residential care setting for older people with dementia: Experiences from the Netherlands and the United States. In B. Resnick, L. P. Gwyther, & K. A. Roberto (Eds.). *Resilience in aging: Concepts, research, and outcomes* (pp. 289–304). New York: Springer.

Verbeek, H., Van Rossum, E., Zwakhalen, S. M. G., Kempen, G. I. J. M., & Hamers, J. P. H. (2008). *Kleinschalig wonen voor ouderen met dementie. Een beschrijvend onderzoek naar de situatie in de provincie Limburg* [Small scale living for older people with dementia. A descriptive study to the situation in the province of Limburg]. Maastricht: University Press Maastricht.

Vieth, R., Kimball, S., Hu, A., & Walfish, P. G. (2004). Randomized comparison of the effects of the vitamin D3 adequate intake versus 100 mcg (4000 IU) per day on biochemical responses and the well-being of patients. *Nutr J, 3*(1), 8.

Wagnild, G. (2003). Resilience and successful aging. Comparison among low and high income older adults. *J Gerontol Nurs, 29*(12), 42–49.

White-Chu, E. F., Graves, W. J., Godfrey, S. M., Bonner, A., & Sloane, P. (2009). Beyond the medical model: The culture change revolution in long-term care. *J Am Med Dir Assoc, 10*(6), 370–78.

Wilkins, C. H., Sheline, Y. I., Roe, C. M., Birge, S. J., & Morris, J. C. (2006). Vitamin D deficiency is associated with low mood and worse cognitive performance in older adults. *Am J Geriatr Psychiatry, 14*(12), 1032–40.

Woolf, S. H. (2009). A closer look at the economic argument for disease prevention. *JAMA, 301*(5), 536–38.

Yennurajalingam, S., Atkinson, B., Masterson, J., Hui, D., Urbauer, D., Tu, S. M., & Bruera, E. (2012). The impact of an outpatient palliative care consultation on symptom burden in advanced prostate cancer patients. *J Palliat Med, 15*(1), 20–24.

Yoon, D. P., & Lee, E. J. (2007). The impact of religiousness, spirituality, and social support on psychological well-being among older adults in rural areas. *J Gerontol Soc Work, 48*(3–4), 281–98.

Zeisel, J., Silverstein, N. M., Hyde, J., Levkoff, S., Lawton, M. P., & Holmes, W. (2003). Environmental correlates to behavioral health outcomes in Alzheimer's special care units. *Gerontologist, 43*(5), 697–711.

CHAPTER 14

Epilogue

I N THIS BOOK I have described the current state of resilience research and highlighted evidence-based theory, research, and clinical developments. I also have summarized psychosocial and neurobiological characteristics and models of resilience, as well as emerging interventions to enhance resilience.

Although resilience researchers have been struggling with different definitions and diverse approaches, now is the right time to provide this summary of what is already known and to outline future research directions. This inventory can help clinicians and students of geriatrics and gerontology to choose and integrate measures of resilience and spirituality and to direct their traditionally illness-oriented practices toward emphasizing positive aspects of aging and prevention. It is also timely because of the characteristics and needs of aging Baby Boomers, who are more self-deterministic in directing their healthcare and more inclined to be involved in preventive care compared to prior generations of older adults.

Resilience is a dynamic characteristic of the interaction between individuals and their environments. It is clear that resilience can be fostered in older and younger individuals. Adaptive and coping skills can be taught and enhanced across age spans, which will lead to better outcomes for the medical and mental disorders that come with aging. Thus, applying positive psychology and positive mental-health approaches to health and resilience in clinical practices can promote successful aging and ensure productive contributions to society by millions of aging baby boomers.

On the personal level, to develop resilience, individuals need to accomplish two key adaptive tasks across the life span. First, they must *build* knowledge and skills responsive to the changing requirements for personal adjustment, given their personal physiological, physical, psychological, and behavioral characteristics in the context of their environment and life circumstances. Second, they must establish and enhance a foundation for *sustaining* the cognitive and behavioral skills needed for survival and thriving. To accomplish these two goals, executive cognitive skills and emotional responses need to be coupled with the actions required for turning life goals into reality and thus into successful personal adjustment and adaptation.

During later years of life, seniors need to adjust all responses and expectations to changing neurological, cognitive, emotional, somatic, and behavioral characteristics within the key context of their lives—including families, peer groups, and communities. Mental health specialists working with older adults can facilitate these complex processes.

On the societal level, to achieve societal cohesion and happiness, we need to change the perception that the ever-increasing aging population is a negative social phenomenon. Instead, we should create a society where elderly people can enjoy a healthy, prosperous life through participation and contribution. Factors that hamper the elderly from leading such healthy lives include various psychological and social problems occurring with older age, as well as a high incidence of disease. Therefore, we can promote health among the elderly by the study of social welfare, psychology, environment, and social systems. Accordingly, the field of geriatrics—which focuses on healthcare for older people and carries out research, education, and practices to promote health in the elderly—is becoming more important.

Another urgent societal need is the development of a comprehensive education system for healthcare professionals, so that they are well trained to deal with the "aging tsunami." Thus, we should now recognize the importance of gerontology and geriatrics; also, we should insist on a concomitant reform of healthcare services to cope with the aging society. To solve these problems, we need integration and cooperation among federal and state programs, industries, educational institutions, administrative bodies, and community organizations, through an interdisciplinary approach that includes medical science, nursing science, and nursing care. Researchers must continue to pursue related studies of social welfare, social science, engineering, psychology, economics, religion, and ethics.

Programming on the federal and state levels should include the development and promotion of systems that enable elderly people to participate in and make a contribution to society. Such programs can profit from interdisciplinary approaches among medical sciences—including nursing science and nursing care—along with studies of social welfare, social science, psychology, economics, religion, and ethics. Agencies can promote social participation and contribution by elderly people through adjusting and modifying expected workforce trends, predicted to result from low birthrates and high life expectancy. Many older adults will have sufficient physical health to remain fully or partially employed as long as they have access to re-education, vocational retraining, and options to work at varied types of jobs. This trend and the opportunities it encompasses will likely benefit total financial systems and will also decrease the number of elderly people in need of care.

Another important future task is to increase the eldercare workforce via promotion of gerontology, which will entail the reform and enhancement of geriatrics in undergraduate, postgraduate, and life-long educational and infrastructural development, in addition to the promotion of home-based care and multidisciplinary care. In a geriatric clinical setting, healthcare professionals should be aware of the physical traits of older people, who often develop not only dementia but also geriatric syndromes such as late-life depression, anxiety, insomnia, chronic pain, falling, and urinary incontinence. This will require a holistic approach that considers complementary and alternative medicine along with nursing care. Promoting home-based and multidisciplinary care can reduce the length of stays in acute hospitals and meet the demand of older people who prefer to remain in their own homes. We will inevitably find that multidisciplinary care is increasingly needed to meet various demands in the medical care and welfare of the elderly.

On the professional level, as medical practitioners begin to appreciate the importance of wellness and positive psychosocial factors in the management and prevention of pathology, positive psychology and psychiatry will be an increasingly important component of healthcare. Research and education will change the current stereotyping and ageism prevalent in society and healthcare.

Treatment trials have shown the beneficial effects of behavioral and lifestyle strategies that boost resilience, change attitudes toward aging, or incorporate meditation on outcome measures such as alcohol consumption, biological response to stress, and mortality rates in older adults. Emerging evidence increasingly suggests that prevention strategies in later life can be practical and cost-effective. For example, depression following strokes, myocardial infarction, and bypass surgery can be treated, and even prevented, leading to a significant reduction in morbidity and mortality. Likewise, interventions aimed at altering partially malleable risk factors, such as social isolation, physical disability, and sleep problems, can prevent, or at least delay the onset of, depression. Similarly, the risk of older victims of natural disasters, wars, or tragic events developing post-traumatic stress disorder can be decreased with appropriate counseling together with optimal use of pharmacotherapy and behavioral interventions, including cognitive-behavioral therapy, work rehabilitation, and intergenerational programs to enhance everyday functioning.

For researchers, an exciting area of investigation will be identifying and then trying to enhance coping skills and resilience. Developing biological treatments focusing on such processes may help enhance these positive traits in people with neuropsychiatric disorders. Another critical need in the field today is for psychotropic medications that are efficacious, safe, and affordable for older adults with serious mental illness.

Similarly, well-designed and implemented resilience-building preventive strategies have the potential to improve health outcomes and reduce morbidity and mortality. The current example of late-life depression-prevention research has shown robust success in employing indicated and selective prevention models in high-risk groups, even as opportunities for universal prevention in general populations have been little explored. Thus, future prevention studies would ideally examine possibilities for expanding these findings into universal prevention paradigms. Large-scale public-health-promotion efforts (e.g., involving modifiable behaviors such as physical activity or exercise, social activity, and dietary factors) can provide such "natural experiment" opportunities. Finally, collaborative, interdisciplinary care approaches utilizing a central "hub" of primary care, along with an extended network of providers with community ties or remote contacts with patients, could conceivably be employed to test the value of universal screening for late-life mood and cognitive disorders, with the idea of early detection and prevention of adverse outcomes via early interventions.

To sum up, through resilience research and clinical practice, we are learning the remarkable fact that human beings can adapt to nearly all life *and* death situations very successfully. Surprisingly and encouragingly, we are finding that there is no one place, one definition, one right or wrong situation, or one chronological age that can prevent even life's most daunting challenges from being seen as—and converted to—valuable and growth-inducing lessons.